The Founders of Operative Surgery

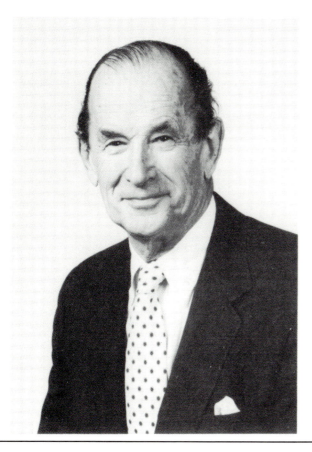

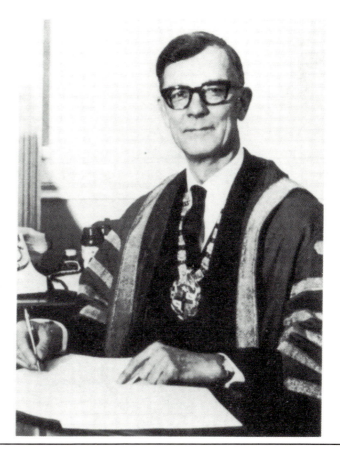

Charles Granville Rob MC, MChir, FRCS, FACS
Professor of Surgery, Uniformed Services University of the
Health Sciences, E Edward Hébert School of Medicine,
Bethesda, Maryland
Quondam: Professor of Surgery, St Mary's Hospital Medical
School, London 1950–1960
Professor and Chairman, Department of Surgery, University of
Rochester, New York, 1960–1978
Professor of Surgery, East Carolina University, 1978–1983

Lord Smith of Marlow KBE, MS, FRCS, Hon DSc
(Exeter and Leeds), Hon MD (Zurich), Hon FRACS,
Hon FRCS(Ed), Hon FRCS (Glas), Hon FACS, Hon FRCS(Can),
Hon FRCSI, Hon FRCS(SA), Hon FDS, Past President, RSM
Honorary Consulting Surgeon, St George's Hospital, London
Quondam: Surgeon, St George's Hospital, London,
1946–1978
President of the Royal College of Surgeons of England,
1973–1977

Rob & Smith's
Operative Surgery

General Editors

Hugh Dudley ChM, FRCS(Ed), FRACS, FRCS
Emeritus Professor, St Mary's Hospital, London, UK

David C. Carter MD, FRCS(Ed), FRCS(Glas)
Regius Professor of Clinical Surgery, Royal Infirmary, Edinburgh, UK

R. C. G. Russell MS, FRCS
Consultant Surgeon, Middlesex Hospital, St John's Hospital for Diseases of the Skin and Royal National Throat, Nose and Ear Hospital, London, UK

Rob & Smith's
Operative Surgery

Head and Neck   Part 2

Fourth Edition

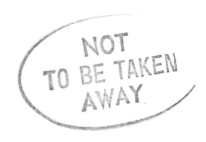

Edited by

Ian A. McGregor ChM, DSc, FRCS(G), FRCS(Eng), Hon FRACS, Hon FRCSI, Hon FRCS(Ed), Hon FACS
Formerly Director, Plastic and Oral Surgery Unit, Canniesburn Hospital, Glasgow, UK

David J. Howard FRCS, FRCS(Ed)
Institute of Laryngology and Otology, Royal National Throat, Nose and Ear Hospital, London, UK

Butterworth–Heinemann
Oxford   London   Boston   Munich   New Delhi   Singapore   Sydney   Tokyo   Toronto   Wellington

Butterworth–Heinemann Ltd
Linacre House, Jordan Hill, Oxford OX2 8DP, UK

 PART OF REED INTERNATIONAL BOOKS

OXFORD   LONDON   BOSTON
MUNICH   NEW DELHI   SINGAPORE   SYDNEY
TOKYO   TORONTO   WELLINGTON

First published 1992

British Library Cataloguing in Publication Data

Rob & Smith's operative surgery. – 4th ed.
  Head and neck.
  I. McGregor, Ian A.   II. Howard, David J.
  III. Rob, Charles, *1913-*   IV. Smith, Rodney
  Smith, *Baron, 1914–*
  617.91

  ISBN 0-7506-0298-8 set
  ISBN 0-7506-0296-1 part 1
  ISBN 0-7506-0297-X part 2

Library of Congress Cataloging-in-Publication Data
(Revised for vol. 14)

Rob & Smith's operative surgery.

  Rev. ed. of: Operative surgery. 3rd ed. 1976–
  Includes bibliographies and index.
  Contents: [1] Alimentary tract and abdominal wall.
1. General principles, oesophagus, stomach, duodenum,
small intestine, abdominal wall, hernia/edited by
Hugh Dudley — [13] Orthopaedics/edited by
George Bentley, Robert B. Greer — [14] Head and neck/
edited by Ian A. McGregor, David J. Howard.
  1. Surgery, Operative.   I. Rob, Charles.   II. Smith
of Marlow, Rodney Smith, Baron, 1914–
III. Dudley, Hugh A. F. (Hugh Arnold Freeman)
IV. Pories, Walter J. V. Carter, David C. (David
Craig). [DNLM: 1. Surgery, operative. WO 500 061 1982]
RD32.06 1983   617'.91   83-14465
  ISBN 0-407-00651-6 (v. 1)

Composition by Genesis Typesetting, Laser Quay, Rochester, Kent
Printed and bound by Butler and Tanner Ltd, Frome, Somerset

Volumes and Editors

Alimentary Tract and Abdominal Wall

1 **General Principles · Oesophagus · Stomach · Duodenum · Small Intestine · Abdominal Wall · Hernia**

Hugh Dudley ChM, FRCS(Ed), FRACS, FRCS
Emeritus Professor, St Mary's Hospital, London, UK

2 **Liver · Portal Hypertension · Spleen · Biliary Tract · Pancreas**

Hugh Dudley ChM, FRCS(Ed), FRACS, FRCS
Emeritus Professor, St Mary's Hospital, London, UK

3 **Colon, Rectum and Anus**

Ian P. Todd MS, MD(Tor), FRCS, DCH
Consulting Surgeon, St Bartholomew's Hospital, London;
Consultant Surgeon, St Mark's Hospital and
King Edward VII Hospital for Officers, London, UK

L. P. Fielding FRCS
Chief of Surgery, St Mary's Hospital, Waterbury, Connecticut, USA;
Associate Professor of Surgery, Yale University, Connecticut, USA

Cardiac Surgery

Stuart W. Jamieson FRCS, FACS
Professor and Head, Cardiothoracic Surgery,
University of Minnesota, Minneapolis, Minnesota, USA

Norman E. Shumway MD, PhD, FRCS
Professor and Chairman, Department of Cardiovascular Surgery,
Stanford University School of Medicine, California, USA

The Ear

John C. Ballantyne FRCS, HonFRCSI, DLO
Consultant Ear, Nose and Throat Surgeon,
Royal Free and King Edward VII Hospital for Officers, London, UK;
Honorary Consultant in Otolaryngology to the Army

Andrew Morrison FRCS, DLO
Senior Consultant Otolaryngologist, The London Hospital, UK

General Principles, Breast and Extracranial Endocrines

Hugh Dudley ChM, FRCS(Ed), FRACS, FRCS
Emeritus Professor, St Mary's Hospital, London, UK

Walter J. Pories MD, FACS
Professor and Chairman, Department of Surgery, School of Medicine,
East Carolina University, Greenville, North Carolina, USA

Gynaecology and Obstetrics

J. M. Monaghan FRCS(Ed), FRCOG
Consultant Gynaecological Surgeon, Head of the Regional
Department of Gynaecological Oncology, Queen Elizabeth Hospital,
Gateshead, Tyne and Wear, UK

The Hand

Rolfe Birch FRCS
Consultant Orthopaedic Surgeon, PNI Unit and Hand Clinic,
Royal National Orthopaedic Hospital, Stanmore, Middlesex, and
St Mary's Hospital, London, UK

Donal Brooks MA, FRCS, FRCSI
Consulting Orthopaedic Surgeon, University College Hospital,
London and Royal National Orthopaedic Hospital, Stanmore,
Middlesex, UK; Civilian Consultant in Hand Surgery to the Royal Navy
and Royal Air Force, UK

Head and Neck

Ian A. McGregor ChM, DSc, FRCS
Formerly Director, Plastic and Oral Surgery Unit, Canniesburn
Hospital, Glasgow, UK

David J. Howard FRCS, FRCS(Ed)
Institute of Laryngology and Otology, Royal National Throat, Nose
and Ear Hospital, London, UK

Neurosurgery

Lindsay Symon TD, FRCS
Professor of Neurosurgery, Gough-Cooper Department of
Neurological Surgery, Institute of Neurology, National Hospitals for
Nervous Diseases, London, UK

David G. T. Thomas MRCP, FRCSE
Senior Lecturer and Consultant Neurosurgeon,
Institute of Neurology, National Hospitals for Nervous Diseases,
London, UK

Kemp Clark MD, FACS
Professor of Neurosurgery, Division of Neurological Surgery,
Southwestern Medical School, Dallas, Texas, USA

Nose and Throat

John C. Ballantyne FRCS, HonFRCSI, DLO
Consultant Ear, Nose and Throat Surgeon,
Royal Free and King Edward VII Hospital for Officers, London, UK;
Honorary Consultant in Otolaryngology to the Army

D. F. N. Harrison MD, MS, FRCS, FRACS
Professor of Laryngology and Otology,
Royal National Throat, Nose and Ear Hospital, London, UK

Ophthalmic Surgery

Thomas A. Rice MD
Assistant Clinical Professor of Ophthalmology,
Case Western Reserve University School of Medicine,
Cleveland, Ohio, USA; formerly of the Wilmer Ophthalmological
Institute, The Johns Hopkins School of Medicine, Maryland, USA

Ronald G. Michels MD
Professor of Ophthalmology, The Wilmer Ophthalmological Institute,
The Johns Hopkins University School of Medicine,
Maryland, USA

Walter W. J. Stark MD
Professor of Ophthalmology, The Wilmer Ophthalmological Institute,
The Johns Hopkins University School of Medicine,
Maryland, USA

Orthopaedics

George Bentley ChM, FRCS
Professor of Orthopaedic Surgery, The Institute of Orthopaedics,
University of London; Honorary Consultant Orthopaedic Surgeon,
The Royal National Orthopaedic Hospital, Stanmore, Middlesex, and
The Middlesex Hospital, London, UK

Robert B. Greer III MD, FACS
Professor and Chairman of Orthopaedic Surgery, Pennsylvania State
University College of Medicine, Hershey, Pennsylvania, USA

Paediatric Surgery

L. Spitz PhD, FRCS(Ed), FRCS(Eng), FAAP(Hon)
Nuffield Professor of Paediatric Surgery, Institute of Child Health,
University of London; Consultant Paediatric Surgeon, London, UK

H. Homewood Nixon MA, FRCS(Eng), FRCSI(Hon), FACS(Hon), FAAP(Hon)
Consultant Paediatric Surgeon, The Hospital for Sick Children,
Great Ormond Street, London and St Mary's Hospital, Paddington,
London, UK

Plastic Surgery

T. L. Barclay ChM, FRCS
Consultant Plastic Surgeon, St Luke's Hospital,
Bradford, West Yorkshire, UK

Desmond A. Kernahan MD
Chief, Division of Plastic Surgery,
The Children's Memorial Hospital, Chicago, Illinois, USA

Thoracic Surgery

The late J. W. Jackson MCh, FRCS
Formerly Consultant Thoracic Surgeon, Harefield Hospital,
Middlesex, UK

D. K. C. Cooper MD, PhD, FRCS
Department of Cardiac Surgery, University of Cape Town
Medical School, Cape Town, South Africa

Trauma Surgery

Howard R. Champion FRCS(Ed), FACS
Chief, Trauma Service; Director, Surgery Critical Care Services, The
Washington Hospital Center, Washington DC; Professor of Surgery,
Chief of Division of Surgery for Trauma, Department of Surgery,
Uniformed Services University of the Health Sciences, Bethesda,
Maryland, USA

John V. Robbs ChM, FRCS(Ed)
Professor of Surgery; Head, Metropolitan Vascular Services;
Head, Division of Surgery, University of Natal, Durban, Natal, South
Africa

Donald D. Trunkey MD, FACS
Chairman, Department of Surgery, University of Portland, Portland,
Oregon, USA

Urology

W. Scott McDougal MD
Professor and Chairman, Department of Urology,
Vanderbilt University Medical Center, Nashville, Tennessee, USA

Vascular Surgery

James A. DeWeese MD
Professor and Chairman, Division of Cardiothoracic Surgery,
University of Rochester Medical Center, Rochester, New York, USA

Contributors

Hugh F. Biller MD
Professor and Chairman, Department of Otolaryngology, The Mount Sinai Medical Center, New York, NY 10029-6574, USA

Patrick J. Bradley FRCS
Consultant Otolaryngologist and Head and Neck Oncologist, Department of Otolaryngology, University Hospital, Nottingham NG7 2UH, UK

A. Cheesman FRCS
Royal National Throat, Nose and Ear Hospital, Gray's Inn Road, London WC1X 8EE and Head and Neck Unit, Charing Cross Hospital, London W6 8RF, UK

Charles B. Croft FRCS
Royal National Throat, Nose and Ear Hospital, Gray's Inn Road, London WC1X 8EE, UK

J. Culbertson MD, FACS
The Emory Clinic, Section of Plastic, Reconstructive and Maxillo-facial Surgery, 25 Prescott Street, N E Atlanta, Georgia 30308, USA

R. J. Cusumano MD
Assistant Professor of Otolaryngology, Albert Einstein College of Medicine, Montefiore Medical Center, Bronx, New York, USA

J. Hochberg MD
Division of Plastic Surgery, West Virginia University, Morgantown, West Virginia, USA

David J. Howard FRCS, FRCS(Ed)
Institute of Laryngology and Otology, Royal National Throat, Nose and Ear Hospital, Gray's Inn Road, London WC1X 8EE, UK

Ian T. Jackson MB, ChB, FRCS(G), FRCS(Ed), FACS, FRACS(Hon)
Director, Institute for Craniofacial and Reconstructive Surgery, Providence Hospital, Southfield, Michigan 48075, USA

M. J. Jurkiewicz MD, FACS
The Emory Clinic, Section of Plastic, Reconstructive and Maxillo-facial Surgery, 25 Prescott Street, N E Atlanta, Georgia 30308, USA

V. J. Lund MS, FRCS
Institute of Laryngology and Otology, Royal National Throat, Nose and Ear Hospital, Gray's Inn Road, London WC1X 8EE, UK

Ian A. McGregor ChM, DSc, FRCS
Formerly Director, Plastic and Oral Surgery Unit, Canniesburn Hospital, Glasgow, UK

R. D. Manderson
Consultant in Prosthetic Dentistry, Stoke Mandeville Hospital, Aylesbury, Buckinghamshire HP21 8AL, UK

A. G. D. Maran FRCS(Ed), FACS
The Royal Infirmary, Lauriston Place, Edinburgh EH3 9YW, UK

Roger Parker MS, FRCS
ENT Department, Royal Berkshire Hospital, Reading, Berkshire RG1 5AN, UK

Bruce W. Pearson MD
Mayo Clinic Jacksonville, 4500 San Pablo Road, Jacksonville, Florida 32224, USA

John S. Rubin MD
Assistant Professor of Otolaryngology, Albert Einstein College of Medicine and Director, Otolaryngology Service, North Central Bronx Hospital, Bronx, New York, USA

Renato Saltz MD
Assistant Professor, Division of Plastic and Reconstructive Surgery, Medical College of Georgia, Augusta, Georgia, USA

O. H. Shaheen MS, FRCS, FRCS(Ed)
Consultant ENT Surgeon, Guy's Hospital, London SE1 9RT, UK

Carl E. Silver MD, FACS
Professor of Surgery, Professor of Otolaryngology, Albert Einstein College of Medicine and Director of Head and Neck Surgery, Montefiore Medical Center, Bronx, New York, USA

Margaret F. Spittle MSc, FRCR
Director, Meyerstein Institute of Clinical Oncology, Middlesex Hospital, Mortimer Street, London W1N 8AA, UK

James Yee Suen MD, FACS
Professor and Chairman, Department of Otolaryngology – Head and Neck Surgery, University of Arkansas for Medical Sciences, Little Rock, Arkansas 72205-7199, USA

A. E. Thompson FRCS
St Thomas' Hospital, London SE1 7EH, UK

Luis O. Vasconez MD, FACS
Professor and Director, Division of Plastic Surgery, University of Alabama, Birmingham, Alabama, USA

Contributing Medical Artists

Patricia Archer FMAA, MAMI, AIMI
Rangemore, 30 Park Avenue,
Caterham, Surrey CR3 6AH, UK

The late Robert Lane MMAA
Medical Illustrator, Studio 19A,
Edith Grove, London SW10, UK

Gillian Lee FMAA, AIMI, AMI, RMIP
15 Little Plucketts Way, Buckhurst Hill,
Essex IG9 5QU, UK

Gillian Oliver MMAA, AIMI
15 Bramble Road, Hatfield,
Hertfordshire AL10 9RZ, UK

Ian Ramsden
Head of Department of Medical Illustration,
Glasgow University, Glasgow, UK

Contents of Part 1
General Considerations, Skin, Facial Structures, Oral Cavity

Contents of Part 2
Pharynx, Larynx and Oesophagus

Preface

Ten years have passed since the 3rd Edition of the Head and Neck volume of *Operative Surgery*, and in the interval there have been major changes in the surgical management of many of the conditions discussed. The previous edition interpreted head and neck surgery widely, but usage of the term 'head and neck surgery' has increasingly come to mean the surgery of tumours in that anatomical region, and it is with that restricted usage in mind that we have endeavoured to interpret our brief.

In rewriting the book in its entirety a real effort has been made to reduce duplication to a minimum by integrating the text more effectively. With authors from both sides of the Atlantic this has not always been easy, but the editorial insertion of cross references has, we hope, been a valuable move in this direction. A criticism of the text in the past has been what is labelled as a 'cookery book' approach, with operative procedures described with a minimum of explanation of the whys and wherefores. In this edition authors have been specifically asked to explain their reasons for advocating the particular techniques they are discussing, the indications for their use and, more important, their limitations and adverse factors, and most important of all, their contraindications. The effect has been to increase the proportion of text to illustrations, but we hope the result is a more rounded and rational product. All the illustrations have been redrawn by a small number of artists aiming for uniformity of style and improved quality. The basis of the illustrations has largely been actual operative sequences and real faces, the object being to add to their overall credibility.

The book does not pretend to describe all the techniques which are available to manage the various problems discussed. Its objective has rather been to describe the techniques which each contributor, an authority in his or her field, has found to be the most effective.

Ian A. McGregor
David J. Howard

Pharyngolaryngectomy: reconstruction by myocutaneous flaps

David J. Howard FRCS, FRCS(Ed)
Institute of Laryngology and Otology, Royal National Throat, Nose and Ear Hospital, London, UK

Surgical treatment of hypopharyngeal tumours

Anatomical and pathological considerations

The hypopharynx is commonly divided into three areas: piriform fossa, posterior pharyngeal wall and postcricoid area. The superior boundary is generally accepted as a horizontal plane drawn at the level of the hyoid bone and the inferior boundary as the cricopharyngeus muscle. The anterior boundary is the posterior aspect of the larynx and the posterior boundary the prevertebral fascia. However, while these anatomical regions are convenient for classification, they are in continuity with each other offering no barriers to the spread of malignancy such as squamous cell carcinoma.

The incidence of hypopharyngeal squamous cell carcinoma varies markedly throughout the world but all major series consist predominantly of advanced lesions affecting several anatomical areas at presentation. While piriform fossa lesions predominate in North America, postcricoid lesions are most common in Northern Europe while in Hong Kong advanced laryngeal carcinoma spreading into the pharynx is the commonest indication for major hypopharyngeal resection and reconstruction.

The hypopharynx and cervical oesophagus should be considered in continuity as submucosal spread of carcinoma is notorious and frequently averages 10 mm when large series of surgical specimens are examined. Many 'early' tumours of the hypopharynx are, in fact, extensive and accurate evaluation of tumour extent rather than the exact site of origin is more important therapeutically.

Lymph node metastases occur early and often from the hypopharynx. The jugulodigastric and mid-jugular nodes are sites of predilection for piriform fossa lesions; the retropharyngeal and mid-jugular nodes for the rarer posterior wall tumours. The postcricoid region, by contrast, drains to the impalpable paratracheal and paraoesophageal nodes.

Direct extension to adjacent sites is not always discernible nor relevant. For example, involvement of the larynx is of considerably less importance than superior oropharyngeal and tongue base extension because complete surgical excision of the latter is less easily accomplished than a total laryngectomy.

The level of the larynx, hypopharynx and cervical oesophagus are variable and, while some patients will have sufficient oesophagus in the neck to allow adequate low resection of advanced postcricoid carcinoma, others will have disease in the thoracic inlet requiring more extensive surgery including oesophagectomy, total thyroidectomy, superior mediastinal dissection and tracheal resection.

It is generally a more rewarding philosophy to treat all hypopharyngeal carcinoma as potentially advanced and it is doubtful whether any patient can be realistically considered as suitable for 'conservation' surgery. There are three commonly used procedures for wide excision of hypopharyngeal carcinoma: partial pharyngectomy with total or near-total laryngectomy, pharyngolaryngectomy, and total laryngopharyngo-oesophagectomy. While the reconstruction techniques for pharyngeal repair continue to interest head and neck surgeons, the over-riding need remains adequate preoperative assessment and excision of the tumour.

Reconstruction by myocutaneous flaps

The earliest methods of reconstruction of the pharynx and cervical oesophagus utilized local skin flaps. In 1942 Wookey[1] described his technique for pharyngeal reconstruction using a laterally based cervical flap. Unfortunately, a large proportion of these patients developed fistulae and stenoses and often required multiple operations, remaining in hospital for a period of many months. In 1968 Bakamjian[2] reported his initial experience in reconstructing the pharynx with a medially based deltopectoral flap. This was a notable improvement on the Wookey technique but still involved a high incidence of postoperative complications including flap necrosis, fistula formation and stenosis.

The superior properties of the myocutaneous island flap, first utilized in the late 1970s, has rapidly led to its application for pharyngeal reconstruction with a single stage procedure, as it provides an alternative to visceral replacement. The most common flap used for this reconstruction is the pectoralis major myocutaneous flap. Other applicable pedicled myocutaneous flaps are the latissimus dorsi and the trapezius. All three flaps can provide large reliable pieces of skin and muscle and can be mobilized to the anterior aspect of the neck. Each flap has its own inherent advantages and disadvantages and the author's preference is the pectoralis major myocutaneous flap. All three can be used tubed to reconstruct the pharynx after total pharyngolaryngectomy; however, if adequate resection margins which leave a lateral or posterior strip of residual pharynx between oropharynx and oesophagus are possible, the myocutaneous repair will have a lower rate of fistula formation and a better long-term functional result. Free microvascular flaps may also be used for pharyngeal reconstruction, and most reports involve the use of the radial forearm flap. The comparative lack of bulk and inherent pliability of this flap make it easier to tube but its use requires microvascular expertise and its reliability is less than that of a pedicled myocutaneous flap. It has not been shown to have superior long-term functional results.

Choice of flap

This is to some extent a matter of the personal preference and experience of the surgeon. The pectoralis major flap is less satisfactory in the female, particularly if the breast tissue is large, as it may result in a flap which is too bulky, particularly when tubed, and gives rise to a greater cosmetic deformity of the chest. The pectoralis major myocutaneous flap does, however, have the advantage over the latissimus dorsi or trapezius that the resection and reconstruction are all undertaken with the patient supine. The latissimus dorsi flap has the advantage of not deforming the breast but the donor site is more troublesome in the postoperative period and primary closure cannot always be achieved when the larger flaps, such as those required for reconstruction of the whole pharynx, are used. Of the three pedicled flaps, the trapezius is least used for this reconstruction, and a satisfactory sized island flap cannot be obtained for this repair if an accompanying radical neck dissection has removed the transverse cervical artery. All three flaps

provide skin and muscle for reconstruction from outside any area of previous head and neck irradiation.

Advantages of a pedicled myocutaneous flap repair

In comparison with repair by major viscera such as stomach, colon or jejunum, myocutaneous flaps have the advantages that: (1) the general medical condition of the patient can be poorer than in the situation where an abdominal viscera is transposed through the chest; (2) additional expertise of an accompanying general surgeon or microvascular techniques are not required; (3) the overall operative procedure may be shorter; (4) through and through defects may be resected and satisfactory neck closure obtained simply with a split thickness skin graft applied to the muscular pedicle of the myocutaneous flap.

Disadvantages

The inferior limit of resection is more limited compared with a situation where the adjacent oesophagus is removed and viscera transposed through the thorax. The flap has potential for single stage reconstruction but is associated with significant postoperative fistula formation and it may be preferable, particularly in irradiated cases, to create a temporary pharyngostome. The donor area of skin may be hair bearing, and donor site healing and deformity may be relevant with the larger flaps required for reconstruction after total pharyngectomy. Functional results in terms of swallowing are notably inferior to those obtained with gastric transposition and microvascular free jejunal grafts. Some patients may remain on a semi-solid diet. Long-term follow-up has shown an incidence of flap to oesophageal stenosis rate of approximately 20 per cent.

Indications

It is of the utmost importance that the surgeon undertaking partial pharyngolaryngectomy or total pharyngolaryngectomy fully understands the surgical anatomy and pathology of carcinoma involving these areas. Generous partial pharyngectomy with total laryngectomy may be required for advanced hypopharyngeal lesions, advanced tonsillar carcinoma, or T4 laryngeal carcinoma with extensive pharyngeal involvement.

All the above may require resection of so much pharynx that primary closure is not advisable and repair and augmentation by a myocutaneous flap is indicated.

Total pharyngectomy may be required for advanced piriform fossa lesions, advanced posterior pharyngeal wall lesions, or postcricoid carcinoma. The last must not have significant cervical oesophageal extension and the surgeon must be certain that the inferior limit of resection is clear and that the lower anastomosis of myocutaneous flap to oesophagus can be accomplished without compromise. For this reason the technique is rarely indicated for hypopharyngeal lesions extending into the cervical oesophagus.

Details of the surgical anatomy of the pectoralis major, latissimus dorsi, trapezius and radial forearm flaps are to be found in the chapter on 'Reconstructive techniques of the skin', pp. 45–103.

Operation

After the resection phase of the partial or total pharyngo-larnygectomy, preoperative assessment of the appropriate reconstruction technique is reassessed. The author's preference is for the pectoralis major myocutaneous flap repair in most patients.

Incision

1

The appropriate surface markings are drawn as a guide to the position of the pectoral branch of the thoracoacromial artery, i.e. a line from the tip of the shoulder to the xiphisternum, and a line at right angles to the clavicle extending inferiorly from its mid point. It is preferable to plan the skin incisions so as not to cross the area of a standard medially based deltopectoral flap; this approach preserves this flap should it be required for future reconstruction, and elevation of the entire deltopectoral flap aids considerably subsequent mobilization of the pectoralis major flap and is to be recommended for the inexperienced surgeon.

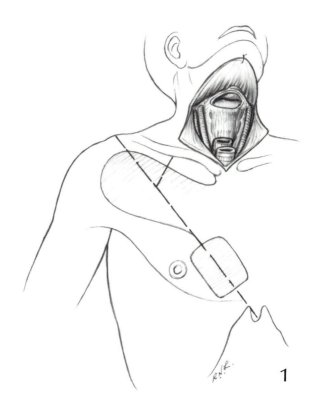

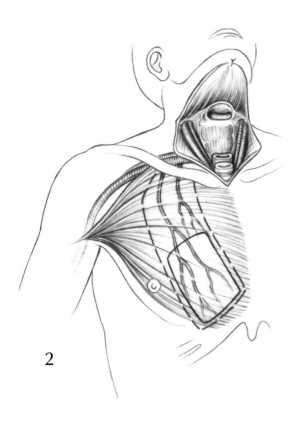

Planning the flap

2

The appropriate size and shape of the cutaneous portion of the flap will vary according to the degree of pharynx to be replaced. After total pharyngectomy it is usually necessary to make the cutaneous portion at least 8 cm wide and it may be necessary to utilize skin which includes the nipple, although the author bases the flap on the most medial aspect of the lower portion of the pectoralis major to avoid including the nipple. In those patients who have had a relatively long vertical section of pharynx removed, it may be necessary to design the skin paddle so that a portion of it extends beyond the inferior limit of pectoralis major and is therefore a random flap based on the myocutaneous element. This random area of skin should not extend more than 2 cm below the inferior margin of the muscle as the chances of necrosis of this portion, which will be anastomosed to the superior aspect of the pharyngeal remnant, are significantly increased. The illustration shows the inclusion of the supreme thoracic artery and the pectoral branch of the thoracoacromial axis. It is not necessary to include the lateral thoracic artery in the pedicle of the flap.

Dissection and transposition of flap

3

After elevation of the deltopectoral flap the appropriate cutaneous portion is isolated by dissection down to and including the pectoralis fascia. Tacking sutures of plain catgut are then placed at regular intervals between the fascia overlying pectoralis major and the dermis of the overlying skin paddle: these prevent any unnecessary shearing of the skin paddle on the underlying muscle as the mobilization and transposition are undertaken. The more experienced surgeon may feel that this is not necessary but it does provide protection to the perforating vessels passing between muscle and skin. These sutures may subsequently be removed when the skin and muscle components are stitched to the pharyngeal remnant or tubed to replace the whole pharynx.

Pectoralis major is then elevated from the chest wall and the underlying pectoralis minor by blunt finger dissection at the lateral edge of pectoralis major to identify the appropriate plane. Dissection along this lateral border continues inferomedially and parallel to the nutrient vessels, which can be observed covered by the deep fascia of the muscle. The vessels usually enter the muscle at the level of the anterior axillary fold and repeated attempts to visualize them below this level in the early stage of the mobilization are unnecessary and cause considerable stretching of pectoralis major. The inferomedial direction of the pectoralis major mobilization is continued, releasing the muscle slips from the fifth and sixth ribs and extending round the inferior aspect of the cutaneous paddle. If an inferior random portion of skin is to be included, the fascia over the external oblique muscle may require mobilization and should be kept on the deep surface of the mobilized flap. The plane of dissection in this area may be less distinct and requires careful attention. The medial aspect of pectoralis major is then detached from the lateral edge of the sternum and the dissection runs in a superolateral direction towards the clavicle. An appropriate-sized pedicle of muscle is lifted (this will vary according to the requirements of the individual patient).

If a radical neck dissection has been performed on the side of the flap mobilization, extra muscle may be incorporated in the pedicle to cover the exposed carotid vessels: this is a considerable advantage of the pedicled myocutaneous technique. As the combined skin and muscle flap is raised above the level of the anterior axillary fold the pectoral vessels will be clearly seen, and further division of the muscle pedicle on its lateral aspect will divide the pectoralis major fibres that run towards the insertion into the humerus. It is important to ligate any bleeding vessels in the excised edges of the muscle pedicle and particularly any that may be running in the deep fascial layer (particularly those communicating between the lateral thoracic and pectoral arteries). Postoperative bleeding and haematoma formation from these vessels can considerably endanger the flap. The muscle pedicle is elevated proximally to the clavicle, but with repair of the pharynx it is very unusual to have difficulty with the length of the pedicle and additional procedures such as resection of the clavicular portion of

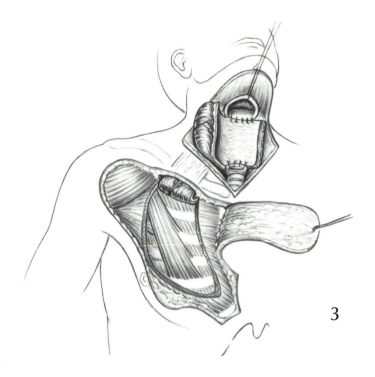

3

the muscle to increase pedicle length are not required.

It is important to handle the myocutaneous flap carefully at all times, avoiding excessive torque, traction and pressure. The flap is transposed superiorly to the surgical defect; marked rotation of the pedicle is unnecessary. The transposition should be gentle and if the pedicle is placed under a skin bridge as depicted in *Illustration 3*, the skin should be elevated widely so that there is no compression of the vessels within the pedicle. If there is any hint of compression related to this bridge, it should be divided and the exposed muscle pedicle simply skin grafted. The flap is positioned in the neck so that it covers any exposed carotid artery. The residual cut edges, both medially and laterally, of pectoralis major are oversewn with a continuous running suture of catgut which provides further haemostasis. The author advocates division of both the lateral and medial pectoral nerves during the elevation so that the transposed flap does not subsequently move and some atrophy of the muscle bulk is assured. Care must be taken when dividing the lateral nerve as it usually lies adjacent to the pectoral artery and vein.

Closure of the chest

Wide undermining of the chest skin can be undertaken without difficulty so that, even with large cutaneous defects, primary closure of the chest wound is almost always possible. This is to be preferred over skin grafting to the anterior thoracic wall, as any graft is directly onto perichondrium and periosteum of exposed ribs and costal cartilage, and its take and long-term viability can be troublesome. Perichondritis has been reported as a complication under these circumstances. Large suction drains or corrugated drains from the inferior aspect of the chest wound are mandatory.

Closure of the pharynx

4

The flap must be carefully positioned, particularly when it is to be tubed for total pharyngeal reconstruction. The skin to pharyngeal/oesophageal mucosa suture is undertaken using interrupted Vicryl 3/0 sutures (Ethicon Ltd, Edinburgh, UK) with both posterior aspects being completed first. Following the anterior suturing any necessary entubation of the flap can be undertaken. This should not bring about any unnecessary tension on the pedicle. A second muscular layer closure is undertaken with 3/0 chromic catgut, but on occasions this is not possible down the vertical line of the flap; because of this the flap is particularly prone to leakage and it is important that, should the suture line of the tubed flap be adjacent to exposed carotid vessels, these should be covered with a levator scapulae or other appropriate tissue.

The incidence of fistulae of the tubed flap, even under satisfactory conditions, may be as high as 30 per cent. These complications are common to all the myocutaneous flaps mentioned. It is of utmost importance that the weight of the entire myocutaneous unit does not bear on the superior and inferior anastomotic lines, and sutures carefully placed between residual neck structures and the pedicle of the myocutaneous flap are placed so as to distribute and balance the weight. The neck skin must be closed without tension and with adequate drainage. If there is any doubt of haemostasis it is better to leave a significant length of the neck wound open in relation to the pedicle of the flap than to risk haematoma formation.

With reconstruction after partial pharyngectomy by means of this flap, nasogastric tube feeding over a period of 10–14 days may be all that is required before healing is complete. However, if most of the pharynx has been resected, or after total pharyngectomy using a tubed flap, the placing of a gastrostomy or jejunostomy is advocated, as healing of these reconstructions may take considerably longer and they have considerable advantages over a nasogastric tube in these circumstances. This point is particulary important in patients whose preoperative condition and nutrition are poor.

Postoperative management

The pedicled pectoralis myocutaneous flap has a high success rate and is generally robust. The most common complication is the loss of a small portion of the cutaneous component, but this can be prevented by careful flap design, attention to suturing techniques and lack of tension within the reconstructions. In the immediate postoperative period prevention of haematoma and correct position of the patient are the most important requirements. Nursing is best carried out in a slightly elevated supine position, with the head and neck positioned neutrally with no excessive flexion, extension or rotation. Any compression of the muscle pedicle is to be avoided and tracheostomy tapes, elastic dressings and

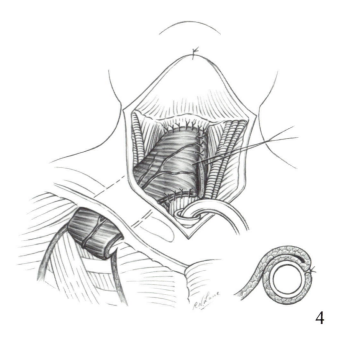

4

bulky bedclothes shoud be avoided. In common with other major head and neck reconstruction the use of perioperative metronidazole and a broad-spectrum antibiotic such as a cephalosporin is recommended. Skilled postoperative and paramedical care are likewise required for all patients and particular attention should be paid to oral hygiene, stomal care, nutrition and physiotherapy. These patients are usually mobilized on the second day after operation and detailed videofluoroscopic examination is undertaken before commencement of swallowing. The advice of a speech and swallowing therapist and the dietitian can be particularly advantageous during swallowing rehabilitation.

References

1. Wookey H. The surgical treatment of carcinoma of the pharynx and upper oesophagus. *Surg Gynecol Obstet* 1942; 75: 499.

2. Bakamjian VY. Total reconstruction of pharynx with medially based deltopectoral skin flap. *NY State J Med* 1968; 68: 2771.

Further reading

Fabian RL. Pectoralis major myocutaneous flap reconstruction of the larynogpharynx and cervical oesophagus. *Laryngoscope* 1988; 98: 1227–31.

Tiwari RM, Snow GP. Evaluation of the role of the pectoralis major myocutaneous flap. In: Ward PH, Berman WE, eds. *Proceedings of the Fourth International Symposium on Plastic and Reconstructive Surgery of the Head and Neck*. St Louis: CV Mosby, 1984: 992–6.

Illustrations by Gillian Oliver

Pharyngolaryngectomy: reconstruction by free jejunal transfer with microvascular anastomosis

M. J. Jurkiewicz MD, FACS
The Emory Clinic, Section of Plastic, Reconstructive and Maxillo-facial Surgery, Atlanta, Georgia, USA

J. Culbertson MD, FACS
The Emory Clinic, Section of Plastic, Reconstructive and Maxillo-facial Surgery, Atlanta, Georgia, USA

Introduction

Indications

The transfer of a segment of jejunum is an effective method of reconstructing the defect following pharyngo-laryngectomy when the resection includes the entire circumference of the pharyngolaryngeal complex, but its lower extent remains above the thoracic inlet. Tumours whose resection may leave such a defect include carcinomas of the larynx, with extension to the pharynx and/or oesophagus, and of hypopharynx with invasion of surrounding structures. The defect following resection of the cervical oesophagus, with or without laryngectomy, may also be suitable for this reconstruction, provided the defect is well above the thoracic inlet.

The method is also available as a back-up reconstruction following the failure of one of the alternative methods of reconstruction, or in the management of radiation necrosis resulting in a large pharyngocutaneous fistula.

The situation may arise when it is not considered necessary to resect the entire circumference of the pharynx and/or oesophagus, but the breadth of the circumference which is left is not sufficient to allow its conversion into a tube. To reconstruct such a partial defect the length of jejunum can be opened along its antimesenteric border and used as a patch to restore the circumferential continuity of the pharynx and cervical oesophagus.

Contraindications

The lower anastomosis of the jejunum becomes increasingly difficult technically as the stump of the oesophagus in the neck becomes shorter, and the technique should not be attempted when the defect extends to, or below, the thoracic inlet. The method is also contraindicated when multiple factors are present which make laparotomy a high-risk procedure, when previous abdominal operations may make the jejunal preparation difficult, or when other abdominal pathology such as ascites or Crohn's disease is present.

Preoperative preparation

Thorough preparation for all aspects of the procedure is the key to a successful outcome. In preparing the patient, optimal achievable nutritional repletion is necessary, particularly in the partially starved patient who has suffered substantial weight loss. Any pathological conditions from which the patient is suffering are corrected as far as possible. The procedure requires a two team approach, and an operating room with ample space is desirable. Prior discussion with the anaesthetist and the nursing staff is essential, so that they have an understanding of the procedure to be carried out, and an awareness of the possible problems which can arise, so that they will be anticipated and prepared for. Equipment must be checked, including the microscope light, appropriate suture material, and the various clamps, intestinal and microvascular. Hydration and warmth of the patient and avoidance of vasoconstrictors are critical.

1

It is often helpful to rotate the operating table to ensure that there is unencumbered access to the patient's head and neck during the extirpative procedure in the head and neck region.

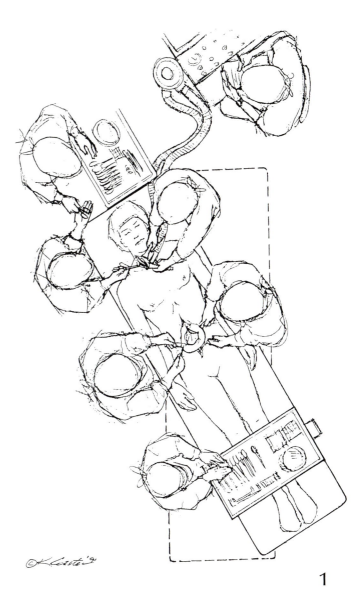

1

Operation

In carrying out the resection, the surgeon should make every effort to preserve a useful recipient vein in the neck, such as the external jugular, as long as its preservation does not compromise the resection. The vein can be dissected free for some distance and preserved ready for future use.

Harvest of jejunal segment

When the resection is nearing completion, and the extent of the resection is known approximately, the second surgical team begins the abdominal exposure. An upper midline or left upper quadrant transverse incision is used, the ligament of Treitz is identified, and a segment is isolated 40 cm distally along the jejunum.

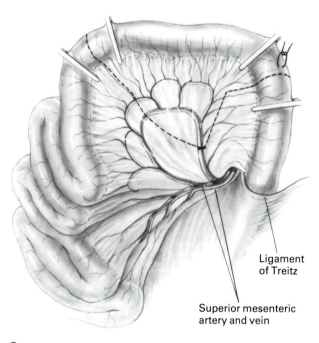

Ligament
of Treitz

Superior mesenteric
artery and vein

2

2

The length of jejunum required for reconstruction averages 8–10 cm in length, its precise length depending on the pharyngeal defect. This is measured in the neck and an appropriate length selected. A reliable radial vascular arcade with its supplying artery and vein is identified within the mesentery, and a suture is used to mark the proximal or distal end of the bowel segment selected to ensure isoperistaltic placement when transferred to the neck.

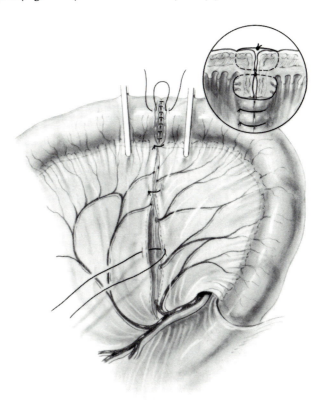

3

3 & 4

The vessel arcade is isolated, vascular branches being ligated as required to ensure an adequate blood supply both to the segment to be transferred and the remaining bowel on each side whose ends will be anastomosed when the segment is removed. In carrying out this part of the procedure, back-lighting of the mesentery and palpation of the vessels are helpful. A wedge of supporting mesentery is divided between silk ligatures, employing a meticulous technique to avoid a mesenteric haematoma. Magnifying loupes are helpful as dissection continues towards the apex of the wedge of mesentery, the veins in particular being quite fragile.

At this stage, vessel loops only are then passed around the single artery and vein of the superior mesenteric vessels supplying the jejunal segment. The segment is divided between clamps, wrapped in a moistened laparotomy pad and allowed to perfuse while preparations are made for anastomosis in the head and neck region. A sutured or stapled anastomosis of the jejunum is then performed, the lumen checked and the mesentery closed.

Proximal jejunum

Superior mesenteric
vein and artery

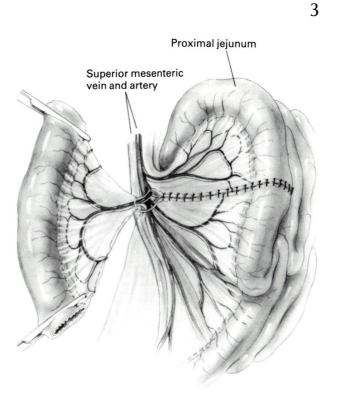

4

Preparation of vessels in the neck

With completion of the ablative procedure in the neck, the defect is measured once more and appropriate vessels, arterial and venous, are identified and prepared for anastomosis in the neck. In making the selection, matching of the vessel sizes is important, as is the location and course of the vessel. Where the ratio of the vessel sizes is greater than 1.5:1, end-to-side anastomosis is recommended. It is rarely necessary to use vein grafts unless there is doubt regarding vessel quality or tension. If the vessels exposed in the ipsilateral neck are unsatisfactory because of extensive inflammation, scarring or atherosclerosis, the contralateral side may be used.

5

Arterial inflow to the transferred jejunal segment is usually provided by one of the branches of the external carotid artery, the superior thyroid, or the transverse cervical artery. Occasionally the common carotid artery has to be used as the arterial inflow, though this is avoided if at all possible.

The artery selected is freed from the surrounding tissue and a soft non-calcified segment is selected as the site of anastomosis. Before a vessel is divided, it is helpful to tattoo the anterior surface of the vessels in preparation for anastomosis to ensure there is no twisting of them later. Neurosurgical vascular clamps seem well suited for these vessels. After the clamp has occluded the vessel selected and the intended position of the final anastomosis has been determined, its adequacy is checked by removing the clamp and documenting strong flow. The vascular clamp is then reapplied.

An appropriate matched vein is selected in the same region, the external jugular or posterior facial regularly being used, or alternatively an end-to-side anastomosis to the internal jugular vein. A vein which is in juxtaposition to the site of the tracheostomy should be avoided. The vein is freed from the surrounding tissue and a vascular clamp applied. If necessary, microvascular suction is placed in the dependent portion of the wound. Vicryl (Ethicon, Edinburgh, UK) or Dexon (Davis and Geck, Gosport, UK) 3/0 sutures can be inserted into the posterior oropharynx to facilitate the subsequent anastomosis.

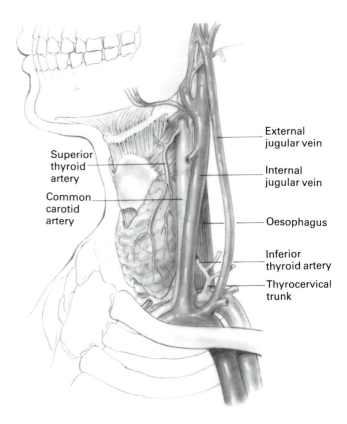

External jugular vein

Superior thyroid artery

Internal jugular vein

Common carotid artery

Oesophagus

Inferior thyroid artery

Thyrocervical trunk

5

Transfer of the jejunal segment

With preparation of the vessels in the neck completed, attention is directed back to the abdomen. The jejunal segment is checked for viability, and the perfusing vessels are divided and ligated with silk ties. The jejunal segment is brought to the head and neck and positioned isoperistaltically. Vessel lengths, contour and size match are checked.

Upper anastomosis of the jejunal segment

6

The proximal oropharyngeal jejunal anastomosis is the first to be performed. Often this is the most difficult portion of the entire procedure. The resection is frequently high as a result of the spread of the pharyngeal carcinoma and suture placement can be difficult, as is proper circumferential matching. This part of the procedure may have to be varied depending on the local situation, including variations in the contour and application of the jejunal segment with occasional oblique cuts or antimesenteric opening of its upper end. The proximal bowel can safely be opened along its antimesenteric border and tailored to fit the defect from tongue to posterior pharynx if necessary. Any of these adjustments may be required to allow adequate anastomosis to a large and irregular pharynx. When a postoperative fistula arises, the upper anastomosis is the most frequent site.

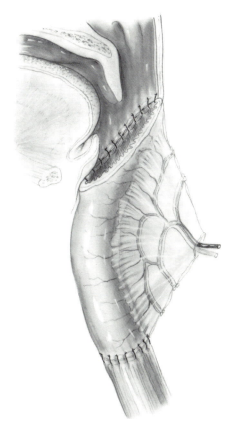

6

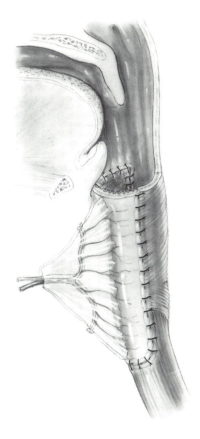

7

7

A further variation is opening of the entire jejunal tube along its antimesenteric border, converting it into a jejunal patch when a portion of the pharynx remains.

Microvascular anastomosis

8

At the completion of the upper pharyngojejunal anastomosis the microscope is brought into the field. The vessels are checked for torsion and contour, and outflow of the artery is again confirmed. The most difficult anastomosis, usually the deeper, is carried out first. The technique of anastomosis is described in the chapter on 'Reconstructive techniques of the skin', pp. 45–103. The more superficial anastomosis is then completed. In the event of an atherosclerotic plaque being unavoidably present in the vessel, it is essential that the needle is passed towards the plaque and outwards in order to avoid dissection of the plaque or intima. With completion of the anastomosis the vascular clamps are removed, vein first, and then artery. Perfusion should be readily apparent, with pulsation of the vessels along the bowel, and bleeding, peristalsis and mucus secretion.

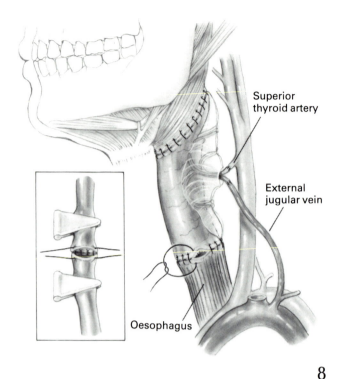

Superior thyroid artery

External jugular vein

Oesophagus

8

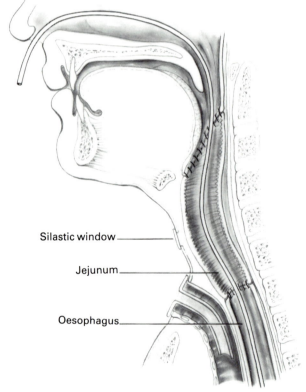

Silastic window

Jejunum

Oesophagus

9

Lower jejunal anastomosis

9

At this point, the length of the jejunal segment is again checked. A frequent mistake is to use a segment that is too long and redundant. The segment is tailored and the distal jejunal oesophageal anastomosis performed with interrupted 3/0 Vicryl or Dexon sutures.

A nasogastric tube may then be passed through the segment on into the stomach. Before the skin flaps are closed, the neck should be put through a full range of passive motion to ensure there is no twisting or torsion of the vessels, and appropriate tacking sutures can be placed to maintain the vessels in a satisfactory position. In addition, the mesentery of the bowel can be appropriately positioned over the carotid vessels with further tacking sutures to provide additional protection. There is usually no difficulty in closure of the skin flaps. Prior to closure of the abdomen, a gastrostomy or feeding jejunostomy distal to the bowel anastomosis is recommended.

Monitoring the jejunal segment

10

Monitoring of the jejunal segment is important and several options are available. One is exposure of an area of the surface of the jejunal segment by making a small window in the anterior neck incision and filling it with a sheet of Silastic film (Dow Corning, Reading, UK) prior to closure of the neck flaps. This allows the state of the jejunum to be monitored visually postoperatively. An alternative is the isolation of a vascular piece of bowel or mesentery on a small pedicle brought out through the wound and observed postoperatively.

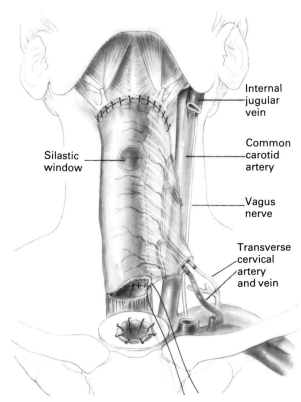

Internal jugular vein

Common carotid artery

Silastic window

Vagus nerve

Transverse cervical artery and vein

10

Postoperative care and complications

It is important that no circumferential tracheostomy tube tapes are placed and that there is no other compression in the vicinity of the vascular anastomosis. Sandbags are also positioned on each side of the neck to control movements of the head.

Cooling of the jejunum prior to revascularization has proved of little benefit, and neither heparin nor dextran has been found of value. We believe the use of aspirin is sufficient when an appropriate surgical technique has been used. Patients routinely receive appropriate perioperative antibiotics, as discussed in the chapter on 'General management and complications' pp. 8–21, and jejunal feeding is begun as soon as they can tolerate it. The viability of the jejunal segment is regularly assessed and, if vessel occlusion is diagnosed, re-exploration is carried out. This can salvage an ischaemic flap.

The nasogastric tube is generally removed 1 week postoperatively and a barium swallow performed. A liquid diet may be instituted if no leak is demonstrated at that time. If a fistula develops, it usually heals by secondary intention and can be managed on an outpatient basis. The abundant production of mucus seen after revascularization gradually subsides, and most patients have recovered with complete healing at 4 weeks, in time to begin radiation therapy as necessary. Effective swallowing is reported in 83 per cent of patients.

Acknowledgements

Illustration 1 is reproduced with permission of Kip Carter, M.S., Fine Medical and Commercial Illustration, Winterville, Georgia, USA.

Illustrations by Robert Lane

Pharyngolaryngo-oesophagectomy: reconstruction by colonic transposition

David J. Howard FRCS, FRCS(Ed)
Institute of Laryngology and Otology, Royal National Throat, Nose and Ear Hospital, London, UK

A. E. Thompson FRCS
St. Thomas' Hospital, London, UK

Introduction

In 1944 Yudin reported resection of the thoracic oesophagus and repair by colon in a series of 80 patients[1]. Goligher and Robin reported in 1954 on the use of colon for reconstruction after pharyngolaryngectomy and cervical oesophagectomy[2]. During the 1960s and 1970s, reconstruction with colon became a widely used technique and is still the procedure of choice in some centres; however, reports show a level of morbidity and mortality greater than that presently experienced following gastric transposition and free jejunal procedures. The higher level of complications appears to be related to the potential problems of three separate anastomoses and the fact that the blood supply of the transposed colonic segment is inferior to that of transposed stomach or free jejunum. However, the choice of procedure will depend on the experience of the surgeon and team rather than on any specific advantages of a particular technique. Colonic transposition may be the best reconstructive method available for patients who have had previous gastric surgery and who have extensive lesions of the cervical oesophagus.

Colonic segment

When choosing an appropriate segment of colon there are two major variables to be considered: the length of segment required and its vascular supply. Portions of the ascending, transverse and descending colon have all been used, based on the marginal artery being supplied by either the middle colic or the left colic vessels. The marginal artery passes along the mesenteric border about 2 cm from the bowel wall but variation is common, and in practice the choice is made at laparotomy following examination of the vascular anatomy by transillumination, palpation and temporary vascular occlusion. The surgeon may elect to raise the ascending colon and transverse colon based on the middle colic or left colic vessels, or the transverse colon and descending colon based on the left colic vessels. The greatest length of bowel available is usually the left half of the transverse colon and the descending colon fed by the left colic vessels.

Route of transposed colon

After resection of the oesophagus the colon may be passed to the neck subcutaneously, retrosternally or through the posterior mediastinum; all three routes have been used and each has its advocates.

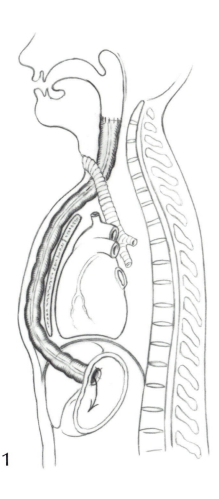

1

1

The subcutaneous route was initially thought to be the safest should necrosis of the transposed segment occur, but it is in fact the longest route, unsightly and more often associated with poor swallowing after the operation.

2

The retrosternal route is shorter than the subcutaneous route and the dissection easily accomplished. The authors advocate removal of a manubrial segment and the medial end of one or both clavicles in order to make the retrosternal transposition easier and safer by preventing any compression of the colonic vascular supply at the thoracic inlet.

Both the above routes are particularly applicable if not all the intrathoracic oesophagus is to be removed.

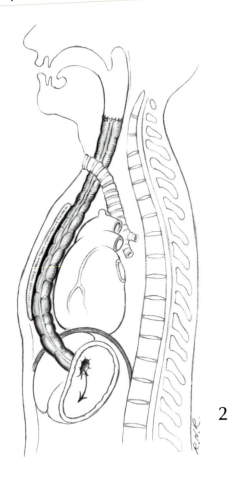

2

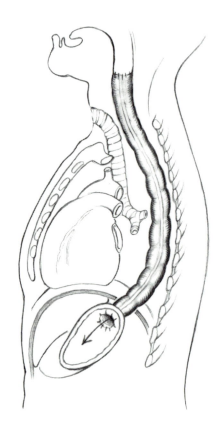

3

3

If the inferior limit of the cervical oesophageal disease is high, division and ligation at the upper end of the thoracic oesophagus may be undertaken, which lessens the morbidity that accompanies blunt dissection of the whole mediastinum. When the whole thoracic oesophagus is removed the colon may be transposed to the neck through the posterior mediastinum, with the advantage that its presence lessens the tendency for bleeding from the posterior mediastinal vessels. However, although this is the shortest route, it is more difficult to perform and any subsequent leakage or necrosis in the mediastinum carries a high rate of morbidity and mortality.

Indications

Advanced hypopharyngeal and cervical oesophageal carcinomas and extensive benign disease of the oesophagus can be treated by this method. However, the use of colon is advocated only when the gastric transposition and free jejunal procedures are unsuitable. Colonic viability is not sufficiently satisfactory to advocate using this method for replacing the pharynx after removing advanced laryngeal carcinoma with base of tongue and hypopharyngeal involvement, or after resection for stomal recurrence.

Preoperative assessment and contraindications

These are as indicated on p. 403 in the chapter on 'Pharyngolaryngo-oesophagectomy: reconstruction by gastric transposition' and are of extreme importance. Inadequate preoperative preparation and lack of attention to detail will substantially raise the morbidity and mortality of the procedure.

Operation

UPPER END OF PHARYNGOLARYNGO-OESOPHAGECTOMY

Anaesthesia and incision

The preferred method of general anaesthesia is via endotracheal intubation; initial establishment of a tracheostomy may compromise the laryngopharyngeal resection and is to be avoided. Where cervical neck nodes are not clinically palpable or suspected, a shallow U-shaped Gluck–Soerensen incision is most suitable and can, if necessary, be extended for neck dissection. Elective neck dissection is not usually advocated, post-operative radiotherapy being the treatment of choice in the high-risk N0 neck. In patients with predominantly postcricoid and cervical oesophageal disease, para-tracheal nodal spread is the main concern, rather than cervical nodal involvement.

Resection

4

The strap muscles are divided flush with the sternum and the root of the neck evaluated to determine the approximate limits of the primary lesion and to confirm resectability. Suspicious lymph nodes may be sent for frozen section review. Manubrial resection and excision of the medial ends of the clavicles is then undertaken, not only to facilitate clearance of the disease but also to allow unhindered transposition of the colonic segment. The details of this procedure are discussed in the chapter on 'Surgery for the prevention and treatment of stomal recurrence', pp. 508–516.

The mobilization of the laryngopharyngeal segment proceeds routinely as described in the chapter on 'Total laryngectomy', pp. 481–493, but in patients with post-cricoid disease includes total thyroidectomy. Care must be taken to include as much paratracheal and para-oesophageal areolar and lymphatic tissue as possible, using the medial aspect of the carotid sheath as the lateral limit of clearance. The superior limit of the resection will depend on the distribution of the primary lesion; colonic

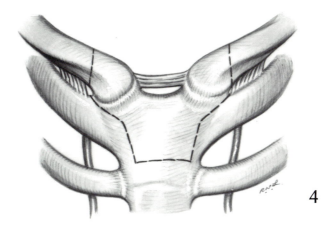

4

replacement is unsatisfactory if the superior limit includes the tongue base or there is oropharyngeal involvement. The propensity for submucosal spread of pharyngeal disease should constantly be borne in mind and maximal mucosal limits of clearance obtained superiorly.

Once the laryngopharyngeal complex is mobilized a decision should be made as to whether the whole intrathoracic oesophagus should be removed. If a satisfactory inferior margin can be obtained, the upper thoracic oesophagus may be divided and the stump closed in two layers with interrupted chromic catgut. Should the inferior limit be in any way doubtful, it is preferable to resect the whole intrathoracic oesophagus by blunt dissection/excision at the gastro-oesophageal junction, which is then closed with two layers of interrupted chromic catgut.

The trachea is transected at an appropriate place below the larynx, cut obliquely if possible but bearing in mind that both lower hypopharyngeal and cervical oesophageal lesions often involve the posterior trachealis by direct spread. The routine manubrial resection allows for as low a division of the trachea as necessary, and the stoma is usually established in the vertical lip of the skin incision which extends in the midline below the Gluck–Soerensen incision. General anaesthesia is continued by means of a new tracheal tube and sterile connections through the stoma.

As with the gastric transposition procedure, the abdominal procedure may be undertaken following pharyngolaryngo-oesophagectomy, rather than synchron-ously. This will depend on the preference of the individual surgeon, the facilities available and experience in any given centre.

CERVICOABDOMINAL PROCEDURE WITH COLONIC TRANSPOSITION

Incision

5

An extended midline anterior abdominal wall incision is used. Laparotomy is performed and metastatic spread in the liver or other intra-abdominal anomalies are established.

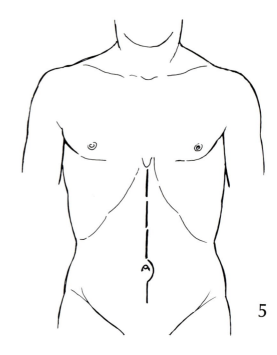

5

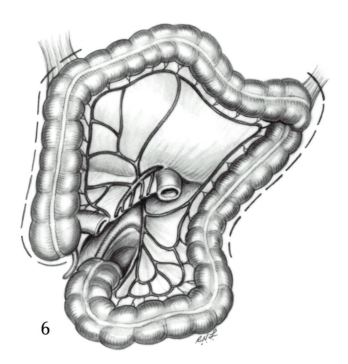

6

Mobilization of colon

6

The whole of the colon is mobilized, using incisions in both paracolic gutters and detaching the omentum from the transverse colon.

7

The vascular anatomy of the colon is studied by transillumination and palpation. The blood supply to be used is carefully planned. The vessels to be divided are carefully exposed, without damage, and bulldog clamps applied to test the adequacy of the blood supply once these vessels are occluded. Care and patience are required at this stage. The surgeon may attend to the retrosternal dissection at this stage, to allow a longer period of vessel occlusion.

The loose areolar tissue between the residual sternum and the pericardium is freed from above, avoiding damage to the innominate vein which is already displayed by removal of the manubrial segment.

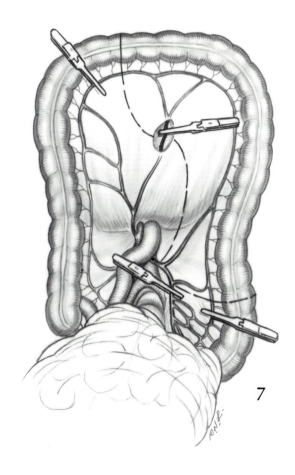

7

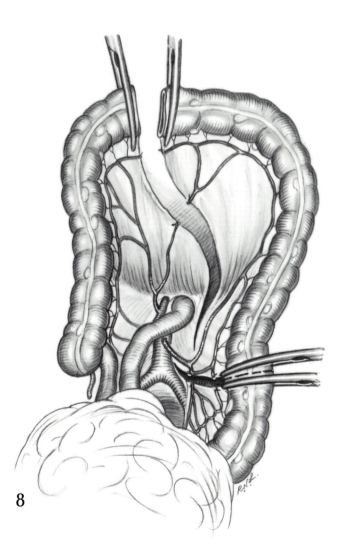

8

8

Both transverse and descending colon are used based on the left colic vessel. The local vascular anatomy may require use of the middle colic artery to supply the colonic segment, with division of the left colic vessel. It is preferable to divide either artery before its bifurcation to the marginal artery, as this allows a secondary vascular arcade around any portion of the marginal artery which may be insufficient. Following vascular isolation, the colon is transected between soft intestinal clamps at appropriate points. Compression of nearby blood vessels must be avoided.

Restoration of continuity

9

Colonic continuity is restored by an end-to-end anastomosis using two layers of sutures in the conventional way: continuous catgut for the all-coats layer and interrupted seromuscular silk externally.

The freed bowel is now prepared for passage through the chest. Any peritoneal bands restricting use of its full length are carefully divided. Damage to vessels must be avoided.

At this stage a pyloromyotomy may be undertaken, as this is necessary after the vagotomy which accompanies an oesophageal excision.

If required, mobilization of the lower part of the oesophagus is carried out by finger dissection through the diaphragmatic hiatus, working synchronously from above and below. Gentle traction on the laryngopharyngeal specimen by the upper operator and temporary deflation of the endotracheal tube cuff are advised during this manoeuvre. The oesophagus is then divided at the gastro-oesophageal junction and removed by gentle upward pulling with additional assistance from below. The gastro-oesophageal junction is closed in two layers with interrupted chromic catgut sutures.

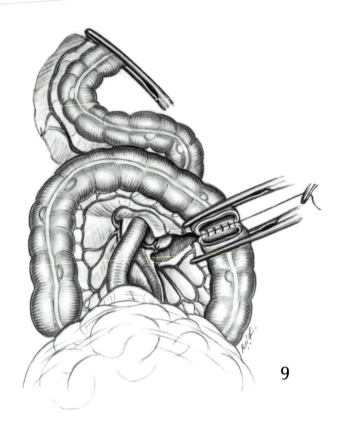

9

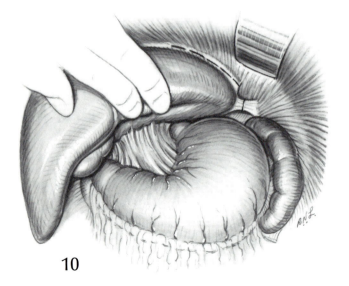

10

10

The attachment of the anterior part of the diaphragm to the chest wall is exposed by division of the triangular ligament of the liver, which allows the left lobe to be retracted to the right.

11

The diaphragm is exposed from below. A liberal hiatus is developed through the central tendon.

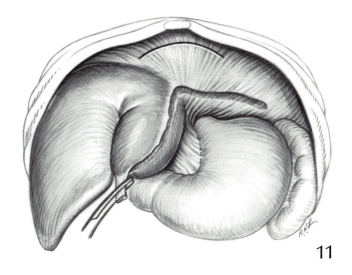

11

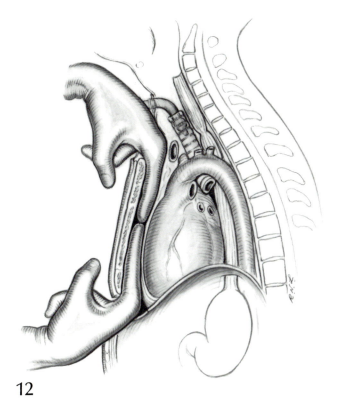

12

12

The space behind the sternum is developed by blunt dissection upwards to meet the space from the neck.

Transposition

13

The colon is passed through this space by gentle traction on a loosely tied piece of Paul's tubing, supplemented by gentle pushing from below. The tubing is removed as soon as possible to avoid pressure on vessels.

At this point an adequate length of colon lying comfortably at the root of the neck and in the upper abdomen should be visible. The feeding vessels must be slack without twists.

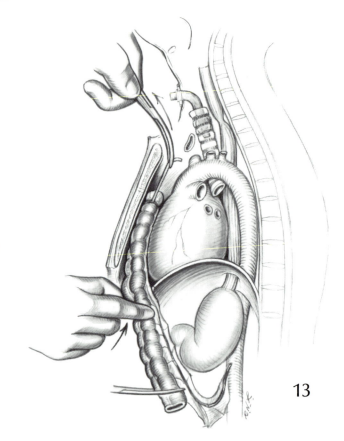

13

Anastomosis

14

The lower end of the colon is anastomosed to the anterior surface of the stomach in two layers, as described for the colon.

The upper end of the colon is anastomosed to the residual pharynx using a similar two-layer closure. It is important to ensure that the vascular pedicle and marginal artery are not twisted or compressed at any point in their passage from abdomen to neck.

Jejunostomy

A jejunostomy is constructed approximately 20 cm from the duodeno–jejunal junction. A Foley catheter is used and the bowel sutured to the abdominal wall at four points by interrupted chromic catgut sutures.

Closure

Following irrigation with noxythiolin the abdomen is closed and drains placed in the left paracolic gutter and subhepatic area. The neck wound is closed over bilateral corrugated drains and an additional small mediastinal drain is placed inferior to the stoma in the vertical component of the incision. The right pleural cavity may be opened inadvertently during retrosternal dissection and a right basal chest drain is advisable.

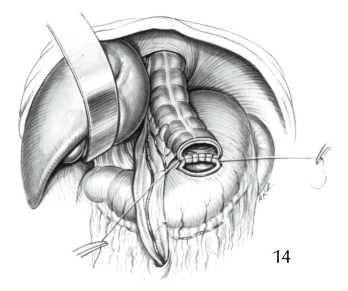

14

Postoperative management

Postoperative care is as described in the chapter on 'Pharyngolaryngo-oesophagectomy: reconstruction by gastric transposition', pp. 402–410, with similar attention to fluid balance, thyroxine and calcium replacement, drains, dressings, stoma care, chest and general physiotherapy.

In contrast to the gastric transposition procedure, there are two intra-abdominal anastomotic suture lines, but jejunostomy feeding can usually be started slowly on the third or fourth postoperative day. However, the pharyngocolonic anastomosis is less reliable than the pharyngogastric anastomosis and before oral feeding is commenced, usually 7–10 days after operation, a videofluoroscopic swallow evaluation should be undertaken. A normal swallow often takes considerably longer to establish after colonic transposition, and although there may initially be less regurgitation than with the stomach, persistent unpleasant thick mucus secretion can sometimes be a problem. Local rehabilitation in these patients is unpredictable, although approximately 20 per cent of long-survival patients will develop a serviceable voice with speech therapy. Experience with Blom–Singer valve type prostheses is limited and no reliable figures are available.

Complications

Respiratory and cardiovascular complications may occur (as with all major surgery); however, the increased mortality and morbidity of the colonic procedure is a consequence of increased graft failure, i.e. colonic necrosis. Anastomotic leakage, particularly from the pharyngocolonic anastomosis, with fistula formation between the anastomosis, skin and/or trachea is more common than with the gastric procedure.

Long-term problems

Recurrence of disease is the most frequent long-term problem; the quality of swallowing is also considerably lower overall than that for transposed stomach or free jejunal transfer. Upper and lower anastomotic stricture formation contribute to dysphagia but the overall transit time of food through the colonic segment is slow.

References

1. Yudin S. Surgical construction of 80 cases of artificial esophagus. *Surg Gynecol Obstet* 1944; 78: 561–3.

2. Goligher JC, Robin IG. Use of left colon for reconstruction of the pharynx and oesophagus after pharyngectomy. *Br J Surg* 1954; 42: 283–90.

Further reading

Griffiths JD, Shaw HS. Cancer of the laryngopharynx and cervical esophagus. *Arch Otolaryngol* 1973; 97: 340–6.

Slaney G, Dalton GA. Problems of viscus replacement following pharyngolaryngectomy. *J Laryngol Otol* 1973; 87: 539–46.

Pharyngolaryngo-oesophagectomy: reconstruction by gastric transposition

David J. Howard FRCS, FRCS(Ed)
Institute of Laryngology and Otology, Royal National Throat, Nose and Ear Hospital, London, UK

A. E. Thompson FRCS
St. Thomas' Hospital, London, UK

Introduction

The literature of the last three decades on head and neck surgery contains a wide variety of treatment regimes for hypopharyngeal and cervical oesophageal carcinoma. Management options such as microvascular free tissue jejunal transfer, colonic transposition and myocutaneous flap reconstruction are covered in adjacent chapters. Although surgical emphasis is often placed on the most effective, safe and rapid means of reconstructing a pharyngeal or pharyngo-oesophageal segment after tumour resection, it is meaningless unless the margins of resection are clear. Failure to eradicate tumour at the primary site is by far the largest cause of patient morbidity and mortality in carcinoma of the hypopharynx and cervical oesophagus. It is therefore of utmost importance that the surgeon undertaking the treatment of disease in this area is fully conversant with the surgical anatomy and the detailed natural history of the pathology of hypopharyngeal and cervical oesophageal cancer. These important details are to be found on pp. 379–380. The gastric transposition procedure is an effective but potentially hazardous method which, if carried out in selected patients by an experienced surgical team, comes close to meeting the requirements of an ideal means of reconstruction. As clearly stated in 1980 by De Santo and Carpenter[1], this involves resection of the cancer and restoration of a swallowing conduit in one stage, employing tissue outside the field of radiation, and allowing healing without troublesome morbidity from complications. Pharyngolaryngo-oesophagectomy allows good margins of excision inferiorly but is limited superiorly to the same extent as all types of pharyngectomy. Gastric transposition through the posterior mediastinum brings fresh healthy tissue up to the level of the soft palate with an excellent, almost trouble-free, anastomosis. There are no absolute guidelines for gastric transposition and each patient must be considered carefully to assess whether this procedure is the most suitable means of offering radical resection with cure or worthwhile palliation.

Indications

Bearing in mind the anatomical and physiological considerations on pp. 379–380, the authors advocate gastric transposition in:

1. Postcricoid carcinoma.
2. Cervical oesophageal carcinoma.
3. Advanced piriform fossa carcinoma.
4. Advanced posterior hypopharyngeal wall carcinoma.
5. Advanced laryngeal carcinoma with base of tongue and hypopharyngeal involvement.
6. Stomal recurrence requiring pharyngectomy or cervical oesophagectomy.

Many other patients with hypopharyngeal disease may be treated by partial pharyngectomy and laryngectomy or by pharyngolaryngectomy with primary closure using myocutaneous flaps or free jejunum.

Preoperative procedures

Assessment

In much of surgery for head and neck cancer the nutritional status and general condition of the patient are relevant to subsequent morbidity and operative mortality. However, these factors unfortunately rarely receive adequate attention. This must not be the case when considering pharyngolaryngo-oesophagectomy and gastric transposition, as mortality and morbidity can become unacceptable, as demonstrated by experience in some centres. Patients with hypopharyngeal and cervical oesophageal carcinoma frequently present after prolonged periods of dysphagia and with weight loss in excess of 10 kg. This is particularly true in failed radiotherapy patients who have residual or recurrent disease. Immediate operation in these patients can have disastrous consequences. The authors advocate 2 weeks of intensive nutrition, preferably by nasogastric tube or jejunostomy but alternatively by intravenous means. This period can usefully be utilized for other essential preoperative measures such as chest physiotherapy, counselling of the patient and family, preoperative introduction to the speech therapist, social service assessment and the other mandatory preoperative assessments outlined below.

Contraindications

Age is a poor guide, but in general patients over 75 years of age are not accepted for this procedure. Other definite contraindications are:

1. Systemic metastases.
2. Bilateral or fixed cervical lymph nodes.
3. Gross local disease with bilateral carotid invasion.
4. Severe emphysema.

Relative contraindications are a previous history of myocardial infarction and severe diabetes. Other major medical conditions may exist which have to be assessed in each patient against a background of the inevitably progressive, unpleasant and fatal primary disease.

Investigations

An exhaustive list of investigations to cover every individual patient is not possible here, but the following are routinely undertaken:

1. Radiographs: chest; video swallow; CT or MRI scans.
2. Blood tests: cross-match six units; full blood count; urea and electrolytes; liver function tests; serum iron and total iron binding capacity; Australia antigen.
3. General tests: electrocardiograph; nose and throat swabs; midstream specimens of urine; respiratory function tests; sputum microbiology.

Fibreoptic and rigid endoscopy under general anaesthesia, with accompanying biopsy, confirm the extent and diagnosis of mucosal tumour. In obstructing lesions a nasogastric tube for preoperative nutrition is inserted at this procedure.

Bowel preparation

All patients undergo preoperative bowel preparation in case colonic transposition is required because of unforeseen difficulties with gastric transposition. Those patients on a normal diet commence laxatives on a regular basis 4 days before surgery and receive phosphate enemas as required. Patients on a low residue or liquid diet require less bowel preparation. All patients are placed on a low residue diet 24 h before surgery.

Prophylactic perioperative antibiotics

High dose metronidazole and cefuroxime are given with the premedication and continued for up to 10 days after surgery.

Operation

UPPER END OF PHARYNGOLARYNGO-OESOPHAGECTOMY

Initial considerations

The preferred method of general anaesthesia is via endotracheal intubation. Initial establishment of a tracheostomy may compromise the laryngopharyngeal resection and is to be avoided. Where cervical neck nodes are not suspected or clinically palpable a shallow U-shaped Gluck–Soerensen incision is most suitable, which can, if necessary, be extended for neck dissection. Elective neck dissection is not usually advocated, postoperative radiotherapy being the treatment of choice in the high-risk N0 neck. Over 70 per cent of the patients treated by the authors using this procedure have postcricoid and cervical oesophageal disease, and spread to paratracheal nodes, rather than cervical nodes, is the main concern. Following division of the strap muscles flush with the sternum, the root of the neck is evaluated to determine the approximate limits of the primary lesion and to confirm resectability. Suspicious lymph nodes may be sent for frozen section review. A decision is made as to whether manubrial resection and mediastinal dissection are required to facilitate clearance of the disease (these are discussed in the chapter on 'Surgery for the prevention and treatment of stomal recurrence' pp. 508–516); if they are, the manubrial excision is performed at this point.

Resection

1, 2 & 3

The mobilization of the laryngopharyngeal segment proceeds routinely as described in the chapter on 'Total laryngectomy', pp. 481–493, but in patients with postcricoid disease includes total thyroidectomy. Care is taken to include as much paratracheal and paraoesophageal areolar and lymphatic tissue as is possible, using the medial aspect of the carotid sheath as the lateral limit of this clearance. The superior limit of the resection will vary according to the distribution of the primary lesion but may involve tongue base or oropharyngeal dissection to obtain reasonable superior clearance. The propensity for submucosal spread of pharyngeal disease should constantly be borne in mind and maximal mucosal limits of clearance obtained superiorly. Following mobilization of the laryngopharyngeal complex the specimen remains attached to the oesophagus, which is later completely removed by division at the gastro-oesophageal junction.

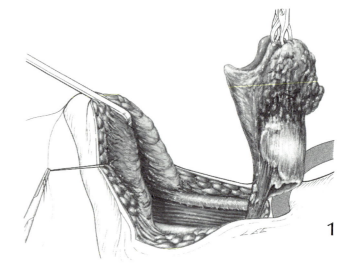

3

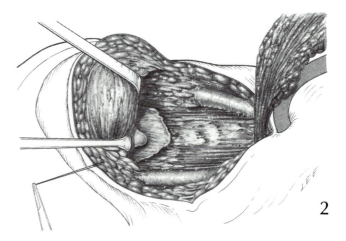

2

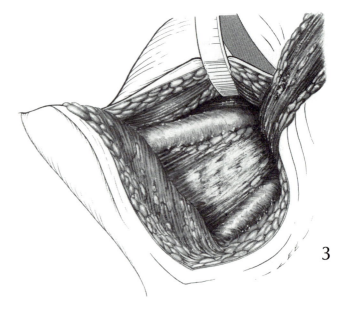

1

Tracheal stoma

The trachea is transected at an appropriate place below the larynx, cutting obliquely if possible but bearing in mind that both lower hypopharyngeal and cervical oesophageal lesions tend to involve the posterior trachealis by direct spread. The tracheal stoma is then established in a new incision below the apex of the Gluck–Soerensen incision and administration of the general anaesthetic gases is transferred to this stoma using a new tracheal tube and sterile connections. The laryngopharyngeal specimen is wrapped in a large, moist pack while the rest of the resection and gastric transposition is completed. Occasionally, if disease involves prevertebral fascia and muscle, additional excision will be required, but care must be taken not to resect the anterior longitudinal ligament nor to injure the vertebral arteries in their lateral position.

Opinions differ as to whether the abdominal procedure can be undertaken synchronously with the cervical resection: it depends on the facilities and experience in any given centre. The authors' preference is for the abdominal procedure to follow the laryngopharyngeal mobilization. Little time is lost by the abdominal team waiting, and indeed both teams tend to operate more quickly without the distraction of the other.

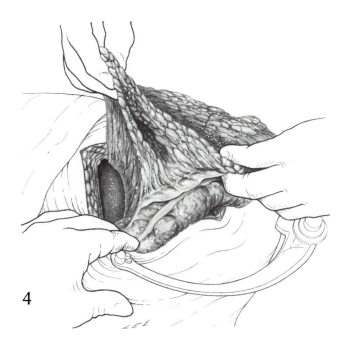

4

LOWER END OF PHARYNGOLARYNGO-OESOPHAGECTOMY WITH GASTRIC TRANSPOSITION

The purpose of this stage of the operation is to mobilize the stomach and allow sufficient length to be taken through the mediastinum into the neck so that the fundus can be anastomosed to the remaining pharynx. The patient undergoes a full bowel preparation before surgery, in case the stomach is not suitable and the colon has to be used as an alternative.

Incision

A midline epigastric incision is used, which allows adequate access to the oesophageal hiatus and to the second and third parts of the duodenum. A preliminary laparotomy establishes that no other intra-abdominal pathology is present. Hepatic metastases secondary to squamous carcinoma of the hypopharynx are uncommon.

Gastric mobilization

The stomach is mobilized on the right gastric and right gastroepiploic vessels. The latter vessels are particularly important and care must be taken not to damage them.

4 & 5

The first manoeuvre is to divide the gastrocolic omentum well away from the right gastroepiploic vessels. The lesser sac is entered at roughly the midpoint of the greater omentum above the colon and must be carefully delineated, for a number of naturally occurring adhesions always tend to obscure the field and need to be carefully divided. One of these adhesions will contain the left gastric vessels and should be clearly identified. Once the lesser sac has been entered and the gastrocolic omentum defined, the latter should be divided between artery forceps.

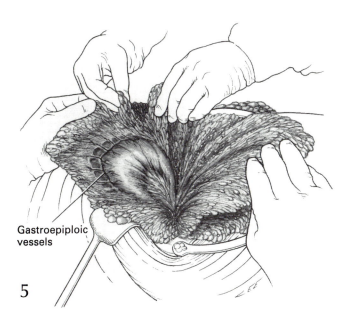

Gastroepiploic vessels

5

6

The line of division is continued distally to the first part of the duodenum and proximally along the hilum of the spleen until all the short gastric vessels have been ligated. In the course of this procedure attention is diverted to the left gastric vessels which are ligated separately with strong ligatures.

The lesser omentum proximal to the right gastric vessels is divided, including the vessels and nerves going into the left end of the porta hepatis. The phreno-oesophageal ligaments and both vagus nerves are exposed and divided.

Duodenal mobilization

Attention is then turned to the distal end of the stomach. The duodenum is mobilized as far as the middle of the third part of the duodenum, entailing a transverse incision above the hepatic flexure followed by downward displacement of the colon. This allows full access to the whole of the second part of the duodenum. Division of the peritoneum and serosal attachments is continued along the proximal half of the third part of the duodenum to allow it to be completely mobilized from the posterior abdominal wall as far as the left side of the aorta. The left renal vein is commonly seen.

Pyloromyotomy and jejunostomy

7 & 8

After this mobilization, the pyloric muscle is divided (pyloromyotomy), taking the whole of the gastric muscle wall down to the mucosa, carefully avoiding the shouldering of the first part of the duodenum. At this stage a jejunostomy is established 20 cm from the duodeno-jejunal flexure. A Foley catheter is commonly used and the bowel sutured to the abdominal wall at four points.

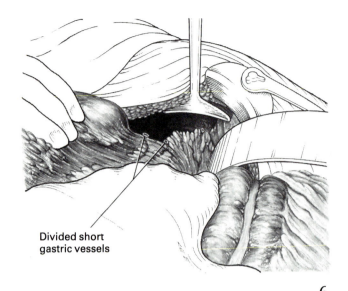

Divided short gastric vessels

6

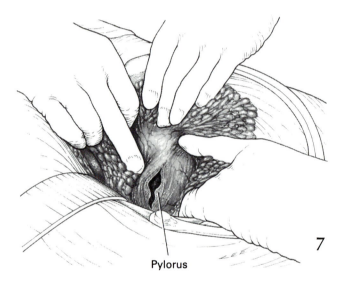

Pylorus

7

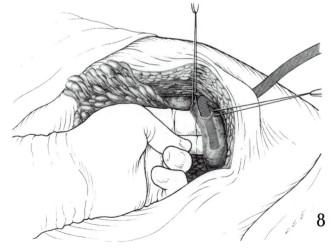

8

Chest drains

9

Bilateral lower chest drains are established by inserting cannulae into the lower part of the chest through a lateral incision, guiding the tip of the trocar/cannula with fingers under the diaphragm. These are connected to underwater seal drains and carefully stitched and taped in place.

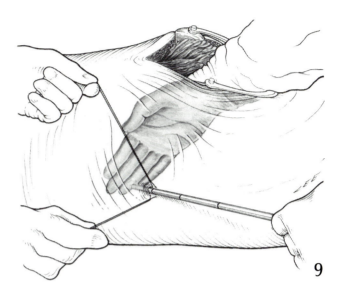

9

Oesophageal mobilization and gastric transposition

10

The oesophagus must now be mobilized, and the procedure involves operators working from both the upper and lower ends. The lower end of the oesophagus is separated from the aorta posteriorly by finger dissection, extending to both sides of the oesophagus and then to the front. Great care must be taken at the level of the bifurcation of the trachea, where some oesophageal muscle fibres run forward onto the trachea. The balloon on the endotracheal tube is deflated at this stage. A bimanual approach, with blunt finger dissection by the operator at the lower end from above and below, is often essential to complete the separation of the oesophagus from the surrounding tissues. When it is free, the oesophagus will be drawn upwards and the mobilized stomach pushed through from below until the fundus can be reached from above. A combination of pulling and pushing brings it into the neck.

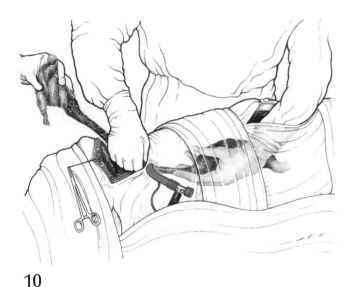

10

Closure

The lower end is now almost complete. Haemostasis is achieved and the hiatus should be carefully examined, as it sometimes needs to be enlarged by stretching to allow mobilization of the oesophagus. Several interrupted sutures may be required to restore a reasonable hiatus. The abdomen is not usually drained, but can be if necessary. The abdominal wall is closed in layers.

PHARYNGOGASTRIC ANASTOMOSIS

Following transposition of the stomach, the surgical specimen comprising the pharynx, larynx and oesophagus is freed from the stomach by division at the gastro-oesophageal junction between non-crushing bowel clamps. The oesophageal stump is closed in a meticulous fashion with two layers of interrupted chromic catgut sutures.

11

If the superior limits of the pharyngeal tumour were high and the excision included oropharynx and/or tongue base, the pharyngogastric anastomosis may be under some tension. This tension can be lessened and distributed more evenly by insertion of a number of horizontal mattress sutures between the posterior wall of the stomach and the prevertebral fascia. The fundus of the stomach is held between Babcock's soft tissue forceps and approximated to the pharyngeal remnant.

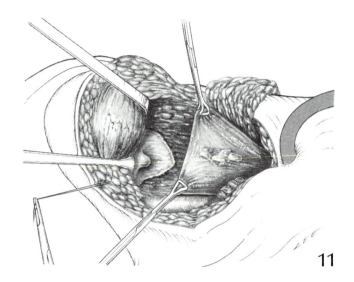

11

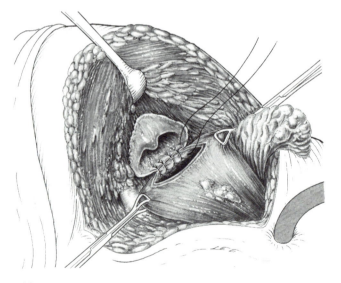

12

12

The outer posterior layer of interrupted catgut sutures at the anastomosis is placed through serosa and muscle prior to opening into the fundus of the stomach. This is done using a No. 15 blade scalpel, and any blood or gastric secretions are carefully sucked from within the stomach to prevent soiling of the neck wound. The second layer of inverted sutures is then begun in the midline on the posterior wall, advancing in a circumferential fashion to complete a water-tight inner layer between pharynx and stomach. These sutures must be placed carefully to distribute tension and generous 5 mm bites are recommended. The width of the anastomosis should be 4–5 cm.

13

An anterior second layer of interrupted sutures completes the anastomosis and, as this is the most likely area for increased tension, it may be preferable for these to be horizontal mattress in type. If sufficient omentum is available and can be approximated without tension, it is used to reinforce the anastomotic suture line.

If a neck dissection has been undertaken, there is often sufficient gastric tissue to cover exposed carotid vessels and on occasions when anterior neck skin is removed as part of the excision, simple direct skin grafting of the anterior stomach wall obviates the need for more complicated flap surgery[2].

The tracheal stoma is placed in either a separate incision below the apex of the Gluck–Soerensen incision or in the vertical limb used when manubrial resection is undertaken. The neck incisions are closed in two layers over bilateral corrugated neck drains and a small central midline drain inferior to the stoma draining the manubrial space. A light but bulky soft gauze dressing is applied to the neck. A cuffed light-weight Silastic tracheostomy tube (Dow Corning, Reading, UK) is inserted at the end of the procedure and the flanges are stitched to the underlying skin for security. Great care is also taken with the security of the chest drains and the connections for underwater sealed drainage. Mobilization of the patient from the operating table to the intensive care unit bed requires skilled cooperation by all concerned.

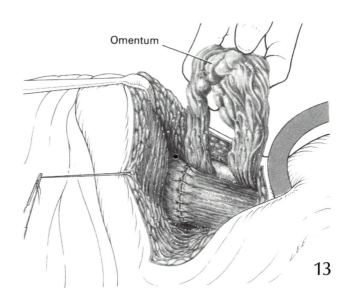

Omentum

13

Postoperative management

These patients require a high level of postoperative nursing skill and medical management. Postoperative ventilation is not routinely employed on our unit and indeed is not without its own risks, particularly to the relatively unsupported posterior tracheal wall as a consequence of the inflated cuff and positive pressure ventilation. All patients require regular and careful monitoring as for any major surgery, bearing in mind the possible respiratory complications and major fluid losses. The patients are normally nursed sitting semi-upright at 45° to the horizontal.

Chest drains

These are mandatory in our experience and their routine use offsets many of the major complications. In addition to preventing problems with pneumothorax, they allow accurate estimation of blood loss within the thorax, which in these patients can be considerable. They are removed in the majority of cases between the second and fourth postoperative day.

Jejunostomy

The jejunostomy provides decompensation and obviates the need for nasogastric intubation in these patients.

Jejunostomy feeding can usually be commenced on the third or fourth postoperative day and is maintained until oral intake is adequate and established.

Oral feeding

The pharyngogastric anastomosis can be tested by videofluoroscopy and the vast majority of patients can begin oral fluids on the fifth to seventh postoperative day. Initial regurgitation occurs in virtually all patients but settles over a period of days to weeks. In the long term all patients are encouraged to eat small, fairly frequent amounts of food and initially they will find it helpful to sit upright when eating and to walk a little after food.

Thyroid and calcium replacement

As a consequence of total thyroidectomy at the excisional stage these patients require thyroxine supplements which are usually commenced on the fifth postoperative day. Calcium is monitored regularly and 20 ml of 10 per cent calcium gluconate added to each litre of intravenous fluid in the early postoperative stage. Subsequently, vitamin D_3 and calcium supplements are given orally, according to needs. Long-term review of these requirements is necessary as small amounts of parathyroid tissue remaining within the mediastinum can give rise to hypercalcaemia as late as 3 years after surgery.

Complications

Undeniably, gastric transposition is a potentially danger-ous operation requiring considerable surgical and nursing expertise, but provided that preoperative preparation and the operative measures outlined above are undertaken, the operative mortality should be below 10 per cent. Respiratory complications remain the highest cause of death and include respiratory failure, bronchopneumonia and pulmonary embolism. Myocardial infarction may occur in these patients as in all major operations of this magnitude. The pharyngogastric anastomosis should not be the site of frequent fistula formation and serious stomach wall necrosis has occurred in less than 1 per cent in our series of 150 patients.

Long-term problems

Recurrence of disease is the commonest long-term problem. Despite the introduction of the Blom–Singer valve, vocal rehabilitation to any reasonable degree is only possible in 20 per cent of patients. In contrast to other methods of pharyngeal replacement, the quality of the swallow is excellent and over 90 per cent of patients eat normal food without difficulty at 1 year after surgery, pharyngogastric junction stenosis being rare. Approxi-mately 5 per cent of patients in the long term complain of a recurrent sense of fullness after food.

References

1. De Santo LW, Carpenter RJ. Reconstruction of the pharynx and upper oesophagus after resection for cancer. *Head Neck Surg* 1980; 2: 369–79.

2. Howard D, Lund V. Skin grafting of the anterior stomach wall following pharyngogastric anastomosis. *J Laryngol Otol* 1985; 99: 273–6.

Further reading

Harrison DFN. Surgical repair in hypopharyngeal, cervical and oesophageal cancer. *Ann Otol Rhinol Laryngol* 1981; 90: 372–5.

Harrison DFN, Thompson AE. Pharyngolaryngo-oesophagectomy with pharyngogastric anastomosis for cancer of the hypopharynx. Review of 101 operations. *Head Neck Surg* 1986; 8: 418–28.

Lamb KH, Wong J, Lim SKT, Ong GB. Pharyngogastric anastomosis following pharyngolaryngo-oesophagectomy. Analysis of 157 cases. *World J Surg* 1981; 5: 509–16.

Wei WI, Lamb KM, Choi S, Wong J. Late problems after pharyngolaryngo-oesophagectomy and pharyngogastric anastomosis for cancer of the larynx and hypopharynx. *Am J Surg* 1984; 148: 509–13.

Repair of oral and pharyngocutaneous fistulae

A.G.D. Maran FRCS(Ed), FACS
Department of Otolaryngology, University of Edinburgh, Edinburgh, UK

Introduction

In a wound dehiscence one epithelial surface is lost, but in a fistula two epithelial surfaces are lost and there is a connection with a viscus which will discharge secretions. In repair, two epithelial surfaces must therefore be closed, whether by direct suture or by the introduction of fresh tissue in the form of flaps. Fistula formation of any size from the oral cavity or pharynx may be a serious complication and is sometimes potentially lethal, depending on whether the carotid arteries are exposed and whether or not they have been irradiated.

Nearly all fistulae of less than 2 cm in greatest diameter in non-irradiated patients will be self-healing, but this may take several weeks. The probability of spontaneous closure is greater with fistulae from the oral cavity and subsequent function may be minimally impaired. However, spontaneous closure of a pharyngeal defect with healing of the walls by secondary intention may be associated with some degree of stricture formation and subsequent morbidity such as dysphagia. Fistula formation from a primary pharyngeal repair after laryngectomy will almost certainly lead to narrowing and some degree of stricture formation; likewise a self-healing fistula at a skin mucosa junction, most commonly between a myocutaneous flap and the upper oesophagus, will also often result in stricture formation.

Primary fistula formation within the first 48 h after major head and neck surgery may be due to an inadequate closure or gross flap failure and is basically a surgical error. Secondary fistulae, most commonly occurring several days postoperatively, are due to avascular necrosis. The causes for this may be general, such as diabetes, atherosclerosis or poor nutrition; or local, such as radiation or compromise of the local blood supply. The principles of management of these fistulae are covered in the chapter on 'General management and complications', pp. 8–21.

Once a stable situation has been reached and a permanent fistula persists, treatment planning will depend on the position and overall size of the fistula. No absolute rules can be given but the principle of closure of both epithelial surfaces with the introduction between them of fresh tissue with a good blood supply should be constantly borne in mind. In older text books the use of local flaps of tissue to close the two epithelial surfaces was frequently advocated and described in a variety of situations. These techniques have been almost completely superseded with the possible exception of the closure of a small long established fistula of less than 5 mm in greatest diameter.

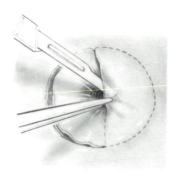

1a

Operations

1a–d

When dealing with small long established fistulae, it may be sufficient to excise the tract and close the epithelial surface either by direct suture or the use of small local flaps. The skin may be closed by turning one semicircular flap over and burying it in a pocket on the opposite side of the fistula. However, even with these small tracts, the success rate will be improved by the introduction of new tissue between the two epithelial surfaces.

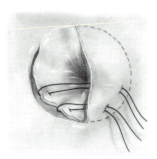

1b

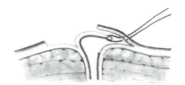

1c

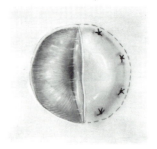

1d

REPAIR OF MINOR AND MODERATE-SIZED FISTULAE

Fistulae of up to 4 cm in their greatest diameter between the oral cavity and the pharynx can be reliably repaired by means of a superiorly-based sternocleidomastoid muscle or myocutaneous flap, if the muscle has not been removed at previous radical neck dissection.

2

The tissues of the fistula tract are excised and sufficient elevation of the surrounding cervical skin undertaken to allow the introduction of the full width of the sterno-cleidomastoid muscle between the internal epithelium of the oral cavity or pharynx and the cervical skin. A sternocleidomastoid myocutaneous flap may be isolated from the clavicle and transposed into the defect carrying an island of skin which can either be rotated into the pharyngeal or oral defect, or more appropriately used to close the cervical skin defect caused by the fistula tract.

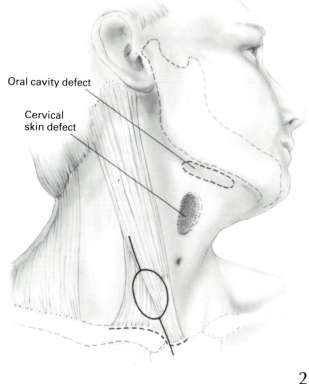

Oral cavity defect

Cervical skin defect

2

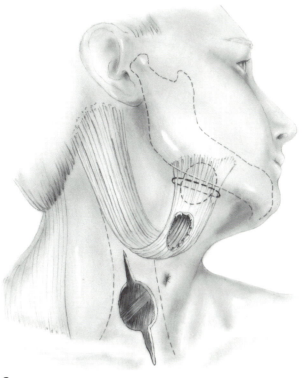

3

3

To undertake this procedure, the inferior attachment of the muscle is released via a lower vertical incision over the mid-point of the muscle and may include an appropriately sized island of skin. Following excision down to the deep layer of cervical fascia covering the superficial surface of the muscle, the dermis of the skin of any island outlined is tacked to this layer of fascia with a small number of appropriately placed catgut sutures. This stabilizes the fragile connection containing the perforating vessels between the underlying sternocleidomastoid muscle and the skin island.

4 & 5

With sufficient elevation and retraction of the skin, the sternoclavicular lower attachment of the muscle can be divided and the muscle, with or without a skin island, mobilized from inferiorly upwards preserving both the superficial and deep layers of cervical fascia which invest the muscle. At its anterior border this mobilization can continue to the level of the hyoid bone but care should be taken not to divide the sternomastoid artery arising higher from the occipital artery at the point where the hypoglossal nerve is adjacent. Posteriorly, the mobilization of the muscle is limited by the accessory nerve. The mobilized muscle is then swung into the defect created by the fistula and most commonly the internal opening to the oral cavity or pharynx is simply tacked with chromic catgut sutures to the internal surface of the muscle. This will readily become covered by mucosa. Externally the transposed skin island may close the cervical skin defect or the cervical skin may also be tacked to the muscle and a split-thickness skin graft used to complete the closure. The inferior incision used to mobilize the lower aspect of the sternocleidomastoid muscle can be closed primarily.

The technique using sternocleidomastoid muscle cannot be used if the muscle is absent following a radical neck dissection, and indeed this is often the case after major head and neck procedures. It may therefore be necessary to use alternative muscle or myocutaneous muscle flaps of which the most commonly used is the pectoralis major, as outlined below. This may bring a relatively large portion of muscle to the small or moderate-sized fistula area, and in itself this is usually of benefit and further ensures the adequacy of closure without the need to use inadequate local skin or muscle repairs. Transposed pectoralis muscle, with or without skin, is outside the field of any previous irradiation and, if necessary, can be used to cover the entire associated carotid artery.

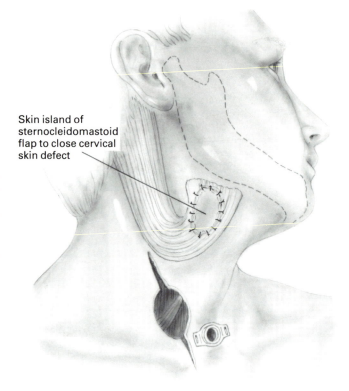

Skin island of sternocleidomastoid flap to close cervical skin defect

4

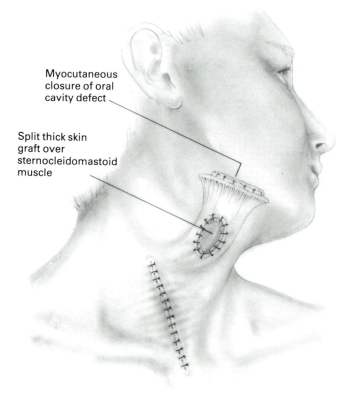

Myocutaneous closure of oral cavity defect

Split thick skin graft over sternocleidomastoid muscle

5

CLOSURE OF MAJOR FISTULAE

Despite the many advances in head and neck surgery and the overall decreasing incidence of fistulae in many major head and neck centres, large fistulae can still occur as a result of catastrophic wound breakdown, particularly in irradiated patients and as a consequence of total necrosis of pedicled or, more commonly, of free flaps transferred with microvascular anastomoses.

In dealing with these major fistulae, the author advocates the use of the pectoralis major muscle or myocutaneous flap as it has proved itself to be a reliable method of repair, even when more sophisticated flaps may have been used for the primary procedure. Following the development of the major fistula, particularly with exposure of the carotid vessels, the surgeon may be tempted to proceed too rapidly with a further flap reconstruction and this may be particularly inappropriate if there is gross salivary contamination and necrotic tissue remaining in the cervical region. Under these circumstances, transposition of the pectoralis major myocutaneous flap may simply be followed by further suture breakdown, flap detachment and continuing problems. It cannot be stressed too strongly that some degree of stability is preferable before carrying out this repair.

The principles of the pectoralis major flap are given in the chapter on 'Reconstructive techniques of the skin', pp. 45–103, but as with the sternocleidomastoid repair outlined above, simple transfer of the muscle flap alone is highly effective and indeed rotation of a bulky myocutaneous flap into the fistula area may be detrimental to the repair.

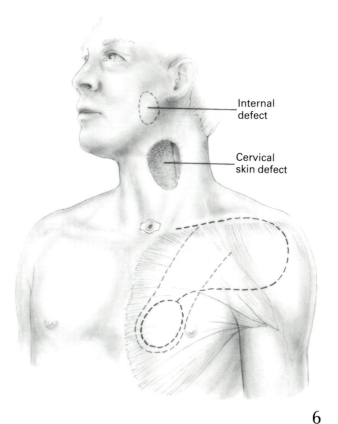

Internal defect

Cervical skin defect

6

6 & 7

The edges of the internal opening from the oral cavity or pharynx may be excised to healthy tissue and tacked with chromic catgut sutures to the adjacent surface of the transposed pectoralis major flap. With large epithelial defects, the surgeon may wish to rotate in a pectoralis major myocutaneous flap or apply a split-thickness skin graft to the muscle so that its edges approximate to those of the epithelial defect in the oral cavity or pharynx. It is important to place the transposed muscle so that it adequately overlaps the edges of both the internal and external openings of any major fistula and, as is commonly required, also covers the adjacent carotid vessels. Tacking sutures carefully placed to adjacent structures are required to evenly distribute the weight of the entire muscle flap. The external defect may either be closed by means of a split-thickness skin graft applied to the pectoralis major muscle or by rotation of the pectoralis major myocutaneous flap such that a transposed skin island closes the external defect.

If the cervical skin is of poor quality following previous irradiation and prolonged fistula damage, a combined pectoralis major myocutaneous flap and deltopectoral flap repair can produce excellent results. These two flaps are complementary in that elevation of the deltopectoral flap aids the elevation and placement of the pectoralis major myocutaneous flap and the deltopectoral flap may be used to replace large areas of cervical skin and may remain transposed into the neck without the need for later division of the pedicle.

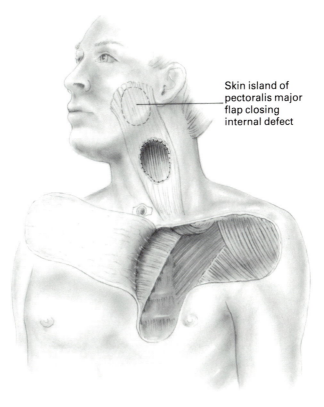

Skin island of pectoralis major flap closing internal defect

7

8

The defect in the shoulder is closed by means of a split-thickness skin graft. If the skin element of the pectoralis major myocutaneous flap is rotated to close the internal defect, this will then give the optimum of full epithelial closure of both internal and external aspects of the fistula with an intervening layer of pectoralis major muscle which has an excellent blood supply.

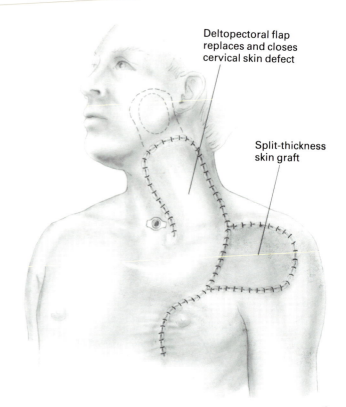

Deltopectoral flap
replaces and closes
cervical skin defect

Split-thickness
skin graft

8

Endoscopy

David J. Howard FRCS, FRCS(Ed)
Institute of Laryngology and Otology, Royal National Throat, Nose and Ear Hospital, London, UK

Charles B. Croft FRCS, FRCS(Ed)
Royal National Throat, Nose and Ear Hospital, London, UK

Introduction

There have been many significant advances in the last three decades in endoscopic evaluation and surgery of the head and neck. Improvements in both rigid and flexible endoscopic equipment continue apace with an ever increasing range of light sources, microscopes, still cameras, video and stroboscopic equipment. The problems confronting the head and neck surgeon vary widely from patient to patient and different types of endoscope are required. It is important that the head and neck surgeon is familiar with this instrumentation.

Larynx

FLEXIBLE NASOPHARYNGOLARYNGOSCOPY

The present-day endoscopes give excellent images of the nasal cavities, pharynx and larynx and, with practice, are easy to use. They have considerably improved patient evaluation under a wide variety of circumstances; one of these improvements has been in outpatient evaluation, and the larynx and pharynx can be clearly visualized in almost all patients in whom indirect mirror laryngoscopy

has been unsatisfactory. Previously a significant number of these patients would have required admission for direct examination under general anaesthesia, and this is now obviated. In contrast to the situation under general anaesthesia, fibreoptic nasoendoscopy in outpatients allows the dynamic function of the larynx and pharynx to be viewed and the nose and nasopharynx can be inspected carefully during the passage of the endoscope. Several nasoendoscopes are now available with high quality optics and small outer diameters of 3–4 mm. They have short distal flexible sections allowing at least 120° of upward movement and 90° downward.

In the majority of people, fibreoptic nasoendoscopic examination is well tolerated under local anaesthesia. It can be carried out with the patient either prone or sitting; at initial nasal inspection the wider side of the nose is chosen and sprayed with 1 ml of 10 per cent cocaine solution. The nose may also be packed with a pledget of cotton wool soaked in a further 1 ml of 10 per cent cocaine. Occasionally, patients with a prominent gag reflex may also benefit from a benzocaine lozenge, 10 mg, sucked slowly over a period of 15 min. These levels of anaesthesia should allow successful examination and the failure rate should be as low as 2–3 per cent. Occasional vagal attacks, vomiting or cocaine reactions have been reported and suction and resuscitation equipment must be available.

1

A right-handed examiner will stand to the right of the patient. Following lubrication and demisting of the objective lens, the endoscope is inserted into the anaesthetized nasal cavity through the middle or inferior meatus, through the posterior choanae, and into the nasopharynx. The distal tip of the instrument is directed by means of the thumb control on the body of the endoscope. Passage past the soft palate, tongue base and epiglottis will allow an excellent view of the larynx in the vast majority of patients. Misting of the objective lens may be counteracted by the patient swallowing, and the vocal folds can be viewed while the patient is speaking or saying 'eee', breathing and coughing. Inspection is continued during withdrawal of the laryngoscope with additional inspection of the hypophyarnx, oropharynx and nasopharynx.

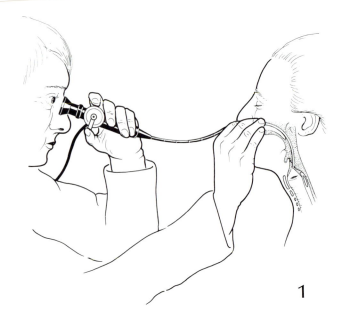

1

Advantages and disadvantages

As indicated above, the procedure is well tolerated and avoids the necessity for general anaesthesia in many patients who fail the mirror examination. The examination itself can be a valuable aid to reassurance in patients with non-organic disease. Excellent 35 mm still photography or video pictures can be obtained with a wide range of cameras attached to the endoscope and these can be used for documentation or teaching purposes. The procedure is not limited by fixation or trismus and is extremely unlikely to injure any aspect of the nose, pharynx or larynx. Nasoendoscopes are now available with suction and biopsy capabilities, but the majority of surgeons still favour later examination by direct laryngopharyngoscopy under general anaesthesia if abnormalities are found at fibreoptic assessment. Anaesthesia and biopsy of the larynx in an outpatient situation remain hazardous because of bleeding or airway obstruction and the biopsies obtained through fibreoptic laryngoscopes are very small, making histological interpretation at times difficult or misleading. Occasionally marked deviation of the nasal airway by septal abnormalities, a large overhanging epiglottis, or an anxious patient with a severe gag reflex, may prevent examination, or an inadequate intralaryngeal view is obtained and the findings misinterpreted. The small objective lens has a 'fish eye' effect and the inexperienced observer may mistake the laryngeal findings. Direct laryngoscopy should be undertaken if there is any doubt. In contrast to this latter examination by rigid instrumentation, the flexible technique does not allow maintenance of the airway, other surgical procedures or assessment of the passive mobility of the cricoarytenoid joints.

RIGID TELESCOPIC PHARYNGOLARYNGOSCOPY

2

The authors use a wide variety of Storz Hopkin's telescopes in their head and neck practice and they are of considerable use in examination of the pharynx and larynx, either as a primary means when they can offer an excellent view – better than that of a flexible nasoendoscope – or especially when still photographic or video recordings are required. Apart from the improved view, they also have advantages of speed, ease and economy when compared with the flexible nasoendoscope. However, as they must be passed through the mouth they are often not tolerated by patients who have failed indirect mirror laryngoscopy. Even when tolerated by the patient, abnormalities of the epiglottis may preclude good visualization of the larynx in outpatients. These rigid telescopes come in many different lengths and viewing angles, ranging from 0° to 120°. The largest diameter 70° and 90° angled laryngeal telescopes make good general instruments for indirect laryngoscopy.

Rigid telescopes are also used at operative endoscopy. They allow improved visualization of the laryngeal ventricles, vocal folds and subglottis when inserted down a rigid Negus laryngoscope. They will allow evaluation of the entire tracheobronchial tree and are particularly useful in paediatric practice.

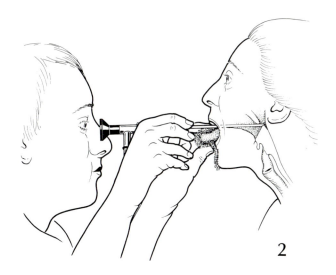

2

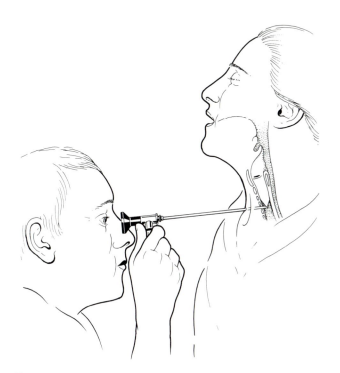

3

3

They can be passed into a tracheostome to allow evaluation of the glottis, subglottis and trachea.

Modern liquid light guides may improve photographic results when coupled to these rigid telescopes but are, in themselves, less flexible.

STROBOSCOPY

More accurate assessment of the vibration of the vocal folds can be obtained by examination with a stroboscopic light source coupled to either the rigid or fibreoptic instruments described above. However, this evaluation has not become generally established in the diagnosis of vocal fold carcinoma.

DIRECT LARYNGOSCOPY AND MICROLARYNGOSCOPY

Rigid system endoscopy has been the standard method of diagnosing disease of the upper respiratory and gastrointestinal tracts throughout this century. Despite a recent increase in flexible endoscopy, rigid endoscopic techniques remain the most important in head and neck surgical units. Personnel must be available who have expertise in their use. Direct laryngoscopy under general anaesthesia allows thorough laryngeal evaluation, appropriate biopsies, removal of foreign bodies and benign lesions, assessment of cricoarytenoid ability, and active movement of the vocal folds and sphincters of the larynx may be observed at the termination of the procedure. Microlaryngoscopy allows further accurate study of the surface and extent of laryngeal pathology, and controlled and accurate surgical procedures using microsurgical instrumentation and lasers.

Instrumentation

There are many modifications of the operative laryngoscope. The authors prefer the Storz and Negus rigid endoscopes and use these for all routine direct endoscopy. For microlaryngeal surgery with suspension laryngoscopy we use the Royal National Throat, Nose and Ear Hospital patent laryngoscope and the Dedo–Pilling modified anterior commissure laryngoscope. These allow binocular vision through the operating microscope and yet are narrow enough to be used in most patients, even those with large incisor teeth or a narrow mandibular arch.

Suspension is achieved using a Lewy's support. We do not put the heavy support directly onto the patient's chest (which is particularly inadvisable in children). It rests on a small metal table positioned above the patient's chest and is attached to the operating table. Suspension in this way minimizes movement of the system due to respiratory excursions of the patient, which is particularly important during microsurgery, laser surgery and photography. A 400 mm objective lens in the operating microscope is necessary for most endoscopic surgical procedures. We no longer use cryosurgery endoscopically, but still retain the Pracy suction diathermy apparatus for occasional laryngeal and tracheal use.

Many instruments have been designed and recommended for both direct endoscopic and endolaryngeal microsurgery. While personal preferences may prevail, the set of instruments should be as small as possible and with increasing experience fewer, rather than greater, numbers of instruments are required. It is not appropriate to describe the vast range of instruments available in the surgical catalogues. For microlaryngeal surgery, double cup forceps with 3 mm jaws (straight, curved to right and left and upcutting) are routinely used, complemented by scissor and alligator forcep versions. A sickle knife,

peeler, diathermy probe, Coulidge swab carrier and a variety of suction tubes complete the set.

Anaesthesia

Until the 1950s most laryngoscopy was performed under local anaesthesia. This technique allowed an unobstructed view of the larynx, but the procedure could be uncomfortable and difficult to perform without patient cooperation. Today, the risks of general anaesthesia are probably fewer than those of local anaesthesia in an anxious patient without control of the airway.

General anaesthesia allows pan-endoscopy, a wide variety of precise surgical techniques, photography, teaching and a comfortable patient. Many techniques available require close cooperation between surgeon and anaesthetist, each being familiar with the procedure. No single technique is suitable for all patients. Preoperative assessment of the patient's airway should be made by both anaesthetist and surgeon so that problems may be discussed, and it is our practice that the surgeon is present at induction with the necessary equipment available in difficult cases should a tracheostomy be required. The choice of premedication may vary in individual patients, but atropine is used in most circumstances. Topical anaesthesia of the larynx and trachea is usually secured by a 4 per cent lignocaine spray which minimizes unwanted reflex activity.

The following techniques are commonly used:

1. *Apnoeic oxygenation*. This may be satisfactory for short diagnostic examinations, with operating time lengthened by insufflation of oxygen via a Harris catheter.
2. *Spontaneous respiration*. This is employed for simple diagnostic procedures and is often chosen in children or when vocal fold mobility or laryngomalacia is being assessed.
3. *Endotracheal intubation*. Small-bore microlaryngeal endotracheal tubes combined with muscle relaxants and controlled ventilation allow an unhurried examination of the larynx. As the majority of laryngeal pathology occurs anteriorly, the tube is rarely a nuisance and fold mobility may be observed on extubation.
4. *Venturi jet techniques*. These are commonly used by the authors when undertaking microsurgery, in particular when using the carbon dioxide laser. The Venturi system maintains oxygen at pressures up to 60 p.s.i., the rate being controlled by the anaesthetist using either a hand-operated valve apparatus or a jet ventilation machine. The patient is continually monitored by an oximeter and this allows periods of anaesthesia up to and beyond 1 h using repeated doses of short-acting intravenous agents.
5. If the Venturi technique is not appropriate for laser work in a given patient, an Oswald–Hunton endotracheal metal tube may be used. This is a non-cuffed tube, but with simple packing using moist neurosurgical patties an adequate airway seal can be produced. The use of other cuffed tubes wrapped in aluminium foil tape can cause trauma to the nose and vocal folds from the edges of the tape and potential hazards from the cuff, even if filled with saline. These latter techniques are no longer used.

Confidence in direct laryngoscopy and microlaryngoscopy procedures comes only with experience and a number of pitfalls await the inexperienced surgeon.

Position of patient

4

Correct position is a prerequisite for a satisfactory view of the larynx. The head should be well extended on the atlas and the neck flexed. This position is commonly known as 'sniffing the morning air'. This position may be achieved by means of a head ring and adjustments of the head piece of the table, or by placing a pillow folded so that the main bulk of the pillow lies beneath the occiput and the head extends over the upper pillow edge.

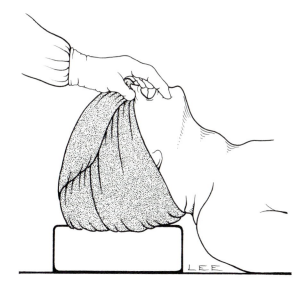

4

Drapes

Endoscopy is not a sterile procedure and although head towels are routinely employed, we do not recommend draping the chest which should remain fully visible to both surgeon and anaesthetist. In small children where cooling may be of importance, the lower half of the body may be blanketed appropriately.

Choice of laryngoscope

The largest laryngoscope which can be comfortably introduced into the patient's pharynx and larynx should be used. This should allow maximum width of vision and manoeuvrability. The shape and length of the patient's neck, state of dentition, mobility of jaw and neck, age and general condition will all have a bearing on this choice. The patient's head should not hang at any point during the procedure and care must be taken when manipulating the head and neck of all patients, but particularly elderly patients with cervical osteoarthritis. No pressure should be necessary. Sometimes a satisfactory view of the larynx can only be obtained with an anterior commissure laryngoscope. A bronchoscope may be passed via the Negus laryngoscope following removal of the sliding blade.

Paediatric endoscopy has its own particular problems. The anatomy differs from the adult with a more curved and mobile epiglottis, anterosuperiorly placed larynx, and an increased tendency to laryngospasm. The use of endoscopes which are too large leads to trauma (especially of the subglottis with bronchoscopy), resulting in postoperative oedema.

5

Rigid Hopkin's telescopes passed through endoscopes allow further visualization of the laryngotracheobronchial tree.

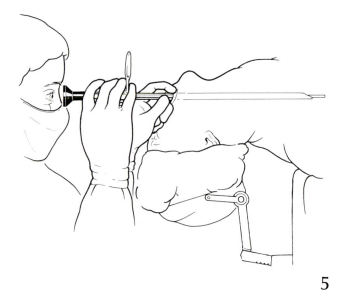

5

Protection of the patient

A variety of metal dental trays and rubber or plastic guards for teeth and gums are available. It is important to assess dentition preoperatively. Most damage is caused by attempts to increase extension of the head by levering the laryngoscope against the teeth. Trapping lips and tongue should also be avoided, as should trauma from the tip of the laryngoscope if used too forcefully.

Positioning the laryngoscope

The tip of the laryngoscope should lie in the region of the petiolus of the epiglottis a few millimetres above the anterior commissure to give the best overall view of the larynx. The surgeon holds the laryngoscope in his non-dominant hand, leaving his dominant hand free to use instruments and suction. External pressure on the larynx may be required to visualize the anterior commissure.

Biopsy

Biopsies removed by cupped forceps must be handled carefully and should be transferred directly from the jaws of the punch forceps to the histology specimen container, either by direct transfer to the formalin within the container or by gentle use of a hypodermic needle. This will prevent the histology report being affected by crush artefact.

Assessment of vocal fold movement

During laryngoscopy most adult patients remain paralysed and therefore, if vocal fold movement is to be assessed, the muscle relaxant must be allowed to wear off. A Mackintosh anaesthetic-type laryngoscope should be inserted with the tip in the vallecula and the vocal folds observed without the presence of the Negus laryngoscope behind the epiglottis (this may cause sufficient distortion of the larynx to impair the vocal fold movements). For further details of direct laryngoscopy and microlaryngoscopy, the reader is referred to the chapter on 'Laryngoscopy, microlaryngoscopy and laser surgery', pp. 451–462.

Trachea and bronchi

Anatomy of the tracheobronchial tree

6

It is vitally important that an understanding of normal bronchial anatomy is gained before insertion of either a conventional rigid or a flexible fibreoptic bronchoscope. Use of the flexible instrument relies particularly on this and the illustration demonstrates the main segmental branches of the bronchial tree, inverted to show the sequence of branching as found in a supine patient. It should be noted that a wide range of normality exists, particularly in the division of the left main stem bronchus and the divisions of the segmental bronchi in the right lower lobe. Practice using a lung model is highly recommended.

7

Rigid bronchoscopy allows inspection of the orifices of the third bronchial division, whereas use of the fibreoptic flexible bronchoscope allows routine inspection of the fourth and sometimes fifth bronchial divisions. The illustration shows the range of the flexible fibrescope.

The bronchoscopist is interested in viewing the walls of the tracheobronchial tree to discern distortion (such as carinal blunting) or reduced mobility; abnormalities of the mucosa with infiltration or ulceration; and the presence of exudate or blood within the lumen.

Indications

Rigid bronchoscopy

1. Removal of obstructing lesion such as foreign body or mucus plug.
2. Diagnostic evaluation of the walls and mucosa of the tracheobronchial tree.
3. Biopsy of a suspected tumour.
4. To secure an airway in upper respiratory tract obstruction, where intubation is difficult or impossible.

Flexible bronchoscopy

1. Diagnostic evaluation of trachea and bronchi third and fourth divisions.
2. Evaluation of haemoptysis, as in post-tracheostomy bleeding.
3. Suction clearance of obstructing mucus plugs in a postoperative or intensive care unit setting.
4. Peripheral lesion diagnosis via transbronchial lung biopsy with radiographic control.

Contraindications

Rigid bronchoscopy is contraindicated in the presence of aneurysms or where there is marked kyphosis.

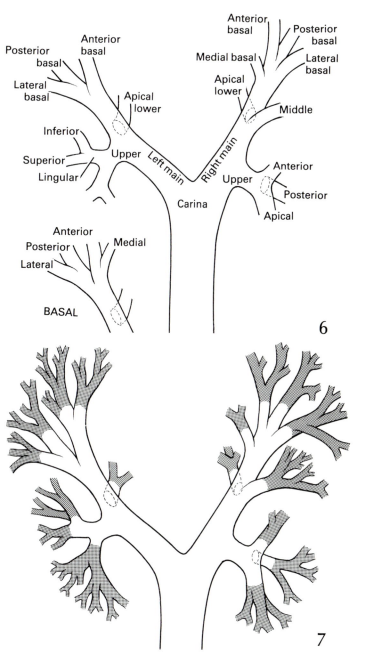

Flexible bronchoscopy is contraindicated where there is a vascular tumour (use rigid scope with balloon and packing ready), and for foreign body removal.

Preoperative preparation

Recent posteroanterior and lateral chest films should be available.

For rigid bronchoscopy standard premedication is given. For fibreoptic flexible bronchoscopy, premedication consists of: atropine 0.6 mg and intravenous diazepam (Valium) 5–10 mg (titration).

An appropriate bronchoscope size is selected. The following diameter sizes are appropriate: neonates, 3 mm; children aged 9–24 months, 3.5 mm; adult women 6 mm; adult men, 8 mm.

RIGID BRONCHOSCOPY

Anaesthesia

General anaesthesia with intravenous suxamethonium and thiopentone is preferred. Ventilation is maintained by the oxygen Venturi system using oxygen at 50–60 p.s.i. (345–414 kPa) (use air at 50–60 p.s.i. if the system is used with the laser).

For children, a reducing valve should be fitted as the smaller bronchoscope sheaths require less pressure for satisfactory ventilation and high pressures can be dangerous.

Position of patient

The patient's cervical spine is flexed and the head is extended (*see Illustration 4*). The eyes are protected. The surgeon's left hand steadies, protects and controls the upper jaw.

Insertion of bronchoscope

8

The bronchoscope is inserted through the right side of the mouth, lifting and following the tongue to the epiglottis. Gentle lateral movements will help identify this if it is not readily visible.

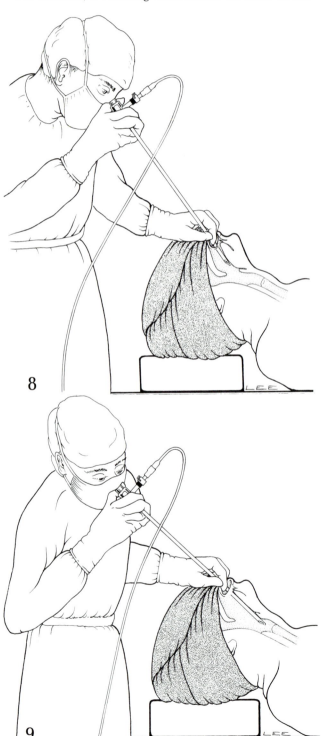

8

Identification of the glottis

9

The tip of the epiglottis is elevated and using the left thumb as a fulcrum the bronchoscope is brought to a more horizontal position, revealing the posterior aspect of the glottis.

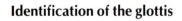

9

Passing the glottis

10

The bronchoscope is passed forward to the glottis and rotated 90° with the tip to the right. The view is centred on the left vocal fold and the instrument is advanced towards this until the beak passes through the vertical axis of the glottis. A gentle twisting movement and further advancement of the bronchoscope allow passage past the larynx.

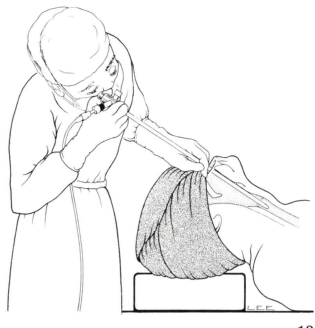

10

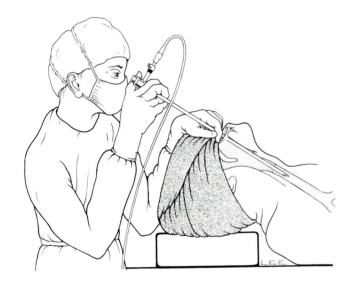

11

Inspection of the trachea and carina

11

Alignment of the bronchoscope and trachea is sought, which may require further extension of the head. The bronchoscope is advanced gently, viewing the tracheal walls until the sharp outline of the normal carina is seen.

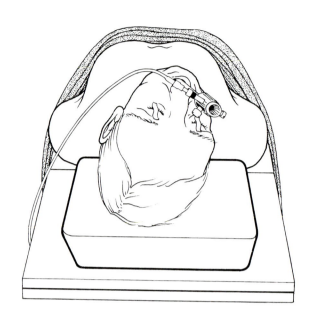

Entry to left main bronchus

12 & 13

This requires particular care as on the left the main bronchus is longer and curved at an oblique angle to the trachea. The bronchoscope is positioned in the right angle of the mouth and the head rotated to the right, bringing the long axis of the instrument and the left main bronchus into alignment and allowing a view of the secondary carina.

12

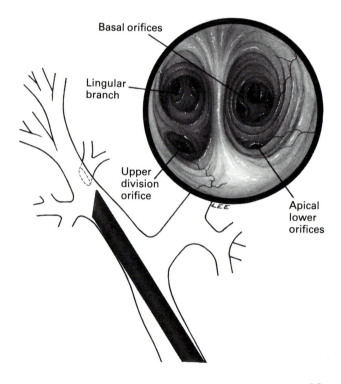

Basal orifices

Lingular branch

Upper division orifice

Apical lower orifices

13

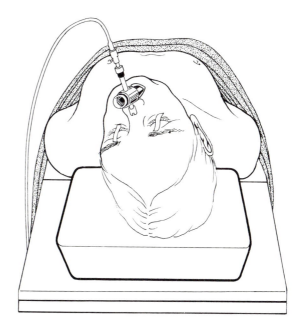

14

Entry to right main bronchus

14 & 15

The right main bronchus is shorter and more vertical and easier to examine. The head and bronchoscope are rotated to the left and the instrument advanced into the bronchus intermedius. The right upper bronchus requires a lateral viewing telescope for adequate inspection.

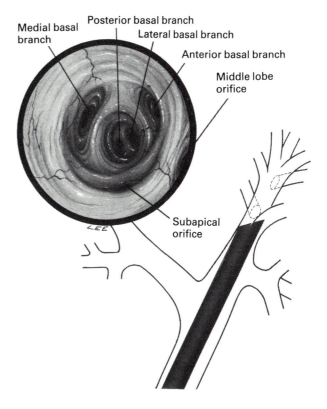

Medial basal branch
Posterior basal branch
Lateral basal branch
Anterior basal branch
Middle lobe orifice
Subapical orifice

15

Taking a biopsy

16

Aspirated material should be collected for (trap) cytology and culture. All suction and manipulation should be performed with the utmost gentleness to reduce the risk of haemorrhage. Endobronchial biopsy should ideally be performed with the bronchoscope close to and giving good access to the lesion. The use of integral telescope and biopsy forceps is highly recommended, allowing delicate and accurate biopsies to be taken.

Removing foreign bodies

Inert

These should be removed after careful inspection, and withdrawn into a bronchoscope of suitable size. If the foreign body is too large it is removed together with the bronchoscope. Aspirated bones and broken pieces of denture are the most frequently encountered. The tracheobronchial tree should be re-examined and cleaned after the foreign body has been extracted.

Irritants

Vegetable foreign bodies such as peanuts rapidly produce mucosal reaction with swelling of the mucosa, partially obscuring the foreign body and making extraction difficult. Telescopic forceps are available and recommended for precise removal in these difficult cases.

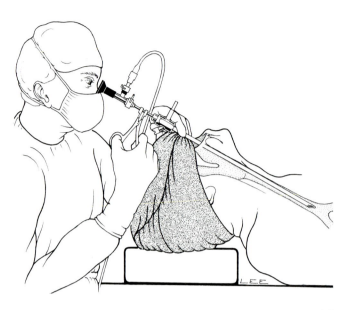

16

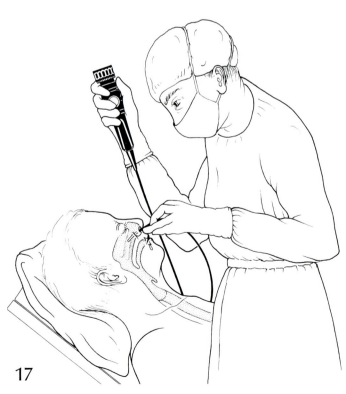

17

FIBREOPTIC BRONCHOSCOPY

Anaesthesia

The local nasal route is preferred, using an oxygen catheter if the patient has obstructive airway disease. The nose, pharynx and larynx are sprayed with topical 4 per cent lignocaine.

Position of patient

17

The patient is semi-recumbent. The operator stands to the right facing the patient, allowing eye contact and reassurance. The right hand controls the instrument housing and the left inserts the fibre bundle through the wider nasal chamber.

Identification of the larynx

18

The instrument is passed above the inferior turbinate and beneath the middle turbinate to the nasopharynx. The patient breathes through his nose, and the tip is deflected down into the oropharynx, allowing a good view of the larynx. The instrument is advanced just proximal to the folds and the two syringes containing 2 ml of 4 per cent lignocaine are injected into the folds and into the glottis. After waiting 2–3 min the tip is advanced through the glottis and into the upper trachea. A further 2 ml of 2 per cent lignocaine is injected down the trachea. The patient may cough briefly but is encouraged and asked to breathe gently until the spasm settles. Further use of 2 per cent lignocaine is required as the major bronchi are entered. The tree is examined, keeping in mind the route taken, as the position of the bronchoscope peripherally can only be ascertained through reference to landmarks already negotiated.

Biopsies

19

The aspirate can be used for cytological examination. Biopsies and brushings taken through the biopsy channel are most useful, even though the specimen is small.

It is important to remember that if the tip is deflected, the biopsy forceps may not pass. In this case the instrument should be withdrawn and tip deflection reduced before biopsy proceeds. The cups should be just in front of the viewing objective for precise manipulation.

Complications

Rigid bronchoscopy

Haemorrhage. Any vascular lesion or friable tumour may bleed briskly. The head should be tilted down and pressure applied with a peanut swab soaked in 1:1000 adrenaline. If ineffective, a larger pack should be inserted or a Fogarty balloon catheter used to tamponade the bronchus. The pack should be left in place for 5 min.

Laryngeal oedema. Use of too large a diameter instrument and prolonged examination, particularly in children, may cause laryngeal oedema and stridor. The use of humidity and steroids is helpful in these cases but avoidance is the best course.

Teeth. Protection of the teeth with a gum shield and using the thumb as a fulcrum for the bronchoscope should prevent damage to the teeth.

Flexible bronchoscopy

As general anaesthesia is avoided, the complication rate should be very low (mortality: 0.01 per cent).

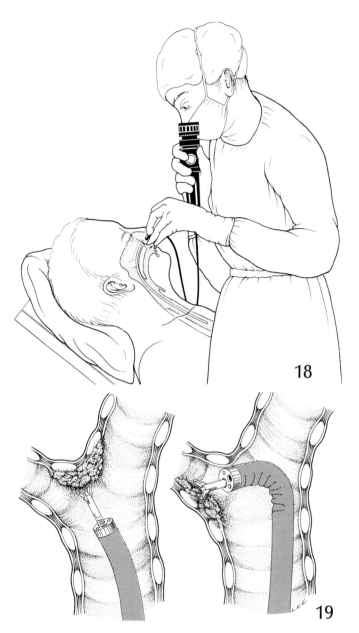

18

19

Haemorrhage. Avoidable if gentle use of the biopsy forceps is achieved. Impacting the instrument tip into a segmental bronchus should be tried if bleeding continues.

Pneumothorax. Pneumothorax occurs in 5 per cent of transbronchial lung biopsies, but is rare in routine flexible bronchoscopy. Postoperative chest radiography is required.

Local anaesthetic reaction. Adherence to recommended doses and lignocaine is the best safeguard.

Oxygen desaturation. A 10 mmHg fall in arterial oxygen tension may occur, and chronic obstructive airway cases should receive oxygen through a nasal catheter during the procedure.

LASER SURGERY OF THE TRACHEOBRONCHIAL TREE

20

The carbon dioxide laser endoscope system can be coupled to a rigid ventilating bronchoscope for endotracheal and endobronchial surgery. It is most useful for the treatment of patients with tracheobronchial papillomas, many of whom have symptoms of airway obstruction. This laser system can also be used for removal of tracheal granulations and minor degrees of webbing and stenosis, although it is only of limited use in the treatment of the latter and may require accompanying dilatation.

Obstructing malignant disease of the trachea and main bronchi can also be readily palliated with the carbon dioxide laser but more recent experience with the Nd-YAG laser transmitted by a flexible fibre and flexible bronchoscope system produces improved access and results. The argon laser can also be transmitted through a flexible fibre but does not have the same power of predictable soft tissue absorption characteristics of the Nd-YAG laser.

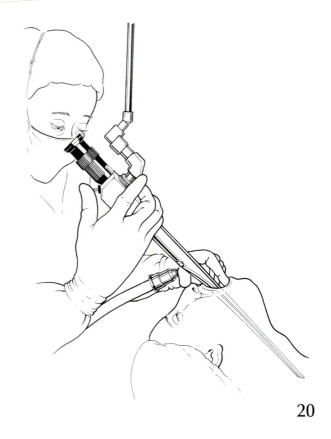

20

Anaesthesia

If the patient has a tracheostomy, general anaesthesia is induced through the tracheostomy tube which is then removed once the bronchoscope has been inserted transorally. General anaesthesia is maintained by inhalation of non-flammable anaesthetic gases through the ventilating sidearm of the bronchoscope or by means of a jet Venturi attachment.

The extent of the disease is then assessed as far as the distal mainstem bronchi. When treating papillomas the distal lesions are vaporized first. This allows better ventilation and a clear view as the procedure progresses proximally. The reverse is required for obstructing malignant lesions which are often friable and vascular, obscuring the normal anatomy, and therefore requiring careful vaporization from proximal to distal aspects. All loose small tumour fragments must be removed and at times it will be necessary to uncouple the bronchoscope from the laser endoscope to remove these fragments by suction.

Preoperative and postoperative chest radiographs, arterial blood gas levels and pulmonary function tests allow objective evaluation of the procedure, and flexible fibreoptic bronchoscopy under local anaesthesia allows continued assessment to determine the need for further laser sugery.

Complications

In selected cases of benign tracheobronchial lesions and stenosis, carbon dioxide endoscope laser surgery can be used with minimal morbidity. However, care is required in patients with advanced obstructing malignant disease. The system provides an excellent means of endoscopic diagnosis as haemostasis at biopsy is usual, but standard surgical and radiotherapeutic techniques should be used to treat the majority of patients. The carbon dioxide endoscopic laser is only indicated for palliation of tracheobronchial obstruction and may then facilitate subsequent radiotherapy by ensuring the patient's comfort with less dyspnoea and possible sepsis. Severe operative and postoperative haemorrhage and perforation have been reported, and there is no doubt that the rigid bronchoscope has a relatively poor proximal optic system when compared with flexible fibreoptic systems.

Pharynx and oesophagus

PHARYNGOSCOPY AND OESOPHAGOSCOPY

Indications

While modern videofluoroscopic studies have markedly improved our diagnosis of all stages through the oral cavity, pharynx and oesophagus, they may still remain an unreliable guide as to the innocence or malignancy of pharyngo-oesophageal lesions. Pharyngo-oesophagoscopy is essential for accurate diagnosis, for by this means alone can the mucosa be directly inspected and biopsies obtained. It is therefore indicated in almost every patient who has dysphagia not of neurological origin. It is also employed in the removal of foreign bodies and the treatment of cardiospasm and in the palliation of both malignant and innocent strictures. Pharyngo-oesophagoscopy should be an integral part of the pan-endoscopic investigation of a cervical node mass containing metastatic tumour. Passage of the oesophagoscope is best carried out under general anaesthesia and it is by no means without surgical risk, demanding both practice and skill. Dohlman's upper oesophagoscopy with a bivalved oesophageal speculum may be used for the treatment of a hypopharyngeal pouch.

In the presence of a suspected malignancy, bronchoscopy is always performed after oesophagoscopy to ensure that the bronchial tree is not the primary seat of a growth and that it has not become secondarily invaded by neoplasm. The commonest site for infiltration and subsequent fistula formation is the posterior wall of the left main bronchus.

Contraindications

These include both local and general factors, the former of which includes gross trismus, hypomandibular development, dental malocclusion with prominent upper teeth and patients with short thick necks. The general condition of the patient may make the examination hazardous and difficult as a result of gross spinal abnormalities, spinal rigidity, aortic aneurysm or left ventricular hypertrophy.

Anaesthesia

Although it is possible to perform the procedure under local anaesthesia using a combination of a 4 per cent lignocaine spray applied to the pharynx, larynx and piriform fossae, it is rarely used nowadays. The superior laryngeal nerve may also be infiltrated externally with Jackson's applicators placed into the piriform fossae. Usually endotracheal general anaesthesia is used after premedication with atropine and scopolamine. It is important to consider deflation of the endotracheal tube cuff when passing the oesophagoscope through the cricopharyngeus.

For flexible fibreoptic gastroscopy, a 10 mg benzocaine lozenge is given 30 min before the start of the procedure followed by intravenous midazolam or diazepam just before commencing the examination.

Instrumentation

21

Rigid instruments are superior for examining the pharynx and lesions close to the cricopharyngeal sphincter, removal of foreign bodies, obtaining large biopsy specimens, and cautery of oesophageal fistulae. Rigid oesophagoscopes with distal or proximal fibreoptic lighting are available in adult and children's sizes.

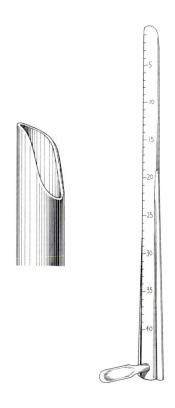

21

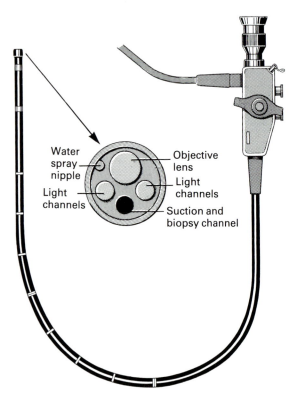

Water spray nipple — Objective lens

Light channels — Light channels

Suction and biopsy channel

22

Modern flexible oesphagoscopes and gastroscopes give a better field of view and greater accuracy of biopsy than the rigid instruments, although the biopsy material obtained is substantially smaller. They are superior for examination of the mid and lower oesophagus, stomach and duodenum. They are far less hazardous for routine diagnostic oesophagoscopy, particularly in the elderly, as they can be used under local anaesthesia as outlined above.

22

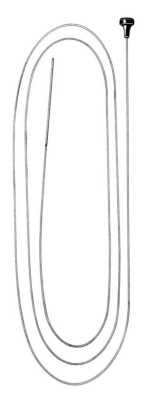

23

23 & 24

They are far safer for negotiating spinal deformities and problems outlined in the contraindications section and may be passed through narrow strictures after guidewire dilatation using Eade–Peusto dilators. Finally, the flexible instruments are superior for photography although rigid telescopic Hopkin's rods can also be passed down the lumen of rigid oesophagoscopes to improve photographic results.

The rigid and flexible instruments are complementary and ideally both should be available. The new younger generation of head and neck surgeons will benefit from training in both techniques. The advent of the flexible instrumentation has certainly decreased the indications for rigid oesophagoscopy.

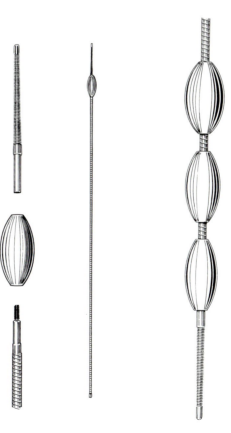

24

25

A multitude of suckers and forceps are available but it is important that the scrub nurse has checked that she has instruments of the appropriate length, which are longer than the pharyngoscopes and oesophagoscopes to be used for rigid examination. Both fine-bore suckers for accurate atraumatic suction and large-bore suckers for removal of any retained food matter above a stricture should be available. Patterson's biopsy forceps or Souttar's cup forceps are recommended. A set of graduated dilators completes the instruments for rigid endoscopy and Chevalier–Jackson gum elastic bougies mounted on rigid wire stems are particularly useful for assessment of an obstruction and dilatation under direct vision.

A wide variety of forward viewing oesophagoscopes and gastroscopes are available with retroflexion and rotation of the distal tip. This allows full examination of the lower oesophagus, cardia, stomach, pylorus and duodenum and aspiration of any obstructing fluid via the suction channel. Separate channels permit passage of biopsy forceps, cytology brushes or guidewires and the water spray clears the distal lens. There are multiple camera attachments allowing still and video photography.

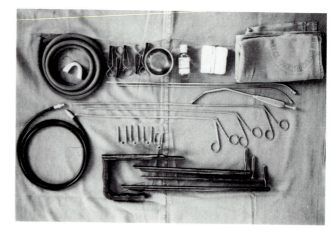

25

26 & 27

A variety of biopsy forceps are available along with cytology brushes for obtaining material for microscopic examination.

With the aid of a guidewire passed under direct vision through narrow strictures, dilatation can often be achieved by graded olivary dilators and inflatable balloon dilators. It may then be possible to take biopsies along the length of the stricture and to pass the flexible instrument distally beyond the stricture.

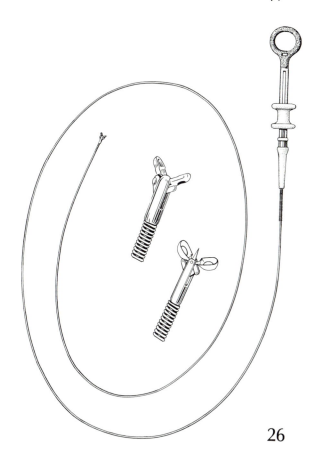

26

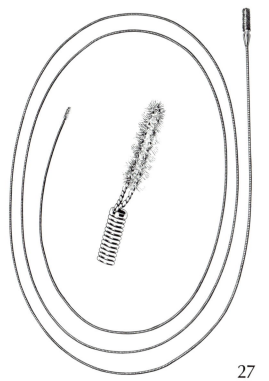

27

Operative technique

Rigid instrument

28

The patient lies supine on the table with the head on a ring on the hinged upper section of the table. The neck is initially flexed forward upon the head rest. The oesophagoscope is held in the fingers and thumb of the right hand for a right-handed surgeon and the left fingers and thumb retract the lips and hold the gum guard over the upper teeth. The lower end of the endoscope is lubricated with water-soluble jelly and the tip of the oesophagoscope is introduced, pointing posteriorly and superiorly, and is then followed through the midline of the palate to reach the posterior pharyngeal wall. The tip of the oesophagoscope now lies behind the epiglottis and the endotracheal tube and may be kept in the midline or passed into the right piriform fossa. All movement should be under direct vision and any pharyngeal contents aspirated through the sucker.

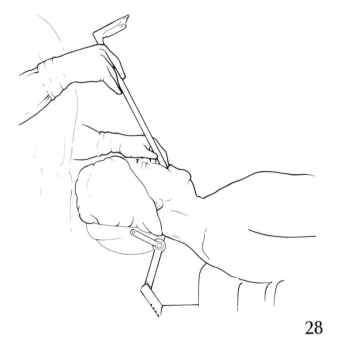

28

29

It is unusual for the oesophageal lumen beyond to be visible for it is guarded by the tone of the upper sphincter and the cricopharyngeus which is about 16 cm from the upper incisor teeth or gums. In order to pass the oesophagoscope through the cricopharyngeus, a number of important points must be borne in mind. The oesophagoscope must never be passed blind, or forced against resistance, as this upper segment is a frequent site of damage and perforation, not only by misdirection but also because the posterior wall of the upper oesophagus may be compressed between the rigid oesophagoscope and the cervical vertebral bodies. The head is now extended at the atlanto–occipital joint by altering the head rest of the operating table. The passage of the oesophagoscope behind the larynx through the cricopharyngeus will be aided by temporary deflation of the endotracheal cuff and the anaesthetist gently lifting forwards the whole larynx. This manoeuvre is often the secret of easy oesophagoscopy. The head may now be extended further as the thoracic oesophagus is explored.

The lumen of the oesophagus should be maintained in the centre of the field of view and continuing suction of secretions and debris should be undertaken to maintain this view. The aortic arch is felt or produces a visible indentation on the left side some 23 cm from the upper incisors and at the level of the fourth thoracic vertebra. The anterior crossing of the left main bronchus is just distal to this point but is not usually seen. Throughout its course the lumen of the thoracic oesophagus expands and contracts with inspiration and expiration and is highly mobile. As the lower end is approached, transposition from oesophageal to gastric mucosa may be observed and the oesophagus passes more anteriorly and to the left so that it is necessary to depress the patient's head to the right to advance the instrument. At approximately 38 cm from the incisor the lumen closes into a mucosal rosette;

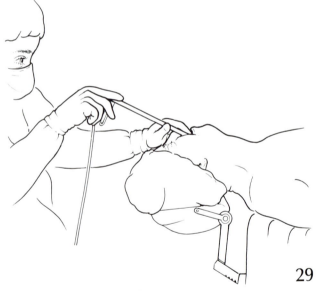

29

this marks the point of tonic contraction of the lower oesphageal sphincter. Gentle pressure with the tip of the oesophagoscope will cause this area to relax, and just beyond the serrated junction of the paler stratified squamous epithelium of the oesophagus with the bright pink columnar transitional epithelium the cardia is usually visible. In the absence of pathology on introduction of the oesophagoscope, further careful inspection should be undertaken as the instrument is withdrawn; this will often give a better view of small lesions. Pharyngoscopy with an oesophageal speculum of the Negus type will provide easier manipulation and an improved view of hypopharyngeal and upper oesophageal lesions. Forward elevation of the larynx while the endotracheal cuff is deflated allows excellent inspection of both piriform fossae, the cricopharyngeal area and post-cricoid region to a degree which is still superior to modern flexible instrumentation.

Flexible instrument

The fibreoptic flexible instrument is usually passed with the patient lying on his side with knees and hips flexed, although it can be used supine or upright. A plastic guard is inserted between the teeth, and the instrument lubricated with water-soluble jelly is then passed in the midline without neck flexion. On reaching the posterior pharyngeal wall, the tip is flexed via the control and the left index finger placed alongside the gag directs the tip over the epiglottis and into the hypopharynx. Resistance is now felt and the patient is instructed to swallow. As the larynx elevates the endoscope is slightly extruded, but as the larynx descends the instrument tip is advanced and will usually pass easily through the relaxed sphincter. Air insufflation of the thoracic oesophagus can now begin and the instrument is advanced slowly under direct vision as the oesophagus is gently distended. If hypopharyngeal or upper oesophageal disease is suspected, or if there is any difficulty, the entrance into the oesophagus must be performed under direct vision. While it is untrue that it is not possible to evaluate this area, rigid endoscopy remains superior in these areas, However, once the lower oesophagus is gained, the flexible fibreoptic instrument comes into its own and complete upper intestinal endoscopy can be carried out.

Diagnosis

Preoperative chest radiographs, posteroanterior and lateral, should be available for postoperative comparison. Prior to rigid endoscopy, elderly and arthritic patients may also require radiographs of the spine. Videofluoroscopy or standard barium swallow are usually undertaken but are particularly important if a pharyngeal diverticulum is suspected, or a lesion causing total dysphagia which may not allow the passage of the oesophagoscope beyond the lesion.

Pharyngeal and oesophageal diverticula are easily missed on both rigid and flexible instrumentation, and the site should be checked on barium swallow radiographs before performing endoscopy.

Ulceration

Superficial erosions may be seen in patients with oesophagal retention or gastro-oesophageal reflux and Barrett's ulcer may form in the lower oesophagus if the muscosa is of the gastric type. Malignant ulcers in the oesophagus are usually squamous, but in the lower third they may be gastric adenocarcinomas invading the oesophagus. Although irregular ulcerating tumours are often easy to detect, their upper edge may form what appears to be a benign stricture. This will require dilatation and the removal of biopsy specimens from multiple sites.

Strictures

These most frequently occur when peptic ulceration develops in relation to a hiatus hernia. Chronic strictures may develop at the sites of anatomical hold-up of the cricopharyngeus, aortic arch and cardia. The hypopharyngeal or upper oesophageal web associated with iron deficiency anaemia dilates easily. Biopsy specimens should be taken. If possible, all areas of a stricture should be biopsied following dilatation either by using bougies through a rigid endoscope or the introduction of a guidewire through the stricture and introduction of a subsequent Eade–Peusto dilator after withdrawal of the fibreoptic endoscope. Cytological brushings of a stricture may be obtained using the flexible instrument with both back and forth and rotation movements. The brush should be immediately wiped onto a microscope slide and sprayed with an aerosol fixative.

Oesophagitis

Oesophagitis is usually related to gastro-oesophageal reflux and bleeds easily on contact with the endoscope. It may also occur in relation to the stagnation of food and fluid above a stricture or in achalasia. Mega-oesophagus is usually seen in achalasia of the cardia.

Hiatus hernia

The rolling type of hernia can be diagnosed by entering the stomach with a flexible endoscope and then reversing the tip to view the fundus. Hiatus hernia of the sliding type is diagnosed when the cardia is met at a higher level than expected and both may or may not be associated with oesophageal reflux.

Varices

Varices are easily recognized at the lower end of the oesophagus where the distended, gorged veins bulge prominently into the lumen and may extend into the cardia.

Therapeutic technique

Dilatation of strictures, biopsies, intubation of strictures, injection of oesophageal varices, and removal of foreign bodies remain the common endoscopic operations. Both flexible and rigid instruments may be required under differing conditions for all these pathologies. Flexible fibreoptic endoscopes can replace the rigid instrument in many instances; a good example is the injection of oesophageal varices, which in many centres is now undertaken via a fibreoptic endoscope without the need for general anaesthesia – an important consideration in patients with portal venous hypertension. However, the removal of foreign bodies is still limited with the fibreoptic endoscope because the channels allow the passage of only fragile forceps and the object cannot be drawn into the instrument. Foreign bodies usually lodge at the anatomical and physiological constrictions of the oesophagus outlined above, and many still require the use of rigid endoscopes so that they may be removed with grasping forceps either whole or piecemeal. The object may be introduced into the lumen of the oesophagoscope with the forceps and both are then gradually withdrawn together. Shears may be required to reduce certain foreign bodies to an appropriate size to allow their safe removal and a variety of ingenious forceps are available, grasping such objects as open safety pins to allow their removal. In some cases, the object should be pushed on into the stomach for natural passage or for subsequent gastrotomy, and occasionally thoracotomy and oesophagotomy may still be required.

Postoperative care

Following oesophagoscopy little analgesia should be required, and if the procedure has been performed under a local anaesthetic the patient should not eat or drink for 4 h. Following rigid oesophagoscopy under general anaesthesia, it is advisable for the patient to take only sterile water until the day after the operation. Postoperative pain, particularly when radiating to the thoracic spine between the scapulae, may indicate that perforation of the oesophagus has occurred during the operation, and it may be accompanied by marked dysphagia, subcutaneous surgical emphysema in the neck or supraclavicular region and by a marked pyrexia. Perforation most frequently occurs at the cricopharyngeus or at the cardiac sphincter. Whenever any manipulation has taken place, the patient's neck should be examined for signs of emphysema and a chest radiograph should be taken. Minor leaks in the neck may be treated conservatively but intrathoracic leakage may demand immediate thoracotomy. Damage to the lips and teeth may occur but, in the event of the latter, dental advice should be sought immediately for, with modern techniques, teeth can often be replaced in a viable state.

Nose and paranasal sinuses

Endoscopy of the nasal cavity and sinuses is not a new technique and a variety of instruments were used and advocated in the 1920s and 1930s. However, the introduction of the Hopkin's fibreoptics and cold light sources in the early 1960s greatly enhanced its popularity. Problems with the depth of field of the telescopes and inadequate illumination have now been overcome, and in modern rhinological practice endoscopy may be used to determine diagnosis, to facilitate surgical techniques and for precise documentation. Direct visualization and biopsy can establish a diagnosis with greater ease and precision than was previously possible. In the presence of an obvious radiological abnormality it can provide confirmation, but it is equally useful where such radiographic evidence is lacking but clinical suspicion is high. Useful documentation of pathology and operative results is possible and endoscopy has an important role in the follow-up of both benign and malignant disease. Endoscopic examination surgery is most often performed on the nasal cavity and maxillary sinus, and while it is technically possible to use a similar technique on the frontal and sphenoid sinuses, the lower incidence of pathology in these areas limits its use.

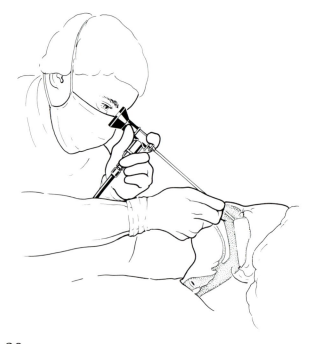

Position and preparation of patient

30

Nasal endoscopy may be performed with the patient sitting or supine with the head slightly elevated at 15°. The procedure may be performed under local anaesthesia or under general anaesthesia as a precursor to other procedures. Local anaesthesia is achieved by spraying the nose with 5 per cent cocaine and then placing two cotton wool pledgets soaked in 5 per cent cocaine hydrochloride in each nasal cavity for 2–3 min.

31 & 32

The maxillary sinus may be viewed by the inferior meatus either by puncture under the genu of the inferior turbinate or through an existing antrostomy, but this does not always give a satisfactory view of the natural ostium and the canine fossa approach may be preferable. This may also be done under local or general anaesthesia using a trocar sheath through which the sinuscope can be introduced. In either case the canine fossa should be infiltrated with 1 per cent lignocaine with 1:200 000 adrenaline. The frontal sinus can be entered with a drill after making a small skin incision usually under general anaesthesia. A custom-made long trocar is necessary for sphenoidal endoscopy.

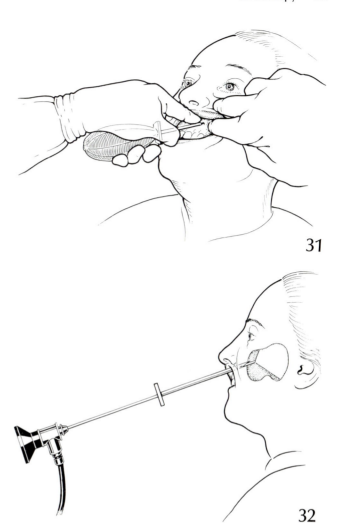

31

32

Light source and instrumentation

The author's preference is for a xenon cold light fountain (350 W); less powerful illumination can be used but necessitates the use of flash full photography. Fluid-filled light cables connect the light source to the Hopkin's telescope and this system provides depth of field, excellent illumination and high resolution. A variety of telescopes are available: a 4 mm 0° instrument allows a range of vision with adequate orientation, while being small enough to fit in the nasal cavity of most patients. Fogging is avoided by using a demisting solution on the distal end of the telescope. A variety of specula, probes, angled forceps and rigid optical biopsy forceps are required. Combined sinuscopes are now available which allow irrigation and suction.

Operative technique

The endoscope is placed gently in the nasal cavity without touching the vestibular skin which is particularly sensitive. Care is also taken to avoid the septum and lateral wall and the patient breathes gently through an open mouth. The maxillary sinus is entered and any contents can be aspirated for microbiological and cytological examination, the condition of the mucosa inspected and the ostium examined. Biopsies under visual control can be taken and ciliary brushings obtained to determine mucosal damage. These techniques can be performed via the canine fossa or inferior meatal approach alone, but a combination of the two routes is sometimes advantageous. On removal of the trocar the resulting small wound heals within 24–48 h.

Anatomy, pathology and therapeutic possibilities

Endoscopy offers the possibility of carefully assessing the normal anatomy in greater detail than is possible by anterior and posterior rhinoscopy. Congenital deformity from mild septal deviation to choanal atresia can be established. The presence of foreign bodies and adhe-

sions can be found and dealt with under direct vision. Mucosal pathology such as hereditary haemorrhagic telangiectasia, and chronic inflammatory processes such as sarcoid, are eminently suitable for such examination. The origin and extent of tumours in the nasal cavity can be assessed and diagnosis established by obtaining an adequate and representative biopsy. In the maxillary sinus in particular, the irreversibility of mucosal damage can be evaluated and obstruction of the natural ostium established. The presence of cysts, dental roots and the results of trauma, for example blow-out fractures of the orbit, can be visualized.

With regard to surgical procedures, instrumentation is too small for major operations and any significant haemorrhage rapidly obscures the view. Functional endoscopic surgery for acute and chronic inflammatory disease is a rapidly growing branch of otorhinolaryngology. The endoscope is extremely useful in the follow-up of patients who have undergone craniofacial, base of skull and sinus surgery operations for both benign and malignant tumours and, apart from close visualization, it allows detailed removal of crusts, granulations and biopsy of possible recurrent disease.

Evaluation and treatment of swallowing disorders in head and neck surgical patients (including cricopharyngeal myotomy)

David J. Howard FRCS, FRCS(Ed)
Institute of Laryngology and Otology, Royal National Throat, Nose and Ear Hospital, London, UK

Introduction

Swallowing is a complex neuromuscular act and functional aberration results in dysphagia and, at times, accompanying aspiration. The causes of dysphagia and aspiration are many but fall into the three broad groups of cerebrovascular accidents, neurological diseases, and the results of major surgery for head and neck tumours. This chapter will deal in the main with the last group, but also includes an overview of the role of cricopharyngeal myotomy and excision of a cricopharyngeal pouch.

Patients who have undergone major resections for tumours of the oral cavity, oropharynx, skull base, hypopharynx and larynx may experience a wide variety of swallowing problems. These may result from partial or total resection of structures, loss or incoordination of peristaltic and sphincteric functions, loss of sensory or motor nerve supply and, finally, persistent oedema, fistula formation and scar tissue in the operative site. Additional factors such as pain, psychological and emotional problems and post-irradiation changes may all influence swallowing. The rehabilitation of swallowing disabilities remains a major challenge in head and neck surgery. The surgeon requires an understanding of the mechanism of normal swallowing, of the preoperative and postoperative changes associated with the disease and surgical resection, and of the adaptive and compensatory mechanisms that may be developed by patients. These patients can be considerably aided by the surgeon, radiologist, speech and swallowing therapist, nurse and dietician, working as a team. While the detailed study of swallowing has for long been of interest to a small number of physiologists and doctors using cineradiographic and manometric techniques, it is only in the last 15 years with the increasingly widespread use of modern videofluoroscopy that the range of swallowing disorders associated with head and neck surgery is beginning to be evaluated and understood.

Normal swallowing

1

The act of swallowing is commonly described as consisting of three stages: oral, pharyngeal and oesophageal. Radiographical evaluation of the passage of a bolus from the mouth, through the pharynx into the oesophagus is based on the identification of specific anatomical landmarks and the integrated motion accomplished by the oral and pharyngeal muscles during swallowing. A total of over 20 muscles and five cranial nerves must be coordinated to allow the safe transfer of liquids and solids from the mouth into the oesophagus and, while a full discussion of the anatomy and physiology will not be given here, some details of the complex pharyngeal anatomy and physiology are appropriate.

Muscle groups participating in the oral and pharyngeal phases of swallowing are those of the lips, cheeks, soft palate and pharyngeal isthmus, the tongue and hyoid bone, the pharyngeal constrictors, and those which elevate the larynx.

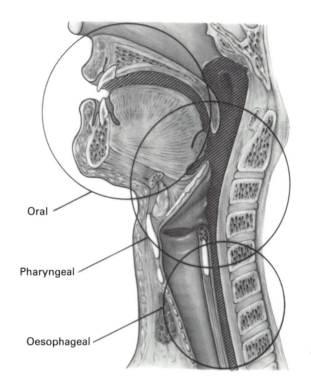

2

A dorsal view of the pharynx reveals the three pharyngeal constrictors (superior, middle and inferior) which overlap like tiles on a roof and insert into a dense collagenous sheet of multidirectional fibres – the buccopharyngeal aponeurosis. In the upper pharynx this fascia is joined to the prevertebral fascia by a median raphe, but inferiorly the constrictor wall is mobile in relation to the prevertebral fascia.

The cricopharyngeal sphincter at the junction between the pharynx and oesophagus includes fibres of the inferior pharyngeal constrictor – both thyropharyngeal and cricopharyngeal muscles – as well as the circular muscle fibres of the upper cervical oesophagus. This segment, which is closed between swallows, is 3–5 cm long and corresponds to an area of high pressure identified by intraluminal manometry. In the literature it is often referred to as the 'upper oesophageal sphincter'. Maintenance of an elevated cricopharyngeal sphincter pressure at rest is necessary to protect the pharynx from exposure to regurgitated oesophageal or gastric contents and to prevent passage of air into the oesophagus during respiration. During swallowing the sphincter relaxes in advance of the descending bolus and laryngeal elevation and closure assures separation of the airway from the pharynx. Since swallowing is both an airway protective reflex and alimentary supportive reflex, there is necessarily an interplay between the respiratory and swallowing centres.

In the oral phase of swallowing the lips, cheeks, tongue, floor of mouth, teeth and palate participate in preparing the food. The food is held in the oral cavity, lateralized for mastication and then formed into a bolus. The tongue propels the formed bolus posteriorly into the oropharynx. In the involuntary pharyngeal phase, the soft palate is elevated to prevent nasopharyngeal escape and the lateral and posterior walls contract to propel the food down-

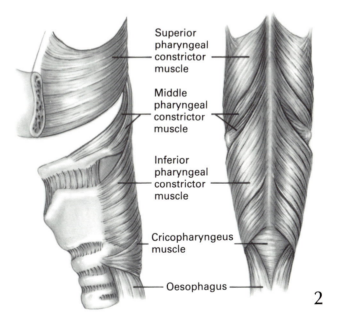

wards. The larynx moves upwards and forwards as the posterior tongue moves backwards and downwards. The larynx is protected by two sphincter units, one consisting of the epiglottis, aryepiglottic folds and false folds, and the other of the true folds. As the food enters the piriform sinus there is anticipatory relaxation of the cricopharyngeal sphincter and the food enters the oesophagus. Oesophageal peristaltic waves convey the food down the oesophagus. Gravity aids both the pharyngeal and oesophageal phases of swallowing and the so-called buccopharyngeal squirt mechanism acts to propel liquids quickly through the pharynx and into the oesophagus.

Evaluation of swallowing

While history and examination remain essential and helpful in all swallowing disorders, they do not allow assessment of the patient's swallowing physiology in sufficient detail to determine the exact cause or degree of dysphagia and will often not identify aspiration nor its cause. Currently available procedures to examine swallowing include manometry, videofluoroscopy and forms of ultrasonography. While manometry has a long history and nowadays is coupled in many centres with videofluoroscopy, there is still considerable debate over this form of measurement and it gives no information concerning aspiration or the function of the oral cavity or larynx which are critical components of the swallowing mechanism. Videofluoroscopy is the only available investigation that allows direct observation of the aerodigestive tract during all stages of swallowing.

Videofluoroscopy and the modified barium swallow

The standard long-established barium swallow procedure was introduced primarily for the study of oesophageal pathology and is inappropriate for examination of head and neck surgical patients or those with neurological diseases who are having severe problems and are at risk of aspiration. The modern modified barium swallow technique allows examination of the oral cavity and pharynx radiographically as these areas present different problems from those encountered when examining the oesophagus. In a standard barium swallow procedure the oesophagus must be filled with barium to be viewed and the patient lies in a supine position. However, in order to view the oral cavity and pharynx they must not be filled with large amounts of barium material as this obliterates their structure and masks their function. In addition, the patient with an oral or pharyngeal swallowing disorder at risk of aspiration may have great difficulty in handling a large bolus of barium. Thus the modified technique involves the use of only small amounts of material, generally one-third to one-half of a teaspoon per swallow. A variety of materials of different consistencies may be used other than liquid, and most commonly these consist of barium paste or biscuits coated with barium paste or with barium baked into their contents. This variety of food consistencies allows overall evaluation as some patients may experience difficulty in swallowing liquids, but not heavier food.

3

The modified barium swallow is undertaken with the patient seated upright in a normal eating position. In patients with dysphagia the physiology of the oral cavity and pharynx in the normal eating position must be established first and then, if desired, the patient's position can be changed and the postural effects on swallowing noted. The procedure is initially undertaken in the lateral plane with the fluoroscopy tube defining the whole oral cavity and pharynx. The anteroposterior view is taken following the lateral assessment and the overall evaluation allows definition of the oral and pharyngeal motility during swallowing, the presence of aspiration, the oral and pharyngeal transit times compared with normal, and the effect of any positional changes on the overall swallowing performance. Further oesophageal assessment can be completed as necessary.

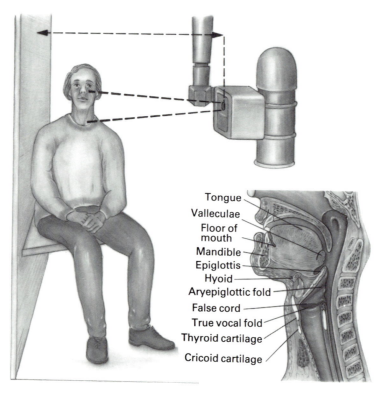

Tongue
Valleculae
Floor of mouth
Mandible
Epiglottis
Hyoid
Aryepiglottic fold
False cord
True vocal fold
Thyroid cartilage
Cricoid cartilage

3

Swallowing disorders following head and neck surgery

Surgical resection may be performed at any level in the upper aerodigestive tract and consequently can affect any phase of the swallowing function. However, certain practical generalizations are possible because postoperative swallowing difficulties can be classified in terms of the phases disturbed. Because of the accumulative effects, problems encountered in patients having wide resection and reconstruction are often complicated and severe. A patient with difficulties involving the oral, pharyngeal and laryngeal levels may have significant aspiration problems and salivary incontinence.

Oral phase dysfunction

The problems here include difficulty with the preparation for swallowing with an impaired ability to hold food or to lateralize the material for mastication. Trismus and dentition problems further complicate the issue and bolus formation and transport through the oral cavity may be severely compromised by tongue and floor of mouth resections. There is then a tendency for the material to remain in the anterior or lateral sulci or to adhere to the hard palate. Disturbance of tongue propulsion may alter the ability to hold the bolus within the oral cavity, leading to premature swallowing and aspiration. The overall results may be a prolonged oral transit time and hesitant and piecemeal swallowing patterns.

Pharyngeal phase dysfunction

Problems here include inadequate initiation of the pharyngeal constrictor wave, delayed soft palate elevation and inadequate velopharyngeal closure with regurgitation into the nasopharynx and nasal cavities, abnormal pharyngeal motility patterns with prolonged pharyngeal transit time, stasis in the valleculae and/or piriform fossa and laryngeal dysfunction. Laryngeal dysfunction may be due to delayed or reduced laryngeal elevation or to ineffective laryngeal closure and may be an extension of pharyngeal phase dysfunction. These effects are particularly seen after vertical hemilaryngectomy and supraglottic laryngectomy. Aspiration may be the predominant symptom in these patients and may also trouble those with bilateral recurrent laryngeal nerve paralysis, with or without superior laryngeal nerve paralysis.

Oesophageal phase dysfunction

A bolus of food material may not progress into the oesophagus because of pooling in the hypopharynx as a result of cricopharyngeal hypertonicity, spasm or incoordination. Impairment of the oesophageal phase results from a wide variety of disorders, most commonly oesophageal obstruction or stenosis.

Radiotherapy

Treatment of head and neck malignancy by radiotherapy often affects swallowing, but the symptoms vary greatly in duration and severity from patient to patient and in some cases may not appear for many months after the completion of a full course of radiotherapy. There is little in the way of detailed study in the literature on this subject. There is no doubt that in the short term radiotherapy to the oral cavity and pharynx markedly decreases salivary flow and mucus formation and may lead to oral and pharyngeal oedema. The swallowing reflex may be delayed in both the oral and pharyngeal phases of swallowing and may be prolonged for many months, even when the gross anatomy remains unchanged and the disease is cured.

Operations

The overall effect on swallowing will depend on the site and size of the resection, the general status and age of the patient and the type of reconstruction. Research into these swallowing problems is continuing apace, but considerable areas of debate with regard to specific surgical procedures still exist and the following is a brief overview of those where the author feels there is general agreement.

Oral cavity

Within the oral cavity the tongue is undoubtedly the most important component, being responsible for the majority of the preparation and the propulsion during the oral phase. It is therefore a simple but important requirement that for cancer of the tongue and floor of mouth a resection and reconstruction should be undertaken in order to permit as much range and coordination of residual tongue movement as is possible. If this important concept is kept in mind, it alone will significantly improve the surgeon's functional results in patients with oral cavity disease. Depending on the size of the defect, reconstructive measures such as split-thickness skin grafting with or without quilting, and thin pliable myocutaneous flaps such as the radial free forearm, have much to commend them in the way of functional results within the oral cavity. In the case of hemiglossectomy and floor of mouth resection, with or without an accompanying radical neck dissection, reconstruction of the floor only, leaving an elevated and mobile residual hemitongue, gives a better functional result than attempted reconstruction of both floor and tongue bulk.

Oropharynx

Surgery of the tongue base, tonsil, retromolar trigone, lateral oropharyngeal wall and soft palate directly affects the swallowing reflex which triggers the pharyngeal phase and may significantly impair tongue mobility during oral preparation and the oral phase of swallowing. It may also damage the attachments of the pharyngeal constrictors, thus reducing pharyngeal peristalsis. Utilization of the remaining tongue for closure can further reduce the swallowing capabilities, and reconstruction of the area with thick bulky myocutaneous flaps may interfere with the functioning of the pharynx, tongue and remaining normal tissues. Thin pedicled or free myocutaneous flaps will give improved functional results. If a pedicled myocutaneous flap is contemplated for the reconstruction, for example the pectoralis major, it may be preferable to raise the flap as a simple myofascial unit without the overlying subcutaneous tissue and skin. The defect is then closed with this myofascial unit and, if necessary, a split-thickness skin graft can be applied on the internal surface of the defect closed by the muscle flap. This technique considerably lessens the bulk of such pedicled flaps and improves the functional results.

TOTAL GLOSSECTOMY

Advanced tumours of the tongue base may, in addition to total glossectomy, also require total laryngectomy. Reconstruction is most commonly by pedicled myocutaneous flaps, although a variety of free flaps have also been used for this purpose. The bulk of the pedicled myocutaneous flap, or the larger free myocutaneous flaps, on this occasion is frequently useful in allowing a satisfactory height and sloping of the reconstructed floor of mouth. Care should be taken not to narrow the pharyngeal inlet and to create a progressive slope downwards and backwards from the anterior incisor aspect of the mandible to the pharyngeal constrictors. This results in surprisingly good swallowing when food is placed into the oral cavity and the head tipped backwards allowing the food to slide into the pharynx. The combination of gravity and pharyngeal constrictor movement will pass the food material into the oesophagus.

The situation is more difficult when the larynx remains in place because of loss of the laryngeal support. This loss of support produces a high rate of aspiration and is a major factor in delaying rehabilitation of swallowing following total glossectomy. In order to overcome this problem it is necessary to resuspend the larynx upwards and forwards. This is undertaken by insertion of strong sutures or wire through the perichondrium and cartilage near the midline of the anterior thyroid lamina and the inferior thyroid notch followed by approximation of these sutures to a wire loop placed through the symphysis of the mandible. The sutures should be under sufficient tension to raise the larynx approximately 2 cm and with careful application and tension of the inferior notch sutures a laryngeal tilt of approximately 45° can be produced. This secures the laryngeal inlet beneath the base of the reconstructed floor of mouth and enlarges the hypopharyngeal tunnel facilitating pharyngeal transit. A partial epiglottopexy with two mattress sutures between the aryepiglottic folds and lateral aspects of the epiglottis may provide an additional degree of protection by partially covering the laryngeal inlet.

MANDIBULAR RESECTION

Resection of any component of the mandible may have a significant effect on the oral and pharyngeal phase of swallowing. Major resection of the anterior arch or hemimandibulectomy may cripple the oral phase to such a degree as to make any form of normal diet almost impossible. There is no doubt that in the recent past far too many mandibular segments have been sacrificed and more limited resection of part of the mandible as outlined

in the chapter on 'Reconstruction of the oral cavity', pp. 215–240 with preservation of a rim of mandible is to be preferred. These conservation resections of the mandible rarely compromise the radical nature of the excisional surgery but have far-reaching consequences in terms of preservation of function. They are to be preferred to any form of mandibular reconstruction using either titanium, stainless steel plates or free bone grafts and osteomyocutaneous flaps. Debate continues with regard to the advantages of the various forms of mandibular reconstruction with the above, when it is absolutely necessary to resect mandible, but the improved success rates of all techniques in recent years are more related to the improved vascularity of the soft tissue defect repair than of the exact material used to restore continuity of the mandible. As with the obvious case of restoration of swallowing following excisional surgery of the upper jaw, expert prosthodontic advice may also benefit the functional rehabilitation of patients when used after total glossectomy or mandibular resection (see chapter on 'Prosthetics in head and neck surgery', pp. 576–592).

Pharynx

PARTIAL PHARYNGECTOMY

If the neurophysiological damage or surgical resection involves only one side of the oropharynx or hypopharynx, patients can usually be taught positional changes which facilitate swallowing on the unoperated and less damaged side. Rotation of the head to the damaged side closes the piriform sinus on that side and thus directs food down the more normal side. Alternatively, the patient may tilt the head towards the more normal side which facilitates food transit down the stronger side. However, as in the oral cavity, the nature of the reconstruction, particularly the inert bulk, may interfere with function on the unoperated side so that even with variations of position the patient is unable to swallow satisfactorily, and if the additional changes of radiotherapy are added, aspiration and severe disability may result.

TOTAL PHARYNGECTOMY

When total pharyngectomy has been undertaken, three groups of reconstructive methods are now available. These are the various free and pedicled myocutaneous flaps, free jejunal transfer with microvascular anastomosis, and the gastric or colonic transposition procedures. Details of these methods are given in the individual chapters in this volume, but there is no doubt that, from the point of view of rehabilitation of swallowing, the results of tubed myocutaneous flaps and colonic transposition procedures are markedly inferior to those obtained by means of a free jejunal transfer or gastric transposition.

In a large series of patients published from various parts of the world, aside from the other considerations, the best long-term swallowing results were obtained with the gastric transposition method. Free jejunal transfer is still associated with motility problems of the transferred jejunal segment and stenosis at the anastomotic areas to a greater degree than is the gastric transposition procedure.

Following pharyngeal resection, the author has seen problems with myocutaneous flap repairs in terms of stenosis and dysphagia occurring as late as 7 years after the initial procedure. More than one-third of patients having reconstruction with tubed myocutaneous flaps are able to swallow little if any form of normal diet, and remain on liquids and semi-solids for the remainder of their life. The incidence of anastomotic or flap stenosis following this latter form of repair exceeds 25 per cent.

Larynx

PARTIAL LARYNGECTOMY

As with the oral cavity, the extent of both resection and reconstruction is important in determining how quickly and how well the partial laryngectomized patient can commence and continue oral feeding. Partial laryngectomy interferes with laryngeal elevation, the laryngeal sphincter mechanism and pharyngeal transit. In vertical hemilaryngectomy disturbance of the laryngeal sphincter and, occasionally, pharyngeal contraction are the obvious problems; however, most patients regain normal swallowing in a relatively short period of time after vertical hemilaryngectomy, especially if an organized programme of swallowing therapy is begun 10–14 days postoperatively. In contrast, horizontal supraglottic laryngectomy is associated with marked swallowing difficulties and all the large series reported in recent years indicate problems with aspiration to a varying degree in up to 70 per cent of patients. Indeed, in the initial stages of rehabilitation all these patients can be shown to aspirate fluids if detailed videofluoroscopic studies are undertaken. Details of both these operative procedures are given in the chapters on 'Vertical partial laryngectomy', pp. 494–501 and 'Horizontal partial laryngectomy', pp. 502–507.

Factors not related to the actual operative technique of supraglottic laryngectomy, but which nevertheless contribute to aspiration, include stricture of the oesophagus, poor pulmonary function, paralysis of one or both vocal folds, pharyngeal dysfunction and tumour recurrence. Cricopharyngeal myotomy at the time of the operative procedure has been advocated by many, although definite evidence in its favour has not been demonstrated. Likewise resuspension of the residual larynx in the manner described under total glossectomy (p. 444) has also been advocated but is not routinely undertaken by many surgeons performing this procedure. However, attempts to lessen laryngeal ptosis by suturing the laryngeal perichondrium to the base of tongue are not always successful. Loss of the supraglottic sphincteric mechanism is partially overcome by the tight apposition of the residual true vocal folds and by the shielding effect of the base of the tongue in its posterior position. Not only does the tongue provide a protective ledge, but in some cases it clears trapped food at the inlet by compression against the folds and arytenoid eminences. However, if any form of vocal paralysis occurs, aspiration is inevitable and also accompanies any major resection of the tongue base or damage to one or other hypoglossal nerve.

Swallowing therapy

As mentioned previously, many of the problems associated with partial laryngeal procedures can be overcome if an organized programme of swallowing therapy is commenced before removal of the nasogastric tube. Removal of the temporary tracheostomy varies enormously in these patients and cannot be undertaken until the airway is adequate. The tracheostomy site should be allowed to close before commencing oral feeding and this is usually between 7 and 14 days after surgery, earlier in the vertical hemilaryngectomy group than in the horizontal supraglottic laryngectomy group.

Swallowing therapy requires a team approach and before commencing oral feeding the dietician should inform the patient about the type of diet necessary with advice about the consistency, rationale and expected progression of the diet. This will relieve much of the patient's anxiety. Feeding should begin with solid and pureed foods without liquids. Attempts at swallowing clear liquids, particularly after supraglottic laryngectomy, frequently produce aspiration. Cold carbonated beverages have been shown to be by far the best clear liquid to introduce once swallowing is established. These impart a much improved sensation to the patient and stimulate the swallowing reflex in a much more satisfactory manner. It is important that the diet progresses and that a positive approach is maintained to keep the patient's confidence. To improve the protection afforded by the residual larynx, the swallowing and speech therapist can give instructions with regard to approximation of the vocal folds and development of subglottic pressure by means of breath holding. The patients, under guidance, follow a step by step sequence of placing the food in the mouth, chewing, taking a deep breath and holding it, swallowing, coughing to clear the vocal fold surface, swallowing again, and then breathing out. Aspiration may be completely avoided. This type of guidance and instruction may be beneficial in a wide variety of swallowing problems already discussed which have aspiration as an integral part of the overall problem.

TOTAL LARYNGECTOMY

A vast amount has been written on vocal rehabilitation after this operation – the largest group of patients undergoing major surgery and radiotherapy for head and neck cancer. What has not been adequately realized and investigated until recent years is that a high proportion of these patients have postoperative dysphagia and that this, rather than acquisition of voice, may be the most limiting factor in their subsequent rehabilitation. Recent detailed videofluoroscopic studies from a number of centres have shown dysphagia produced by short-term and long-term pharyngeal stenosis, gross pseudo-epiglottic formation and neuromuscular incoordination. While much has been written, the situation still remains to be clarified with regard to the best form of pharyngeal closure and the possible benefits of cricopharyngeal and upper oesophageal myotomy. What is not in doubt is that problems of dysphagia in this group of patients are markedly increased should they have concurrent disability of the oral phase of swallowing, most commonly produced by damage to one or both hypoglossal nerves. Dysphagia may also be the early sign of pharyngeal recurrence and it is important to evaluate the overall quality of swallowing in the postoperative follow-up of total laryngectomy patients.

Swallowing dysfunction associated with tracheostomy

It is a well established fact that a small proportion of patients who have a tracheostomy for the treatment of lower respiratory tract pathology, and who have an otherwise normal oral cavity, pharynx, larynx and oesophagus, will nevertheless have considerable swallowing difficulties which may include aspiration. The exact cause of these difficulties is multifactorial and, while numerous studies have been performed using manometric, cinegraphic and, more recently, videofluoroscopic techniques, it is not always possible to be sure in the individual patient as to the exact factors responsible. The situation is further complicated in those patients who have a tracheostomy and additional pathology and/or surgery of the head and neck.

Establishment of the tracheostomy, particularly with a cuffed tube, immediately alters respiratory dynamics. It prevents the establishment of a positive intralaryngeal pressure and strong expiratory cough and produces relative fixation of the laryngotracheal complex. Simple removal of the tracheostomy tube is often essential in the rehabilitation phase of swallowing after head and neck surgery, the obvious example of supraglottic laryngectomy having already been discussed above. Further impairment of swallowing may be produced by the direct pressure effect of an overinflated tracheostomy tube cuff causing compression of the cervical oesophagus. However, this is easily remedied and videofluoroscopic studies would suggest that it is the least important of the factors.

4 a–c

Long established tracheostomy can cause marked fixation of the anterior aspect of the trachea to the neck skin with fibrosis and scar tissue formation around the tracheostomy tract. This may markedly limit elevation and anterior rotation of the larynx during the second stage of swallowing and appears to have an inhibitory effect on relaxation of the cricopharyngeal sphincter causing further incoordination of the swallow. This may be the major factor giving rise to swallowing and aspiration difficulties in these patients. Changes in the pharyngolaryngeal reflex from the position at rest and on deglutition and the inhibitory effect that a tracheostomy has on these movements are shown in the illustration.

Bearing these details in mind, the use of tracheostomy in an attempt to safeguard the airway in patients with aspiration and swallowing difficulties seems inappropriate and at times is detrimental. The idea that a cuffed tube will protect the lower respiratory tract from the entrance of liquids aspirated is, of course, untrue. When the problems of aspiration are serious and likely to be long term, as is the case with major cerebrovascular incidents and neurological disease, far more definitive procedures may be required and the reader is referred to the chapter on 'Surgical management of vocal fold paralysis'.

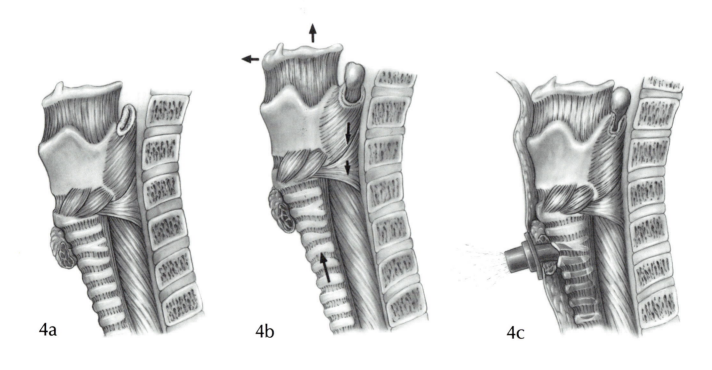

4a   4b   4c

Cricopharyngeal myotomy

Cricopharyngeal myotomy has been widely reported as an effective treatment for dysphagia and aspiration resulting from neurological disease and surgical procedures. However, indications for this procedure are only recently becoming defined. We still have only a limited understanding of pharyngo-oesophageal physiology in normal individuals and the wide variety of disease states, and the functional alterations brought about by a myotomy. Success rates of 60 per cent are commonly quoted for the procedure, but long-standing results and detailed measurements are rarely presented. The relatively low morbidity and mortality rates associated with the procedure have encouraged a liberal indiscriminate use for almost any problem of dysphagia and this is an unsatisfactory situation.

Modern manometric measurements are less controversial than in the past, and certainly the length of the upper oesophageal sphincter manometrically incorporates the lower inferior constrictor muscle of the pharynx, cricopharyngeus muscle and the initial oesophageal circular fibres varying in length from 2.5 to 6.5 cm. This is an important point when cricopharyngeal myotomy is considered as the myotomy must divide the whole of the upper oesophageal sphincter. Data from normal subjects reveal that during swallowing relaxation of the upper oesophageal sphincter should be complete, preceding pharyngeal contraction and terminating thereafter. Disturbances of this sequence give rise to dysphagia.

The initially postulated and still widely held view that spasm of the cricopharyngeus gives rise to dysphagia and the formation of a posterior pharyngeal pouch (Zenker's diverticulum) has been shown to be untrue. While even with modern manometry the situation is not clear, many patients with posterior pharyngeal pouches, for example, demonstrate normal relaxation of the cricopharyngeus in relation to swallowing. Others, however, have been shown to have incomplete pharyngeal relaxation, early cricopharyngeal contraction and abnormalities of the pharyngeal contraction wave in combination with abnormal cricopharyngeal function. Videofluoroscopic studies using the modified barium swallow technique enable the most thorough evaluation of the causes of dysphagia and recent studies have emphasized the necessity of demonstating, with or without additional manometric evidence, definite abnormality of the function of the cricopharyngeal area.

Cricopharyngeal myotomy should be reserved for patients who have a failure of pharyngeal peristalsis and marked cricopharyngeal incoordination. There are two notable exceptions to this. First, the posterior pharyngeal pouch (Zenker's diverticulum) in which an abnormality may not always be detected in the region of the cricopharyngeal sphincter but where the general consensus is that cricopharyngeal myotomy is an essential part of surgery for this condition, and that the recurrence rate, either in terms of symptoms or of the pouch itself, is markedly reduced in patients who undergo myotomy. For further details of pharyngeal pouch surgery the reader is referred to the chapters entitled 'Excision of pharyngeal pouch' and 'Diathermy of pharyngeal pouch' by H. Bernard Juby, pages 245–251, Nose and Throat volume of *Operative Surgery*, 4th Edition. The second exception is dysphagia associated with pronounced oesophageal reflux. This will generally resolve with restoration of distal oesophageal sphincter competence. Indeed cricopharyngeal myotomy in these patients may be detrimental, allowing reflux into the hypopharyngeal area with possible subsequent aspiration.

Operative technique

The procedure may be performed on its own or in addition to one-stage diverticulectomy for treatment of pharyngeal pouch. A left-sided cervical approach is recommended, bearing in mind that the cervical oesophagus is often situated to the left of the midline and the left recurrent laryngeal nerve lies more securely within the tracheo-oesophageal groove. A single posterior myotomy is used by the author as the variations reported such as double myotomies, removal of varying portions of the muscle and total excision of cricopharyngeus have not been shown to offer any definite advantages.

5

The operation is performed under general anaesthesia with the patient placed in a supine position with a small sandbag under the shoulders, the head hyperextended and turned to the right. Thyroid and cricoid cartilages are clearly felt in slim patients and a longitudinal incision along the anterior border of the left sternocleidomastoid gives the widest exposure. A transverse skin crease incision may also be used and may give better cosmesis, although this may be of minimal importance in most of these patients. The incision along the anterior border of the left sternocleidomastoid muscle is definitely recommended for the less experienced surgeon.

After division of the subcutaneous tissues and platysma in the line of the incision, the sternomastoid muscle is freed by a combination of sharp and blunt resection to expose the omohyoid muscle and associated strap muscles.

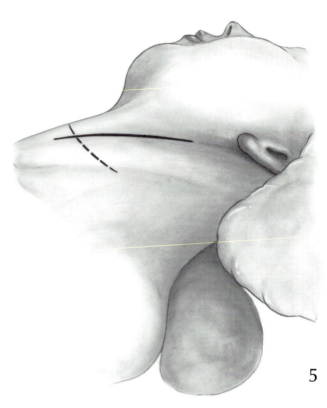

5

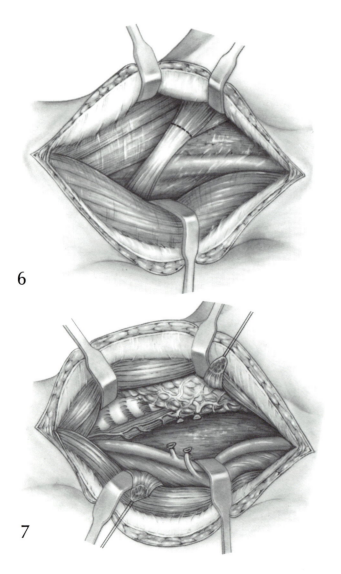

6

7

6 & 7

The sternocleidomastoid muscle and carotid sheath are retracted laterally and the trachea and larynx medially. The anterior belly of omohyoid muscle and middle thyroid vein, when present, are divided allowing further retraction of the thyroid towards the midline. The inferior thyroid artery is found and ligated well laterally where it disappears behind the carotid sheath. This ensures protection of the recurrent laryngeal nerve which is not actively displayed during this procedure. If the retropharyngeal space is entered above the inferior cornu of the thyroid cartilage, there is no risk to the recurrent laryngeal nerve.

8

This illustration shows a cross-section of the neck at the level of the thyroid isthmus showing the planes of access to the posterior aspect of the hypopharynx and cervical oesophagus. The operating surgeon either uses the non-dominant hand to retract the posterior border of the thyroid cartilage, thereby rotating the larynx so that the posterior aspect of the pharynx and oesophagus are clearly seen. Alternatively, this can be done by the assistant.

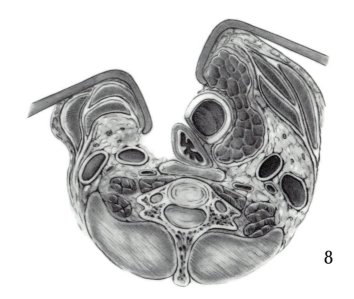

8

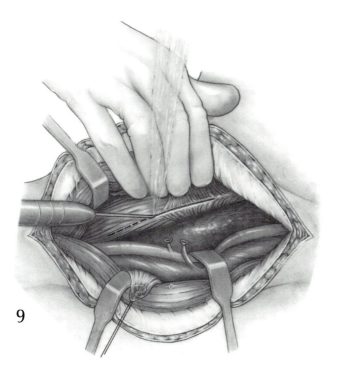

9

9

A variety of instruments have been advocated for undertaking myotomy and there are many ways to facilitate the myotomy by introducing large bougies or Foley catheters into the oesophageal lumen or placing artery forceps between the submucosa and the crico-pharyngeus muscle from above, so that when the blades are opened a knife can be used to divide the fibres which are stretched between the jaws of the forceps. The author uses low intensity needle diathermy as this controls any bleeding from the muscle layers. The myotomy is begun superiorly, dividing 1–2 cm of the inferior constrictor muscle of the pharynx and continuing distally, dividing the muscle fibres of cricopharyngeus and the cervical oesophagus for a length of 4–5 cm. A Lahey swab can be used to produce lateral traction on the muscle until mucosa is displayed and bulges freely through the whole length of the myotomized muscle. There must be no restriction by small fibrous bands and indeed some surgeons have advocated use of the operating micro-scope. If the mucosa is inadvertently damaged it is carefully repaired with interrupted catgut sutures.

10

When a posterior pharyngeal pouch is present it is carefully freed first from the overlying areolar tissue and fascial planes to expose clearly its neck and the underlying pharyngeal constrictor muscle.

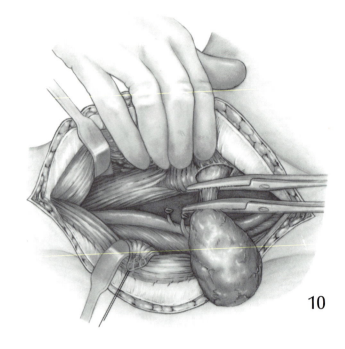

10

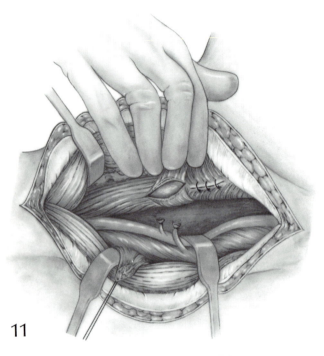

11

11

The fibres of the cricopharyngeal muscle located inferiorly to the neck of the diverticulum are most easily divided down to the mucosa while gentle retraction is maintained on the neck of the sac before diverticulectomy is carried out.

12

The initial cause of dysphagia for which the operation is carried out and additional procedures such as diverticulectomy will determine whether or not a nasogastric tube is placed at the time of the operative procedure and how long it will remain in place postoperatively. The cervical wound is closed over a single suction drain.

Postoperative management

Postoperative progress will, of course, depend again on the reasons for and additional procedures carried out at the time of the myotomy, but in the uncomplicated single procedure oral feeding may commence the following day and discharge from hospital may be as early as the second or third day. Antibiotics are not routinely required and the only significant long-term morbidity from the procedure is either lack of success with regard to relieving the patient's symptoms or progression or recurrence of the previous pathology.

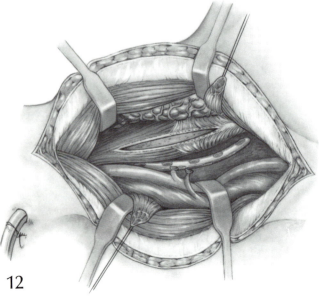

12

Laryngoscopy, microlaryngoscopy and laser surgery

Roger Parker MS, FRCS
ENT Department, Royal Berkshire Hospital, Reading, Berkshire, UK

Introduction

This chapter describes endoscopic procedures for the diagnosis and treatment of laryngotracheal tumours with special emphasis on laser surgery.

Anaesthesia

Diagnostic laryngoscopy

Anaesthesia for diagnostic laryngoscopy is of short duration and the anaesthetist should aim to provide operating conditions with no laryngeal movements. The patient is anaesthetized, where possible, without an endotracheal tube, which hampers the surgeon's view. Recovery from such anaesthesia should be rapid with the early return of the cough reflex.

Premedication with a short half-life benzodiazepine will allay apprehension. Induction with an agent such as intravenous thiopentone should be followed by paralysis with the depolarizing muscle relaxant suxamethonium. At induction, intravenous atropine should be given to counter the tendency of suxamethonium to produce bradycardia, especially if multiple doses are given, together with a small dose of an intravenous non-depolarizing muscle relaxant to reduce the possibility of postoperative suxamethonium muscle pains. The patient should be ventilated with 100 per cent oxygen by mask, and with the onset of paralysis a 16 gauge polyvinyl catheter is inserted through the larynx to lie with its tip just above the carina. Ventilation with 100 per cent oxygen by mask is continued until the surgeon is ready. At this point the catheter is connected to a source of oxygen with a flow rate of 2 litres/min.

Anaesthesia is maintained with intravenous doses of thiopentone and paralysis with small doses of suxamethonium. Oxygenation is maintained by diffusion. As carbon dioxide is not eliminated under these circumstances, the carbon dioxide tension in the blood increases by 4 mmHg/min, therefore procedures using this apnoeic oxygenation technique should be limited to 10 min. Further operating time may be gained by using the injector ventilation technique (see below). At the end of the procedure ventilation by mask with 100 per cent oxygen is resumed until the patient is awake and breathing spontaneously.

Vocal fold mobility is assessed during the recovery phase, while continuing with apnoeic oxygenation. Care should be taken not to vent the injector, if in use, when the vocal folds are adducted.

Therapeutic laryngoscopy

Therapeutic laryngoscopy for longer procedures such as stripping of vocal folds or injection of polytetrafluoroethylene (Teflon, E.I. du Pont de Nemours and Company, UK) still requires an immobile larynx with an unobstructed surgical view. Attempts to produce these conditions with techniques involving spontaneous ventilation, local analgesia to the larynx and anaesthesia maintained by intermittent intravenous injections or tracheal insufflation of inhalational anaesthetics through a catheter were far from ideal, as immobility could not be guaranteed and the anaesthetist had no control over the airway.

There are now two preferred techniques; both involve premedication with a short half-life benzodiazepine.

Injection technique

Anaesthesia is induced with intravenous thiopentone and an appropriate dose of atropine if suxamethonium is to be used to maintain paralysis. Alternatively, paralysis can be maintained by a short-acting non-depolarizing muscle relaxant (e.g. atracurium). Anaesthesia is maintained with intermittent intravenous thiopentone. The patient is ventilated with 100 per cent oxygen by mask until laryngoscopy.

When the laryngoscope is satisfactorily positioned a 16 gauge injector is affixed to the laryngoscope and jet ventilation is commenced using oxygen from a 60 p.s.i. source together with a manually controlled valve or a suitable ventilator, e.g. Penlon 200 (Penlon Ltd, Abingdon, Oxon, UK). This technique may be used in children but a smaller gauge injector must be used.

At the end of the procedure the effect of any non-depolarizing muscle relaxant is reversed with atropine and neostigmine and mask ventilation is continued until the patient is awake and breathing freely.

Endotracheal technique

It is possible to undertake most therapeutic procedures on the larynx with an endotracheal tube if it is not too large. A 5 mm microlaryngoscopy cuffed endotracheal tube has proved quite satisfactory when used with controlled ventilation, provided that the ventilatory pattern allows sufficient time for adequate expiration.

Anaesthesia is induced as before, except that a non-depolarizing muscle relaxant is used. Intubation may be either by the oral or nasal route, depending on circumstances. Anaesthesia is maintained with intermittent positive pressure ventilation with oxygen, nitrous oxide and a suitable inhalational agent. Muscle relaxation is reversed at the end with atropine and neostigmine.

Direct laryngoscopy

Instrumentation

1

The present generation of laryngoscopes has been added to the long established instrument (Chevalier–Jackson). The modern versions have the popular shape of large proximal and distal openings, with a waisted mid-shaft.

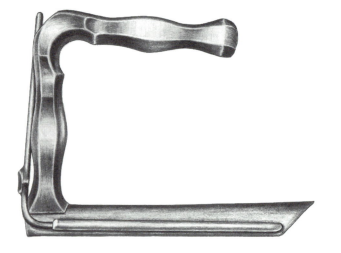

1

Other standard endoscopes required for simple formal direct laryngoscopy include the straight anterior commissure laryngoscope with tapering lumen, which facilitates examination of the anterior commissure and subglottis. The tracheoscope may also be required.

Necessary instruments include those for taking biopsies, for removing foreign bodies and for suction. The variety of such instruments is extensive and has developed further to facilitate the microscopic surgery that can be done. However, for simple biopsies small cup forceps or punches only are used. Suction tubes are plain or fenestrated.

Endoscopic lighting is now fibreoptic. The most modern fibreoptic cables are continuous from power source to the light exit in the endoscope itself, so eliminating light loss at fibreoptic cable junctions.

Finally, fine insulated diathermy instruments are available, including those for suction diathermy. Foreign body extractors, dilating bougies and other less common instruments complete the standard range of endoscopy equipment. The carbon dioxide laser is discussed on pp. 458–461 of this chapter.

Position of the patient

2

The accessibility of the throat to endoscopic examination will depend upon several factors, including the presence or absence of teeth, trismus, a foreshortened jaw, or neck rigidity. Nevertheless, the ideal anatomical position for laryngoscopy is one of neck flexion and head extension; neck flexion is particularly important.

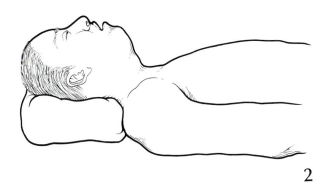

2

Operation

3

On the operating table, the head is towelled and the teeth are protected with a moulded shield of silicone rubber or, occasionally, moulded lead sheeting; the edentulous gingiva can be covered by a lubricated gauze swab. The lips should be lightly lubricated to avoid pinching them as the laryngoscope is passed.

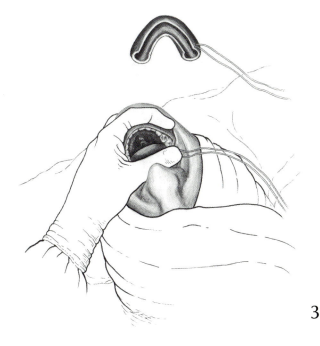

3

4a–d

The laryngoscope passes through the mouth and down into the throat. One hand passes the instrument forwards to obtain the necessary view, while the other keeps the lips free and the thumb of the same hand is used to guide the instrument into the throat. The anaesthetic tube/catheter can be used as a guide if one is in place. It is important to note the anatomical landmarks, namely the uvula (*Illustration 4a*), the epiglottis (*Illustration 4b*) and the arytenoids (*Illustration 4c*), and finally the larynx and vocal folds (*Illustration 4d*).

If anaesthesia has been achieved without intubation a Chevalier–Jackson laryngoscope with detachable slide may be required if an anaesthetic tube/catheter is to be passed subsequently.

The whole of the throat is examined before any biopsy is taken, since disturbing any pathological tissue may obscure bleeding. Ideally the whole of the throat is examined routinely.

It may not be possible to view the anterior commissure with a standard laryngoscope, but the straight-sided anterior commissure endoscope will bring this area into view. This instrument can also be used to move the vocal folds gently sideways for a satisfactory view of the subglottis and upper trachea.

Finally, with the pathological tissue in view, a biopsy can be taken with punch forceps; pedicled lesions can be nipped from the base of the pedicle.

With the operation completed, the anaesthetist should be informed if vocal fold mobility is to be assessed. The surgeon should be aware that muscle relaxant anaesthesia is being used and will prevent interpretation of fold movement.

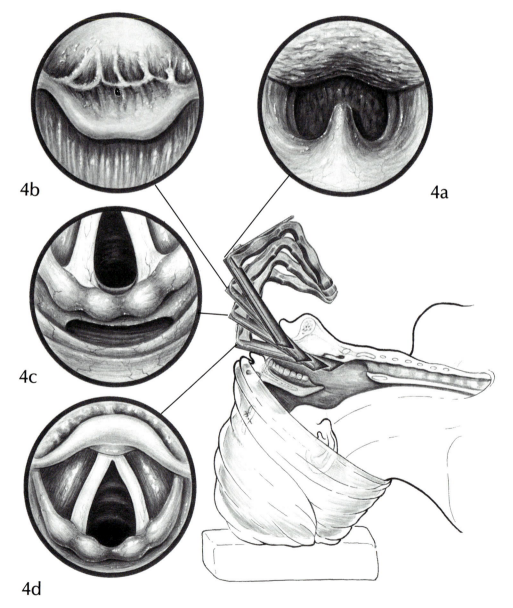

4b

4a

4c

4d

Microlaryngoscopy

This form of laryngoscopy using the operating microscope provides a high power view of pathological tissue and allows fine surgery to the larynx, particularly to the vocal folds where two hands may be required, e.g. Reinke oedema, Teflon fold injection and laser surgery.

Instrumentation

For microlaryngoscopy, the standard operating microscope with a 400 mm objective is used with a wide lumen Kleinsasser laryngoscope suspended from a Lewy pattern suspension apparatus.

The laryngoscope is funnel-shaped in its long axis and oval in section, with a wide opening at the viewing end, allowing a large amount of light to pass down the laryngoscope and provide room for instruments. Such laryngoscopes are blackened to avoid light reflection. With the use of the operating microscope, continuous TV monitoring as well as still photography are possible.

Operation

Exactly the same manoeuvres as described for direct laryngoscopy are employed when inserting this laryngoscope for surgery.

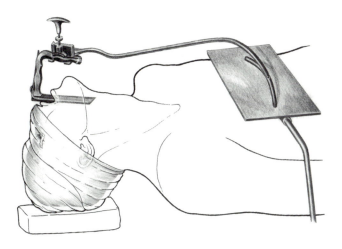

5

5

Once the laryngoscope is in position, it is attached and held by the tightened clamp. The larger suspension key screw is turned to lower the fixing arm to the patient's chest or Mayo table.

With the larynx and pathological tissue in view, the operating microscope is swung into position for use.

Reinke oedema of vocal folds

The precision removal of a vocal fold polyp or Reinke oedema of the vocal folds, and the treatment of vocal fold paralysis are common indications for microsurgery.

6a, b & c

The swollen vocal fold covering is retracted medially so that fine dissecting scissors may detach its superior layer. The inferior membrane is then similarly incised.

Only one vocal fold is dealt with at a time to avoid webbing anteriorly. The other fold may be dealt with some 6 weeks later.

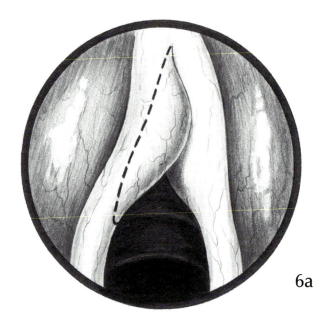

6a

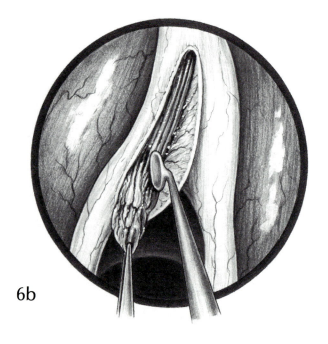

6b

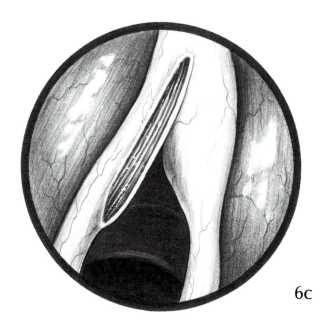

6c

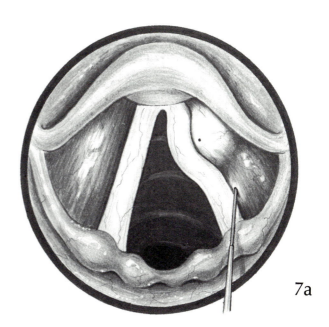

7a

Vocal fold paralysis

7a & b

The paralysed vocal fold is injected with 0.2–0.4 ml Teflon paste 4 mm deep into the lateral portion of the membranous fold at the junction of its middle and posterior third. A Brüning syringe is used.

The paste is seen to expand the fold and subglottis towards the midline. Injection of too much paste may lead to a compromised glottis.

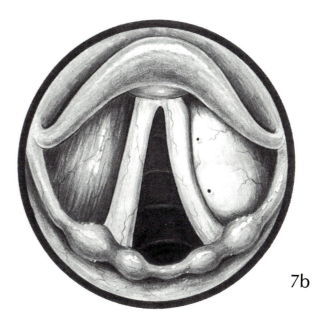

7b

Laser surgery

The use of the carbon dioxide laser for laryngeal surgery has revolutionized the removal of tissue from this area. The technique achieves a bloodless field as the heat of the cutting ray not only vaporizes the area but also seals the ends of associated small blood vessels. Incisions can be made to remove pathological tissue for biopsy of much larger masses, and lesions such as papillomas and leukoplakia can be precisely outlined prior to formal vaporization. Finally, this form of excisional surgery is now being used to remove the early T1 carcinoma of the larynx as the primary and definitive form of treatment.

Anaesthesia

A technique involving endotracheal intubation with a small diameter tube as for direct laryngoscopy is quite appropriate. The difficulty lies in ensuring that there is no risk of fire for the normal endotracheal tube burns when hit by the carbon dioxide laser beam in the presence of high oxygen tension. Special non-metal tubes have now been developed which are treated with a coating of a metal-impregnated material that is resistant to penetration by the laser ray. The cuff of the tube is also vulnerable and should be filled with water (which absorbs carbon dioxide laser light). The tube and cuff should be protected by water-soaked swabs. Also available is a stainless steel malleable endotracheal tube for laser surgery and the high pressure jet injection technique (see p. 452).

Provided the anaesthetist and surgeon are properly trained in laser surgery, the presence of a properly protected anaesthetic tube should be of no more concern than in any other circumstance calling for extreme care in the course of a surgical operation. Every operating theatre employing laser techniques must develop a protocol to ensure that they are used safely.

Instrumentation

The carbon dioxide laser is the most commonly used laser in otorhinolaryngology. The laser energy in the present generation of lasers is produced from a portable independent source, with the laser beam passing down a mobile arm, which is attached to the operating microscope, to be reflected down that optical pathway. As the carbon dioxide laser ray is invisible, there is also in line a visible aiming laser ray (a mixture of helium and neon) that produces a sighting red dot. At this red dot, which itself has no vaporizing power, carbon dioxide laser light will hit the tissue to evaporate it instantaneously when the foot switch is depressed.

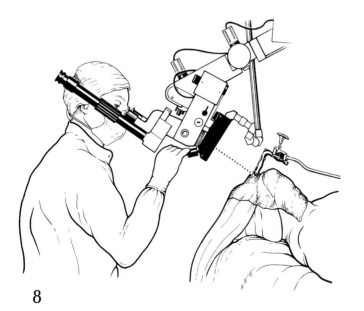

8

8

The amount of power being delivered, the exposure time interval for delivery and the spot size will dictate the width and depth of the laser tissue destruction. The lasering dot is moved about the operative field with a joystick manipulator.

The standard operating microscope is used with a clamp attachment to take the laser that fits over the 450 mm microscope objective. The beam splitter of the microscope allows accompanying side arm attachments including a camera for monitoring or still photography.

9

Because lasered tissue gives off a carbonized steam vapour, suction is required, which can be provided by a standard microsurgical sucker or a fine tube attached to the laryngoscope. If retracting paddles are used, then the paddle handle is the sucker.

Where there has to be retraction of tissue a paddle is used. In the author's experience, a right-angled section paddle and a flat one are all that are necessary for laser surgery. Small thoroughly moistened swabs with retaining threads are used to protect adjacent soft tissue and anaesthetic tubing.

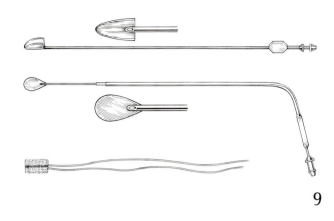

9

10

If the pathology is out of sight, steel mirrors may be used to reflect the laser beam; once again the shaft of the mirror is used for suction. As carbon dioxide laser light will crack glass, the mirror is made from highly polished stainless steel.

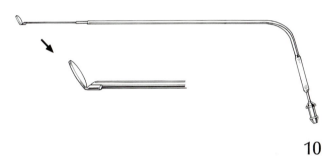

10

Operation

The position of the patient is as for standard laryngoscopy, but the towelling arrangements must include placing a wet eye pad over the eyes prior to the head being covered. Wet gauzes are placed around the laryngoscope once it is in position to protect the circumoral region.

The laryngoscope is passed in the normal fashion with the suspension apparatus attached as for microlaryngoscopy (described above).

With the operating microscope in position the arm of the laser console is fixed to the attachment on the operating microscope. The aiming red dot is then brought into view within the operative field with the joystick manipulator. The joystick moves the reflecting mirror which transfers the laser beam from the attached arm down the optical field of the microscope.

The laser machine can now be switched on and activated for 'standby' with the required dose and duration of laser exposure selected. The carbon dioxide laser normally has timed firing intervals of 0.1–1.0 s and continuous firing is available. With the modern machines, 6 W at the tissue surface is usually sufficient for routine work.

With the laser machine turned to 'ready', laser vaporization can take place.

11a, b & c

Precision laser excision can be used to treat leukoplakia. The diagram demonstrates the pathological tissue outlined by the laser, with a clear margin within which the whole area will subsequently be biopsied or lasered and so vaporized down to the subepithelial layer. Commonly the tissue layers can be identified as the laser removes the superficial layer. Tissue margins remaining can be biopsied for evidence of complete pathological excision if necessary

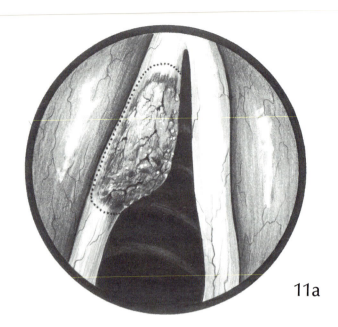

11a

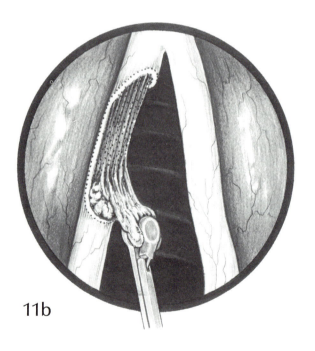

11b

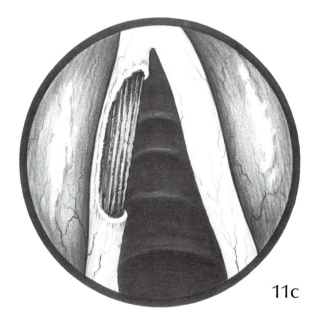

11c

12a–d

The laser can be used to excise an arytenoid granuloma with variable removal of the underlying arytenoid cartilage. As the inflammatory response from the overlying granuloma in this condition may involve the perichondrium and underlying cartilage, the granuloma and underlying perichondrium may be lasered away at the first laser excision. If this is unsuccessful a further removal after several months can be attempted, this time to include part of the underlying cartilage.

An extension of this selective arytenoid surgery is the total removal of the arytenoid to prolapse a vocal fold laterally in bilateral vocal fold paralysis.

Other lesions eminently suitable for laser removal include obstructing laryngeal tumours; provision of a clear airway in such cases may avoid a tracheostomy.

Above all other competitors, the carbon dioxide laser can remove and cure multiple laryngeal papillomas. Where this disease is widespread, several sessions of laser surgery may be required to clear different areas. Treatment should be spaced at 3–6 week intervals at least, if adhesions are to be avoided.

The neatness of carbon dioxide surgery, which leaves a bloodless field, has allowed this cutting tool to supersede conventional endoscopic laryngeal microsurgery.

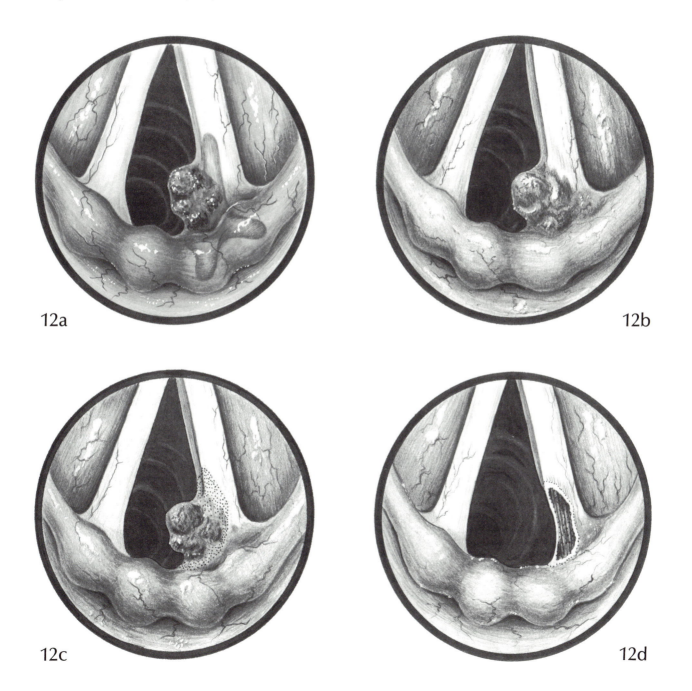

12a

12b

12c

12d

Technical points in laser surgery

Certain technical points should be remembered when lasering. Surface pathology such as leukoplakia is more easily vaporized if the laser beam is defocused to produce a broader and less deep laser removal; the latest carbon dioxide microscopic laser equipment now has an independent focusing delivery that does not require a change of the visual focus of the operator. The hand-held laser can in like fashion be used slightly away from its focal point. These manoeuvres effect surface lasering rather than finer cutting and deeper vaporization.

Carbonization of the laser site should be limited. If the laser is used in an intermittent mode, the foot pedal can be permanently depressed and bursts of laser light of chosen duration only are emitted until the foot is lifted off the pedal; this manoeuvre reduces carbon deposition. This form of intermittent exposure also reduces the heat built up in the neighbouring tissue. By reducing the carbon deposit, even gently removing it by suction, and by limiting heat production, the resulting inflammatory response of the lasered tissue is minimized.

Acknowledgements

I am indebted to Dr Maurus Rimmer for the section on anaesthesia, to Jennifer Southby for her work on the original illustrations, and to Trudy McLoughlin for her help in typing this chapter.

Laryngofissure

Carl E. Silver MD, FACS
Professor of Surgery and Professor of Otolaryngology, Albert Einstein College of Medicine and
Director of Head and Neck Surgery, Montefiore Medical Center, Bronx, New York, USA

John S. Rubin MD
Assistant Professor of Otolaryngology, Albert Einstein College of Medicine and
Director, Otolaryngology Service, North Central Bronx Hospital, Bronx, New York, USA

Introduction

Laryngofissure or median thyrotomy is the oldest surgical procedure for extirpation of laryngeal lesions. Pelletan performed thyrotomy to remove impacted meat in 1778[1]. Desault is believed to have employed thyrotomy for removal of a foreign body in 1810[2,3]. Brauers performed laryngofissure in 1833 to cauterize a warty endolaryngeal growth[3].

American surgeons became interested in the procedure by the mid 19th century. Buck in 1851, and again in 1861, and Sands in 1863 employed laryngofissure for excision of malignant tumours, although none of their patients survived long enough to be considered cured[2,3]. In 1892 Solis-Cohen[4] reported the first documented permanent cure of laryngeal cancer, which he treated in 1868 by laryngofissure. The first laryngofissure in the UK was performed by Duncan Gibb in 1864[3].

For the most part, results of laryngofissures performed in the 19th century were not favourable. Mackenzie noted only a 15 per cent 'complete success' rate in his review of the first 48 non-malignant cases of thyrotomy[5]. He criticized the procedure claiming that excision by laryngoscopy was the preferred treatment for benign lesions, and that piecemeal removal was ineffective for treatment of malignant tumours. Von Bruns, Billroth and Moure also reported poor results[3,6]. By the turn of the century, better understanding of technical requirements, anaesthesia and selection of patients had produced marked improvement in results. Semon, by 1907, had achieved cure rates of 60 per cent[3], while Thomson[7] in 1912 reported 'lasting cures' in eight of ten patients. In 1927, Chevalier Jackson recorded 3-year cures in 29 of 45 patients while Gluck and Soerensen reported 110 of 125 patients cured in 1930[3].

Patient selection

At present the only indication for laryngofissure is the presence of small T1 tumours limited to the membranous portion of one true vocal fold without deep invasion, limitation of movement, involvement of the anterior commissure, or extension onto the vocal process of the arytenoid. Tumours of this nature are amenable to radiation therapy, which remains the treatment of choice at many institutions[8–10]. When surgical therapy is chosen, the smallest such lesions may be managed by endoscopic laser excision[11] while hemilaryngectomy is often employed for larger tumours[12]. Thus, in current practice, laryngofissure is rarely performed for treatment of vocal fold cancer. Cure rates from laryngofissure reported in post-war literature have ranged from 60 to 98 per cent[13–17]. The lower cure rates, for the most part, represent results of treatment following radiation failure.

Quality of voice after laryngofissure varies. The standard technique does not provide for reconstruction of the resected cord. The larynx heals by formation of scar tissue. Bulk and flexibility of this tissue varies from patient to patient, as does quality of voice. LeJeune and Lynch[15] reported 'good' voice in 73 per cent of patients. Sessions et al.[17] reported 'good' voice in 48 per cent and 'fair' voice in 48 per cent. Voice quality after laryngofissure is generally less satisfactory than voice quality after radiation therapy.

Despite a decrease in popularity of this procedure, its place in the modern surgical armamentarium has been nicely defined by Daly and Kwok[13] who noted that 'while specific indications for laryngofissure and cordectomy have declined, the procedure is an effective technique for the control of cordal cancer when, in the judgement of the surgeon, a simple surgical operation is called for'.

Operation

1

A transverse incision is made at the level of the mid portion of the thyroid cartilage.

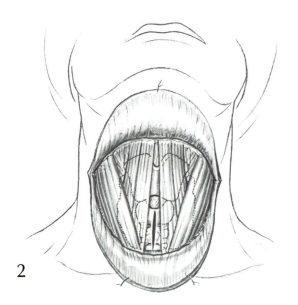

2

Skin flaps are elevated in the subplatysmal plane.

3

Tracheostomy is performed in the usual manner. The infrahyoid ('strap') muscles are separated in the midline. The thyroid isthmus is divided and a window created by excision of the anterior part of the second tracheal ring.

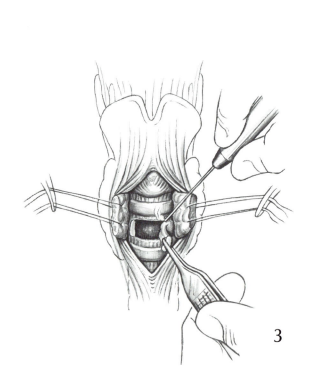

4

The vertical incision between the strap muscles is continued upwards to the hyoid bone. Muscles are retracted, exposing thyroid cartilage. The thyrotomy incision is marked 1–2 mm lateral to the midline of the thyroid cartilage on the contralateral side.

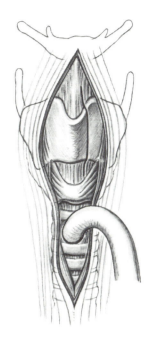

4

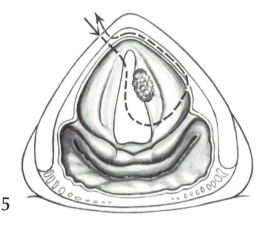

5

5

Transverse section demonstrates the outline of planned resection including true and false vocal folds anterior to the vocal process of the arytenoid, underlying muscle, internal perichondrium of the thyroid ala, anterior commissure and 2–3 mm of the opposite true vocal fold. The tumour, limited to the membranous portion of the right vocal fold, is shown.

6

The thyroid cartilage is divided with an oscillating saw. The thyrohyoid membrane is incised along the superior border of thyroid cartilage for 1 cm on either side of midline. The laryngeal interior is entered through a short transverse incision in the cricothyroid membrane. A vertical incision is made just left of the midline transecting the true and false folds. Retraction of the thyroid alae exposes the laryngeal interior. The resection is indicated by the dotted line. It includes the entire false vocal fold and the subglottic mucosa to the lower border of the thyroid cartilage.

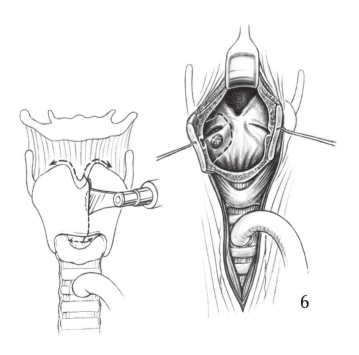

6

7

The specimen is excised by sharp dissection. Injection of lignocaine-adrenaline solution between thyroid cartilage and soft tissue will facilitate dissection. Mucosa and other soft tissues are incised with a cautery knife. A small sharp dissector is used to elevate the internal perichondrium. A pair of curved scissors is convenient for the posterior vertical incision.

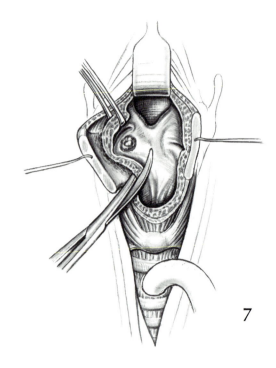

7

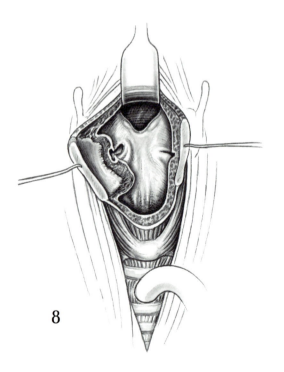

8

8

View of the completed resection. Resurfacing of the mucosal defect is not necessary. The thyrotomy is closed by approximation of overlying muscles and fascia.

9

The endotracheal tube is removed and a cuffed tracheostomy tube is inserted through the previously marked small incision in the inferior flap. A plastic tube with an inner cannula and a high volume-low pressure cuff (Shiley) is preferred.

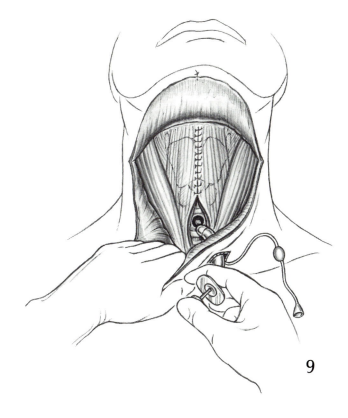

9

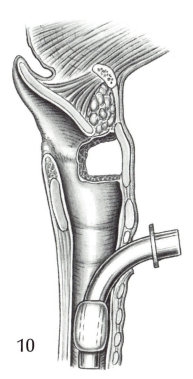

10

10

The sagittal view shows relations of the tracheostomy tube.

11

The skin incision is repaired over closed wound suction drains (Jackson–Pratt). The tracheostomy tube is secured in place with sutures as well as tape.

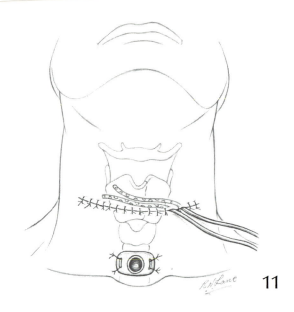

11

Acknowledgements

The illustrations are redrawn with permission from Silver, C. E. (1981) *Surgery for Cancer of the Larynx*, Churchill Livingstone, New York.

References

1. Thorwald J. *The Triumph of Surgery*. New York: Pantheon Books, 1960.

2. Alberti PW. The historical development of laryngectomy. II. The evolution of laryngology and laryngectomy in the mid-nineteenth century. *Laryngoscope* 1975; 85: 288–98.

3. Thomson StC. The history of cancer of the larynx. *J Laryngol Otol* 1939; 54: 61–87.

4. Solis-Cohen J. Two cases of laryngectomy of adenocarcinoma of the larynx. *N Y Med J* 1892; 56: 533.

5. Mackenzie M. *Essay on Growths in the Larynx*. London: J and A Churchill, 1871.

6. Bruns P Von. *Die Laryngotomie zur Entfernung Intralaryngealer Neubildurgen*. Berlin: A Hirschwald, 1878.

7. Thomson StC. Intrinsic cancer of the larynx: operation for laryngofissure: lasting cure in 80 per cent of cases. *Br Med J* 1912; i: 355–9.

8. Lederman M. Radiotherapy of cancer of the larynx. *J Laryngol Otol* 1970; 84: 867–96.

9. Som ML. Cordal cancer with extension to vocal process. *Laryngoscope* 1975; 85: 1298–307.

10. Boles R, Komorn R. Carcinoma of the laryngeal glottis: a five-year review at a university hospital. *Laryngoscope* 1969; 79: 909–20.

11. Vaughan CW, Strong MS, Jacko GJ. Laryngeal carcinoma: transoral treatment utilizing the CO_2 laser. *Am J Surg* 1978; 136: 490–3.

12. Ogura JH, Biller HF. Conservation surgery in cancers of the head and neck. *Otolaryngol Clin North Am* 1969; 2: 641–65.

13. Daly JF, Kwok FN. Laryngofissure and cordectomy. *Laryngoscope* 1975; 85: 1290–7.

14. DeSanto LW. Selection of treatment for *in situ* and early invasive carcinoma of the glottis. In: Albert PW, Bryce DP, eds. *Workshops from the Centennial Conference of Laryngeal Cancer*. New York: Appleton-Century-Crofts, 1976: 146–50.

15. LeJeune FE, Lynch MG. The value of laryngofissure. *Ann Otol Rhinol Laryngol* 1955; 64: 256.

16. McGavran MH, Spjut H, Ogura J. Laryngofissure in the treatment of laryngeal carcinoma: a critical analysis of success and failure. *Laryngoscope* 1959; 69: 44–53.

17. Sessions DG, Maness GM, McSwain B. Laryngofissure in the treatment of carcinoma of the vocal cord – a report of 40 cases and a review of the literature. *Laryngoscope* 1965; 75: 490–502.

Illustrations by Gillian Lee

Near-total laryngectomy

Bruce W. Pearson MD
Mayo Clinic, Jacksonville, Florida, USA

David J. Howard FRCS, FRCS(Ed)
Institute of Laryngology and Otology, Royal National Throat, Nose and Ear Hospital, London, UK

Introduction

The standard conservation operations of vertical and horizontal partial laryngectomy, and their variants, aim to excise tumour while preserving the functions of speech and deglutition and an intact laryngeal airway. However, a considerable number of laryngeal and hypopharyngeal tumours are too extensive to allow complete excision and cure by these conservative procedures. Until the last decade these larger tumours were treated by means of total laryngectomy. This radical procedure results in the loss of both voice and nasal breathing, accompanied by the separation of the upper respiratory and digestive tracts.

The concept of near-total laryngectomy provides a 'missing link' between these two extremes and allows for adequate resection of many of the large tumours with preservation of voice but not an intact airway. It is neither a conservative nor a radical procedure, although principles of both are applied. It is radical in terms of the tumour on the involved side, but conservative in that the patient retains one arytenoid, the posterior portions of the uninvolved false and true fold, and one half of the subglottis. This conserved segment, although not sufficient to act as an airway, does allow the patient to produce a voice by preserving a connection between the airway and the oesophagus. It relies on the dynamic nature of this connection to avoid aspiration by means of activity from the retained recurrent laryngeal nerve on that side. All previously described operations for biological voice rehabilitation (for example, Staffieri[1]) are frequently complicated by aspiration or stenosis, and failure to achieve fistula speech. Employment of the innervated contralateral periarytenoid tissue, preserved in near-total laryngectomy, results in attainment of fistula speech with predictable regularity.

Techniques

Techniques for voice restoration after total laryngectomy using tracheo-oesophageal fistulae maintained by plastic prostheses may provide satisfactory means of voice restoration, but the functional results of such procedures are inferior to those obtained by near-total laryngectomy. Difficulties associated with prostheses include the necessity for cleaning, replacing and managing various fixation devices. These are eliminated by the maintenance-free biological shunt created with the near-total procedure, which is less prone to spontaneous closure or stenosis than are the secondarily created shunts.

Indications

Near-total laryngectomy does not eliminate altogether the use of total laryngectomy, but it can reduce the indication to approximately one-third of patients for whom total laryngectomy would in the past have been recommended. Most patients with a fixed vocal fold are suitable candidates, whether the fold immobility has arisen from involvement of the vocal fold itself or by extension through the paraglottic space from the subglottis, the supraglottic larynx, or the piriform fossa. Fortunately, laryngeal and pharyngeal tumours that are predominantly one-sided are more common than extensive bilateral lesions.

Contraindications

Extensive bilateral intralaryngeal tumours, posterior glottic aryepiglottic or hypopharyngeal lesions involving the interarytenoid and annular subglottic cancers should all be treated by total laryngectomy. Although the near-total procedure has occasionally been used in radiation failures, total laryngectomy is still usually indicated. Radiorecurrent tumour margins are often indistinct and three-dimensional spread is unpredictable in these cases. Therefore, it is far more difficult to ensure that the preserved contralateral arytenoid musculature and mucosa does not contain microscopic disease.

Preoperative considerations

Accurate preoperative laryngeal assessment is essential. Direct laryngoscopy should be undertaken before surgery, to make absolutely sure that the opposite ventricle and posterior interarytenoid region are free from tumour. Computed tomography (CT) and magnetic resonance imaging (MRI) scanning of the larynx and neck are optional. The surgeon and speech therapist must adequately discuss the principles and postoperative course with the patient before operation.

Anaesthesia

During the laryngoscopy general anaesthesia is administered through a cuffed oral endotracheal tube of internal diameter 5.5 mm. Lying between the arytenoid cartilages it helps to separate the vocal folds and give posterior countertraction to the tip of the laryngoscope. The time required for detailed microlaryngoscopy of the glottis and 70° telescopic inspection of the good ventricle and the subglottic margins is assured. When the frozen sections are confirmed, and the surgeon is completely satisfied as to the necessity and feasibility of the excision, the laryngoscope is withdrawn. A nasogastric feeding tube is inserted and the patient is prepared and draped.

The operation itself begins with a separate tracheostomy. The neck should be extended so the tracheal opening can be situated below the thyroid isthmus. An omega-shaped skin excision provides a smoothly continuous margin to which the opening can be sewn. By means of a 'trapdoor' entry into the trachea itself an inferiorly based flap is created for this purpose.

A wire-spiral supported endotracheal tube is sutured into position, taking care to avoid over-advancement. A sterile set of ventilation tubes are connected so the anaesthesia can be switched to their new location, and the oral endotracheal tube is withdrawn.

Operation

The patient shown in the following sequence of illustrations suffered from a right T3 transglottic squamous cell carcinoma. The preoperative evaluation was carefully confirmed by laryngoscopy and, as it had not previously been undertaken, a generous biopsy specimen was removed with cupped forceps from the centre of the lesion and the frozen section diagnosis of invasive squamous carcinoma confirmed. This tumour, like most of those for which a near-total laryngectomy is advised, was invasive and well lateralized, therefore a right comprehensive neck dissection, preserving XI, was completed. The neck was opened through a large apron flap, but it is probably best if the neck incision and tracheostomy incision are kept separate. The subsequent stomocutaneous anastomosis may be difficult to accomplish, but the result enhances the patient's ability to speak. The margin of the stoma will not be notched or creased by any connecting incision, thus a seal will be more easily obtained when the stoma is valved to permit voice.

1

The right thyroid lobe and larynx are mobilized in the same way as in total laryngectomy, with identification and division of superior and inferior thyroid neurovascular pedicles, division of the right infrahyoid musculature and separation of the inferior constrictor and suprahyoid muscles from the right thyroid ala and the hyoid bone around to the left lesser cornu.

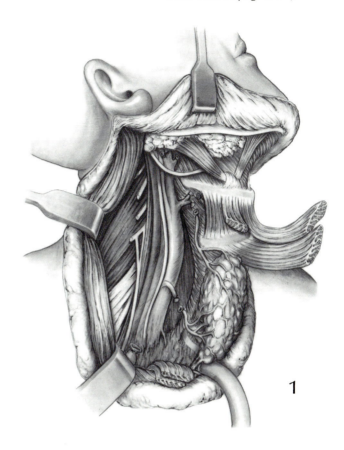

1

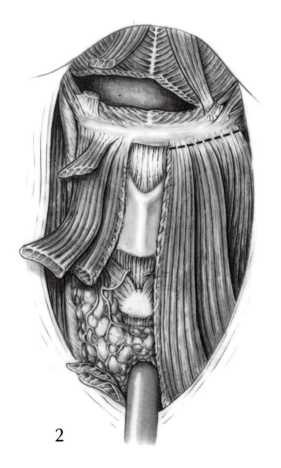

2

2

The surgical techniques that distinguish the near-total laryngectomy begin on the left. The left thyroid lobe is retained but all the prelaryngeal tissues, including the thyroid isthmus, are resected with the surgical specimen. The left strap muscles are cut free from the hyoid bone and reflected laterally to the oblique line, exposing the left thyroid ala, and completing the exposure of the hyoid bone at the left lesser cornu.

3

At the lower edge of the thyroid cartilage, the lateral borders of the cricothyroid ligament and upper medial border of the cricothyroid muscle are defined. The thyroid gland is divided at the junction of the isthmus and the left lobe, and the clearance of the upper trachea is completed by division of all inferior thyroid veins and elevation of the right paratracheal lymph nodes and fat, which are included in the specimen.

Lateral thyrotomy

4

The origin of the left cricothyroid muscle is sharply dissected from the cricoid cartilage and reflected posteriorly. The hyoid is divided at the joint between the body and the greater cornu on the left. A wedge-shaped mid-portion of the left thyroid ala is removed. This lateral thyrotomy is undertaken without disturbing the left thyroarytenoid muscle or the ventricular glands which are visible just above the muscle's superior margin. The angle and anterior third of the left thyroid ala, including the anterior attachment of the thyroarytenoid muscles and Broyle's ligament are therefore kept with the specimen. The posterior third, really the piriform portion of the left thyroid ala, remains.

With these divisions of the framework of the larynx at the hyoid bone and thyroid cartilage completed, the soft tissue resection which separates the larynx into its tumour-bearing and voice-preserving segments can begin. The initial entry into the laryngeal lumen is accomplished through the ventricle, which was shown at laryngoscopy to be free of tumour. This avoids opening into the cancer and does not risk compromising the shunt.

The entry is in the glandular tissue of the saccule over the upper edge of the thyroarytenoid muscle, and it is important that an assistant provides good retraction in this elastic opening with small skin hooks.

These cuts may seem to be better placed if the suprahyoid part of the incision is opened first and then the scissor cut descends the lateral wall of the larynx with the whole tumour under direct vision. However, this method of entry can skirt dangerously close to the supraglottic or vallecular cancer, if present. Lateral thyrotomy forces the surgeon to limit this operation to appropriate cases and to make easy cases a rehearsal for the more challenging. It works from less familiar landmarks, which ultimately become more reliable. The relationship between tumour on the one side and the entry ventricle on the other are clearly defined at direct laryngoscopy; lateral thyrotomy takes advantage of this observation.

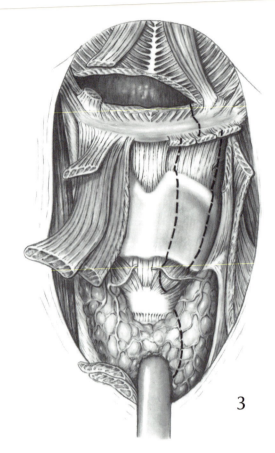

3

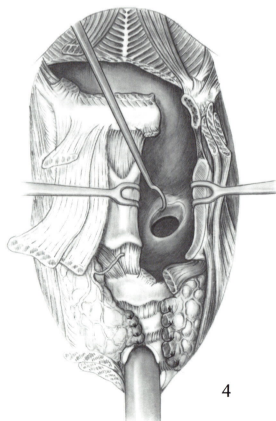

4

5

The opening into the laryngeal lumen on the good side is continued, using scissors inserted upwards through the initial opening to cut across the left false cord and aryepiglottic fold.

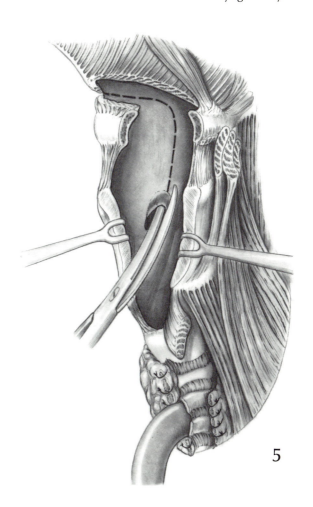

5

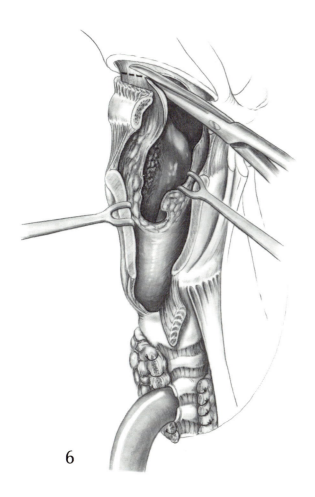

6

Laryngeal resection

6

With the epiglottis under direct vision, the vallecula is transected and the supraglottic laryngeal mobilization completed.

7

With the supraglottic tissues retracted forwards, the remainder of the resection is accomplished under direct vision with an excellent view of tumour on the right side. The initial glottic cut is directed through the true cord on the normal side; the position of this cut is influenced by the extent of the tumour. This means that the width of the vertical strip of larynx remaining in a near-total laryngectomy is not entirely under the surgeon's control but is determined by the extent of tumour. The object is to avoid the tumour, which will usually have crossed the anterior commissure to involve the cordal epithelium on the left side. Resection margins must not be compromised, and to preserve musculature in the posterior portion of the left glottic larynx compromise is not necessary.

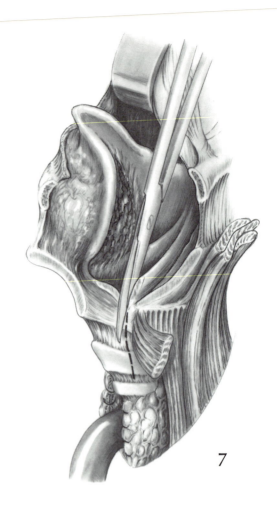

7

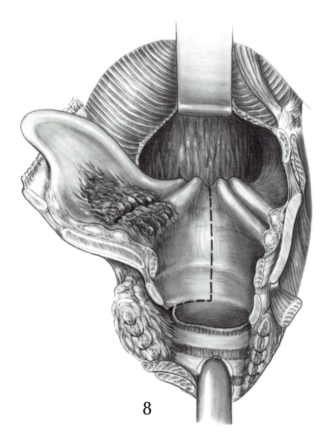

8

8

The cut through the left true fold is carried downwards, then forwards through the subglottic mucosa, conus and cricoid until the lower border of the proposed resection on the right side is reached. It is useful to preserve as much uninvolved subglottic mucosa and trachea as possible, but again, no compromise with the right hemicricoid or lower margin of tumour on the right is implied.

The resection line passes beneath the tumour and then ascends in the midline posteriorly. A number 15 scalpel blade is used to incise the mucosal, perichondrial and cortical layers of the posterior cricoid area vertically.

9

A finger is placed in the pharynx to support the postcricoid region, and the cricoid rostrum is fractured along the previously made vertical incision. The prominent interarytenoid muscle can be seen above this fracture where it is placed under tension for incision. Following incision, the entire specimen and its tumour can be swung laterally and the remaining mucosal attachments in the right piriform fossa placed under tension.

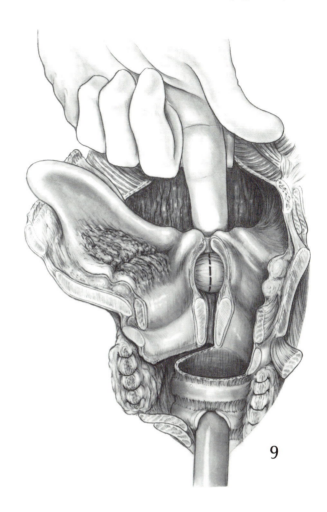

9

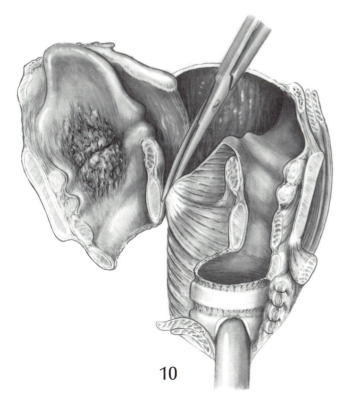

10

10

The removal of the specimen is completed by division through the right piriform sinus, allowing a wide margin of uninvolved mucosa. The specimen consists of the entire right hemilarynx, including the epiglottis, the anterior portion of the left hemilarynx and more than half the cricoid cartilage. With the removal of the right paraglottic space adequate extirpation of the right transglottic carcinoma should have been accomplished. Multiple biopsy specimens from the residual larynx should be checked by frozen section examination to ensure as far as possible that the excision is complete.

Fistula construction

11

While the pathologist studies the specimens, attention should be turned to the residual left hemicricoid cartilage. The fistula which is to be constructed from the residual laryngeal mucosa needs to be 'closed' at rest. In order to aid this, the support of the remaining cricoid cartilage must be destroyed. Subperichondrial dissection is therefore undertaken until sufficient has been removed to allow the subglottic mucosa to be flaccid enough to easily tube. Cricoid cartilage is fragile and should be removed carefully in a piecemeal fashion without trauma to the preserved intrinsic laryngeal musculature and without any disturbance of the region of the left cricothyroid joint, behind which lies the important left recurrent laryngeal nerve.

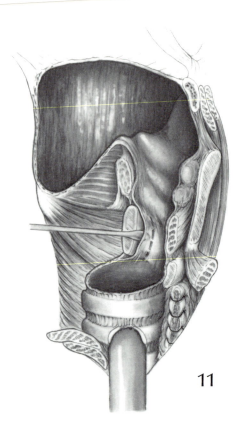

11

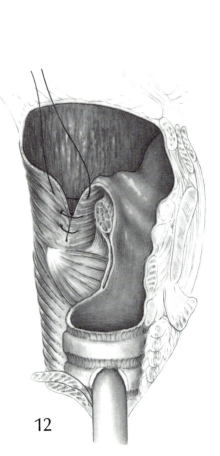

12

12

The right piriform sinus defect is now repaired by interrupted sutures until the reflection of the postcricoid mucosa is reached. The residual laryngeal mucosa must now be flaccid enough to tube, and maintain an unbroken path from the trachea to the pharynx, forming the fistula shunt.

13

In some cases there is insufficient laryngeal mucosa to form a shunt of sufficient diameter. Experience has shown that the mucosal tube fashioned over a 14 Fr rubber catheter is optimal (over 5 mm diameter). The amount of mucosa available for tubing may be augmented by rotation of a flap of mucosa from the pharyngeal defect above the piriform sinus that has just been repaired. The pharyngeal flap of this 'composite' shunt is cut from the edge of the pharyngotomy.

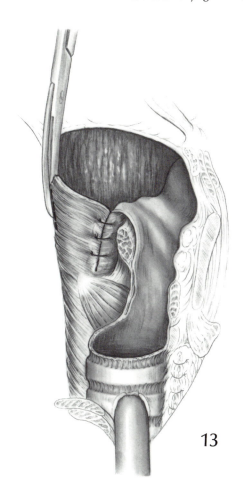

13

14

The flap is then turned down so that its mucosal surface faces the future shunt lumen when it is rotated and sutured to the laryngeal remnant.

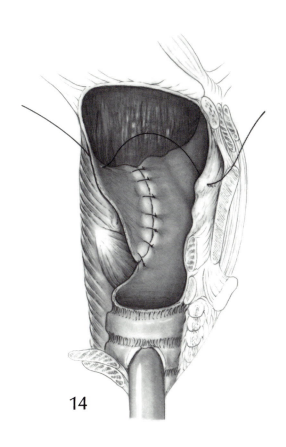

14

15

The tracheopharyngeal strip, augmented if necessary, is then rolled into a tube over a 14 Fr catheter and sutured from below. A small notch may be cut from the second tracheal ring to facilitate closure. The catheter is used only as a template and is removed as soon as the shunt has been fashioned. The suture material used to construct the shunt is 3/0 chromic catgut. In near-total laryngopharyngectomy for piriform cancers, the entire fold on the good side remains and an augmentation, which would not be possible owing to the extent of the pharyngeal resection, proves unnecessary.

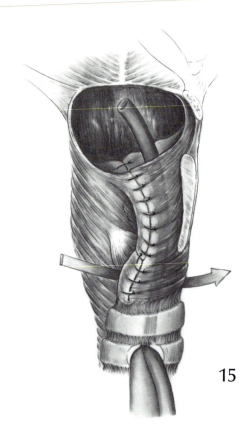

15

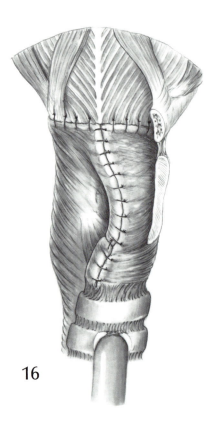

16

Pharyngeal closure

16

The residual pharyngeal defect is closed usually in a 'T' with 2/0 chromic catgut sutures. If the pharyngeal defect is extensive following resection of a piriform fossa, partial posterior wall and/or partial oropharyngeal tumour, augmentation with a pectoralis myocutaneous flap may be required. It is better to augment such a pharynx than encourage a tight closure, with its attendant problems of breakdown or stenosis, or both. The fistula shunt is not being anastomosed to the flap; it flows upwards into the preserved 'good side' piriform fossa. The flap suture lines are to this structure, not the laryngeal remnant.

17

The previously reflected left sternohyoid and thyrohyoid muscles are sewn across the upper portion of the shunt to the suprahyoid musculature and thereby support the closure line. Haemostasis is checked and appropriate suction drains placed, care being taken to keep them away from the pharyngeal closure.

Tracheostomy

The initial tracheostomy was a Bjork inferiorly based trapdoor flap which has already been sewn to the lower margin of the skin incision with 3/0 nylon. The lateral and superior margins of the omega-shaped skin opening are advanced to the tracheostomal margins with nylon sutures, which are vertical mattress in form on the skin side and simple but generous with respect to the trachea. The endotracheal tube is withdrawn and a cuffed disposable tracheostomy tube is inserted in its place. The region under the faceplate is wrapped with an antiseptic ointment-impregnated fine gauze dressing and the tapes are secured around the neck.

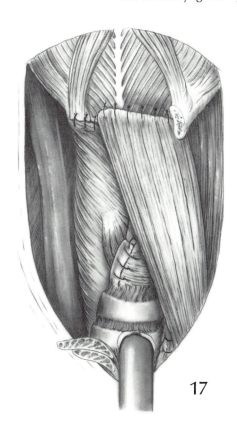

17

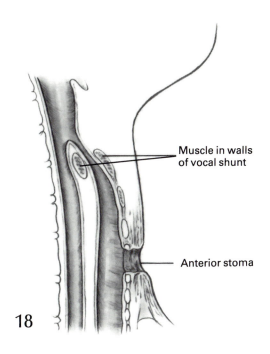

Muscle in walls of vocal shunt

Anterior stoma

18

18

The final relationship of the stoma and fistula is as shown diagrammatically.

Postoperative management

The hospital postoperative management after near-total laryngectomy is the same as after total laryngectomy. Nasogastric feeding is continued to the tenth day, then oral feeding begins. The stoma is fitted with a metal tracheostomy tube on about the fifth day. The patient leaving hospital at 2 weeks should be able to completely change and clean the tube.

Complications

Complications of this operation are generally the same as those of other major head and neck surgery and tracheostomy, but approximately one in five patients have experienced shunt or tracheostomy complications peculiar to this procedure. These include partial shunt stenosis requiring dilatation, aspiration requiring tightening of the upper end of the shunt, or delayed stomal healing indicating the need for better hygiene. By and large the complications are manageable without sacrificing speech.

Voice acquisition

Voice is not a hospital objective, since a healed stable tracheostomy site is required. The patient is simply encouraged to valve briefly at home once or twice a day, when the tube is out for cleaning. Patients report their results at the first postoperative clinical examination, and receive instructions from there. Speech therapists often provide an interim electronic device, then work on stomal valving, encouragement, relaxation and articulation when the first visit, usually about 6 weeks after operation, is completed.

Conclusions

Near-total laryngectomy has proved to be a good primary treatment for cancers which fix the vocal folds. By eliminating the prospect of aphonia it removes one of the major barriers to the patient's acceptance of appropriate curative primary surgery for this disease. With regard to supraglottic cancers it virtually eliminates the prospect of total laryngectomy and avoids the temptation for surgeons to extend the horizontal supraglottic operation beyond its limit, possibly producing inadequate resection margins or persistent aspiration. Supraglottic patients thus require a permanent stoma but retain their voice.

In glottic, transglottic and some subglottic cancers, this technique capitalizes on the remaining functioning con-tralateral posterior laryngeal remnant. For piriform fossa and some tongue base tumours, near-total laryngectomy produces a partial solution to the patient's reluctance to relinquish the larynx when the principal problem is one of swallowing.

Almost all patients achieve voice, and in contradistinction to a wide variety of plastic prostheses, voice, once established, is invariably kept and employed.

Acknowledgements

The illustrations in this chapter have been redrawn after S. Balich, Graphics Department, Mayo Clinic.

References

1. Staffieri M. Laryngectomie totale avec reconstitution de la glotte phonaire. *Rev Laryngol Otol Rhinol (Bordeaux)* 1974; 95: 63–83.

Further reading

DeSanto LW, Pearson BW, Olsen KD. Utility of near-total laryngectomy for supraglottic, pharyngeal, base of tongue, and other cancers. *Ann Otol Rhinol Laryngol* 1989; 98: 2–7.

Dumich PS, Pearson BW, Weiland LH. Suitability of near-total laryngectomy in pyriform carcinoma. *Arch Otolaryngol* 1984; 110: 664–9.

Pearson BW. Near-total laryngectomy. In: Silver CE, ed. *Atlas of Head and Neck Surgery*. New York and Edinburgh: Churchill Livingstone, 1986: 235–52.

Pearson BW. Management of the primary site: larynx and hypopharynx. In Pillsbury HC, Goldsmith MM, eds. *Operative Challenges in Otolaryngology – Head and Neck Surgery*. Chicago: Yearbook Medical Publishers, 1990: 346–76.

Pearson BW, DeSanto LW. Near total laryngectomy. *Operative Tech Otolaryngol Head Neck Surg* 1990; 1: 28–41.

Pearson BW, Keither RL. Near total laryngectomy. In: Johnson JT, Blitzer A, Ossoff RH, Thomas UR, eds. *Instructional Courses. American Academy of Otolaryngology – Head and Neck Surgery*. St Louis: CV Mosby, 1989, 2: 309–30.

Pearson BW, Stell PM, Bowdler DA, Dalley VM. The T3 glottic cancer – diagnosis and management. In Harrison DFN, ed. *Dilemmas in Otorhinolaryngology*. Edinburgh: Churchill Livingstone, 1988: 265–81.

Pearson BW, Woods RD II, Hartman DE. Extended hemilaryngectomy for T3 glottic carcinoma with preservation of speech and swallowing. *Laryngoscope* 1980; 90: 1950–61.

Illustrations by Robert Lane

Total laryngectomy

Carl E. Silver MD, FACS
Professor of Surgery and Professor of Otolaryngology, Albert Einstein College of Medicine and
Director of Head and Neck Surgery, Montefiore Medical Center, Bronx, New York, USA

John S. Rubin MD
Assistant Professor of Otolaryngology, Albert Einstein College of Medicine and
Director, Otolaryngology Service, North Central Bronx Hospital, Bronx, New York, USA

Introduction

History

Development of the operation of total laryngectomy through the first quarter of the 20th century was uneven and marked by occasional spectacular success intermixed with many disastrous results. Billroth performed the first laryngectomy[1–3] in 1873 while Bottini accomplished the first cure of cancer by laryngectomy in 1875[4,5]. Lange performed the first laryngectomy in the United States in 1879[6]. Gluck reported an operative mortality of 54 per cent between 1870 and 1880[6] and Mackenzie could find reports of only three cures in 19 patients compiled in the literature of that era[5]. A two-stage procedure was introduced by Gluck and Leller[7] in 1881. Gluck and Soerensen improved this to a single stage in 1894[6]. By 1922 they had performed 160 laryngectomies, the last 63 consecutive cases without a fatality[6,8,9].

During the period between the two World Wars, however, widespread acceptance of laryngectomy did not occur; many leading institutions employed radiation therapy almost exclusively for treatment of laryngeal cancer. Rapid improvement in radiation techniques occurred during this time, with the larynx considered a 'testing ground' by the radiotherapists[10]. As an example, there were no laryngectomies performed at Memorial Hospital in New York City between 1918 and 1933[11]. Successful and widespread employment of total laryngectomy was eventually made possible by the introduction of antibiotics for control of infection, improvement of anaesthetic agents, blood transfusion and the disappointing results achieved in treatment of advanced laryngeal cancer by radiation therapy alone.

Wide field laryngectomy was described by Jackson and Babcock[12] in 1931. Present day laryngectomy is based on the principles of the wide field operation, but differs from the operation as performed in the 1930s in that it involves more extensive resection of muscle and other perilaryngeal tissues, including the ipsilateral thyroid lobe. The operation is often done in continuity with complete ipsilateral neck dissection.

Indications for total laryngectomy

Total laryngectomy is employed for treatment of advanced laryngeal and hypopharyngeal carcinoma. The 1987 'TNM' system defined by the UICC[13] may be employed as a general basis for determining appropriate treatment for laryngeal cancer. 'Early' (T1 and T2) carcinomas are often amenable to partial laryngectomy or radiation therapy. Such tumours are characterized by mobility of the vocal folds and absence of deep invasion of the larynx. 'Advanced' (T3 and T4) laryngeal carcinomas are characterized by vocal fold fixation, deep invasion of laryngeal structures, cartilage invasion and extralaryngeal spread. Many of these tumours require total laryngectomy for adequate extirpation. The indications for total laryngectomy are summarized in *Table 1*.

Radiation therapy, which is effective for treatment of early superficial laryngeal tumours, is less successful for cure of advanced lesions. Radiation failure may be difficult to recognize at an early stage, while postoperative morbidity is increased and cure rates are lower following 'salvage' laryngectomy after radiation failure. Thus, in our opinion, attempted cure by radiation therapy employed as a single modality is not the preferred treatment for most instances of T3 and T4 laryngeal cancer, if the patient is a suitable medical and psychological candidate for operation. Postoperative irradiation is indicated for patients with cervical lymph node metastases, inadequate resection margins or extralaryngeal spread of tumour.

Table 1 Indications for total laryngectomy

Glottic:
  T3 carcinoma with fold fixation and subglottic extension too extensive for hemilaryngectomy
  T4 carcinoma

Supraglottic:
  T3 tumours with pre-epiglottic space invasion and vocal fold involvement
  T3 tumours with vocal fold fixation
  T4 carcinoma

Subglottic:
  All primary subglottic tumours
  Glottic tumours with fixation and extensive subglottic extension

Transglottic:
  Carcinoma with paraglottic space invasion, particularly with vocal fold fixation

Piriform sinus:
  Carcinoma with involvement of apex of piriform sinus, vocal fold fixation or paraglottic space invasion

All laryngeal carcinomas:
  Following tracheotomy performed as independent procedure prior to definitive resection

Technique of total laryngectomy for endolaryngeal tumours

1

In total laryngectomy for endolaryngeal tumours the mucosa of the uninvolved piriform sinus will be preserved, whereas the entire sinus on the side of the tumour will be resected.

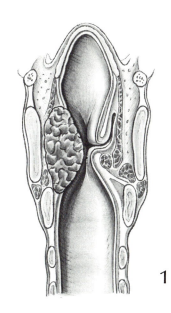

1

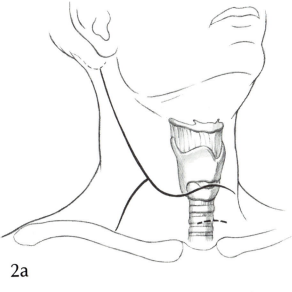

2a

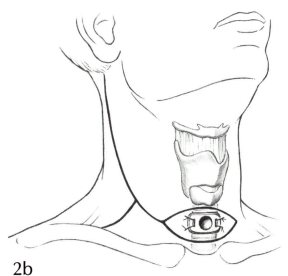

2b

2a & b

A transverse incision situated midway between the hyoid bone and the suprasternal notch is most suitable. The skin incisions and flaps may be extended for neck dissection. The tracheostoma will be placed in a separate incision through the inferior skin flap.

In a patient with an established tracheostomy requiring total laryngectomy, the transverse incision includes an ellipse of skin around the tracheostomy. The tracheostoma will ultimately be placed directly into the transverse incision.

3

At the conclusion of the right radical dissection, the carotid artery is exposed along its length, while the internal jugular vein and sternocleidomastoid muscle are included in the neck dissection. The entire neck dissection specimen is secured within a small bag for convenience and is reflected onto the larynx to which it is left broadly attached.

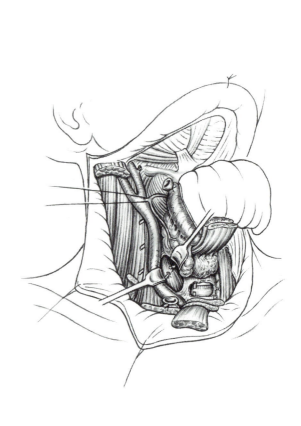

3

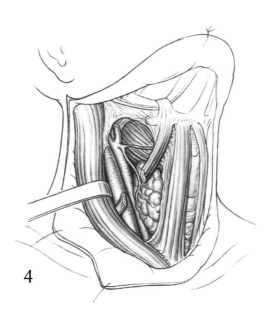

4

4

If a neck dissection is not done, the procedure is started by mobilizing the ipsilateral sternomastoid muscle and separating the jugular vein and carotid artery from the midline structures. The omohyoid muscle is divided.

5

Mobilization of the ipsilateral side is started inferiorly. The sternohyoid and sternothyroid muscles are transected low in the neck, revealing the thyroid gland, trachea and oesophagus. The ipsilateral thyroid lobe will be resected. The inferior thyroid artery is divided, as are the paratracheal structures inferior to the thyroid lobe, including the recurrent laryngeal nerve. Division of the paratracheal tissue brings the trachea into view. Its surface should be skeletonized along the line of resection. If there has been a previous tracheostomy, this step is usually complicated by fibrosis and adhesions. It is then necessary to clear and transect the trachea through uninvolved tissue below the field of the tracheostomy, which will be included in the resection.

5

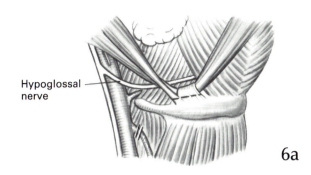

Hypoglossal nerve

6a

6a & b

Mobilization of the ipsilateral side continues superiorly. The superior thyroid artery is divided and the suprahyoid muscles are severed along the superior border of the body and greater cornu of the hyoid bone. As the hyoglossus muscle is separated from its origin on the greater cornu, care must be taken not to injure the hypoglossal nerve which is on the superficial surface of that muscle, and to avoid the lingual artery which is just deep to the muscle. The lesser cornu should be left attached to the hyoid bone. Muscles that originate from the body of the hyoid bone are thick and must be transected completely before the external aspect of hypopharyngeal mucosa is reached. If tumour in the valleculae is suspected, a rim of suprahyoid muscles is left attached to the body of the hyoid bone.

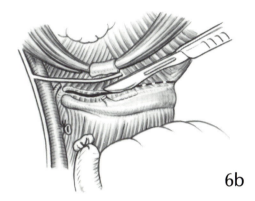

6b

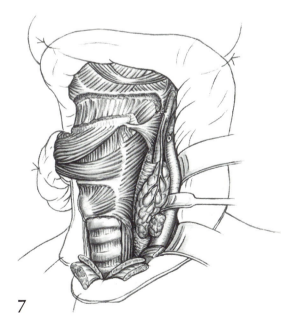

7

7

The contralateral side is mobilized in a manner similar to the ipsilateral side. The thyroid isthmus is divided. The thyroid lobe on this side will be preserved with its blood supply from the superior and possibly inferior thyroid arteries. The thyroid lobe is separated from the trachea, a somewhat tedious procedure because of multiple vascular attachments.

8

If the contralateral piriform sinus is free of tumour, mucosa on this side may be preserved to simplify closure of the hypopharynx. The fibres of the inferior constrictor muscle are incised along the posterior edge of the thyroid ala, exposing the underlying piriform sinus which is dissected from the inner aspect of the thyroid cartilage to liberate as much tissue as possible. The neck specimen and perilaryngeal soft tissues have been removed from the illustration for clarity.

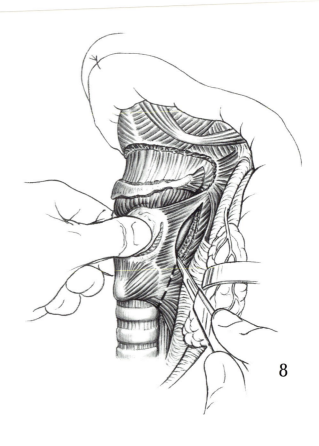

8

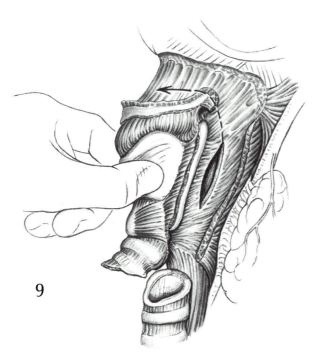

9

9

The larynx has now been completely mobilized. The trachea is transected if possible at least 2 cm below the inferior limit of the tumour or 1 cm inferior to the tracheostomy site. If the resection margin permits, the tracheal incision should be bevelled upwards posteriorly to maximize the size of the tracheostoma. The proximal posterior tracheal wall and cricoid are separated from the oesophagus.

A cuffed endotracheal tube (not shown) is inserted into the distal segment for control of the airway. The hypopharynx is entered through the contralateral piriform sinus. (It can also be entered through the vallecula or through the postcricoid mucosa.) The site of entry should be as far from the tumour as possible.

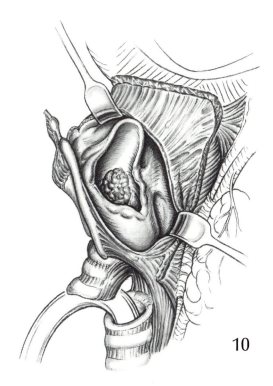

10

The mucosal incision is extended superiorly. As it transects the valleculae, the entire hypopharynx can be visualized and the remaining line of resection planned.

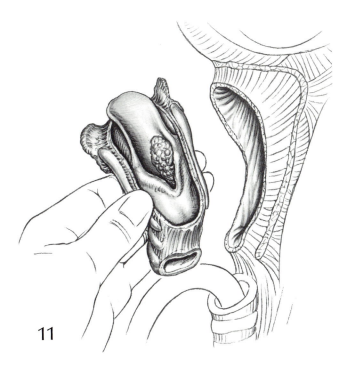

11

The mucosal incision is completed through the post-cricoid region and the remaining attachments of the larynx are severed.

12

Prior to closure, the triangular hypopharyngeal defect is large. A nasogastric tube is passed and secured to the nasal columella with a suture. Flexion of the neck will aid closure and relieve tension on the suture line.

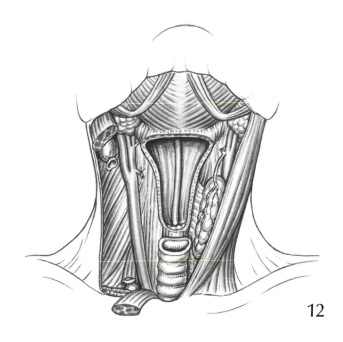

12

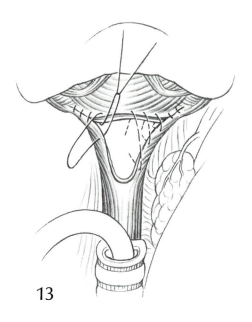

13

13

Closure with interrupted sutures of 00 or 000 polyglactin, knots tied on the inside, is preferred. In order to correct any discrepancy in length between superior and inferior flaps, sutures are placed in close proximity through the superior flap and spaced more widely inferiorly.

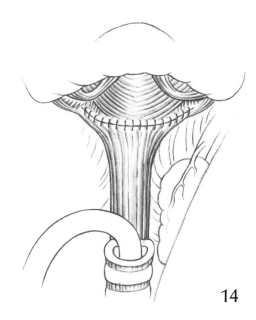

14

In most cases following resection for endolaryngeal tumours, it will be possible to achieve a transverse linear closure. This is preferable to a 'T' or 'Y' closure because of a lower incidence of postoperative fistula. The closure is reinforced by approximating the cut edges of the inferior constrictor to the suprahyoid muscles. A tightly constricting muscular ring should be avoided.

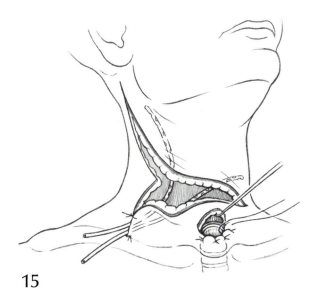

15

The tracheostoma is constructed by suture to the skin edges with interrupted 000 or 0000 nylon. The endotracheal tube is intermittently removed to permit placement of sutures when necessary. The tracheostoma is placed either in the main incision or through a separate small incision in the inferior flap. The latter is preferable, since there is less likelihood of postoperative stricture, but it is usually not feasible if there has been a previous tracheostomy.

Technique of total laryngectomy for piriform sinus tumours

16

This transverse view shows a large tumour in the right piriform sinus. The tumour extends to the apex (not shown) and invades the paraglottic space by penetrating the mucosa anteriorly.

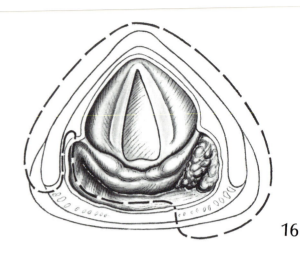

16

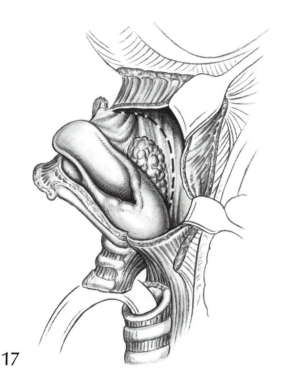

17

17

The initial mobilization of the larynx is similar to the procedure for endolaryngeal tumours (*Illustrations 2–9*). The hypopharynx is entered at a point as remote from the tumour as feasible, usually the contralateral piriform sinus. The tumour mass in the right piriform sinus comes into view as the mucosal incision is enlarged through the valleculae. A wide margin of normal mucosa should be excised with the tumour, extending well into the base of tongue if necessary.

18

Resection is completed and the specimen removed. Resection margins should not be limited by concern for the amount of tissue available for closure of the hypopharynx.

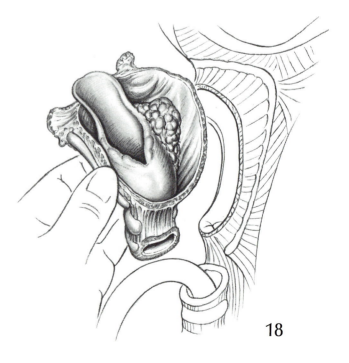

18

19

It is usually possible to reconstruct the hypopharynx by direct suture if no more than 50 per cent of its mucosal circumference has been resected. The defect often extends onto the posterior pharyngeal wall, where closure is commenced by suturing inferior to superior margins of the defect with interrupted sutures of 00 or 000 polyglactin. Closure is aided by flexion of the neck and, occasionally, by cricopharyngeal myotomy. A nasogastric feeding tube is passed before closure.

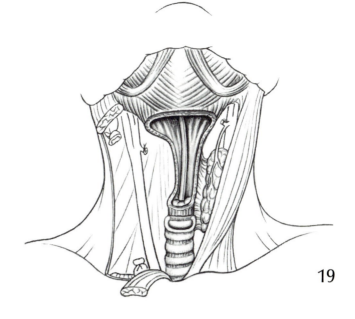

19

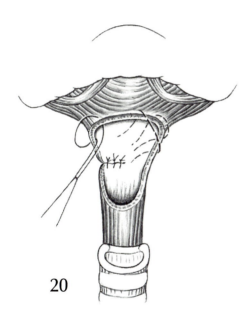

20

20

Closure continues anteriorly, correcting the discrepancy between flaps by appropriate suture placement (see *Illustration 13*).

21

Because more hypopharyngeal mucosa has been resected than is usually required when tumour is confined to the endolarynx, a single transverse closure (*Illustration 14*) often cannot be achieved after resection of a piriform sinus carcinoma. In most cases, an inferior vertical ('T') extension is employed.

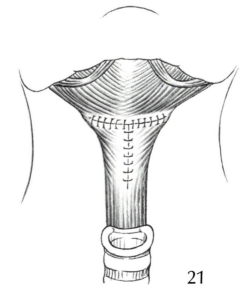

21

22

If mucosal resection has been too extensive to permit primary closure without tension, a mucosal defect remains anteriorly. Mucosal edges of the defect may be sutured to overlying skin edges, thus creating a temporary pharyngostome that is closed at a later date. This two-stage approach is preferable to closure with excessive tension on the suture lines, as the latter will inevitably lead to fistula and infection. Nevertheless, the two-stage procedure, often employed in the past, tends to prolong postoperative disability and hospitalization.

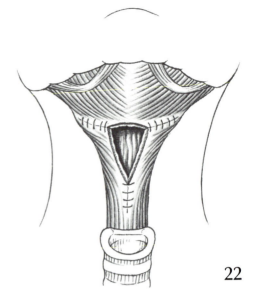

22

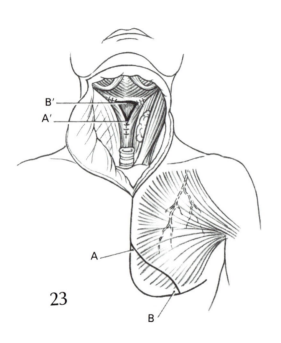

23

23

The pectoralis major myocutaneous flap may be employed for single-stage closure of large hypopharyngeal defects. An appropriate skin 'paddle' is outlined on the parasternal region of the chest and the pectoralis major muscle exposed by elevation of a large flap of overlying skin.

24

After mobilization of the muscle, it is rotated on its vascular pedicle, transferring the skin island to the hypopharyngeal defect. When properly positioned, points AA' and BB' will be approximated.

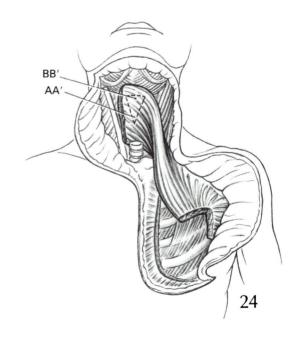

24

25

The donor site on the chest wall can usually be directly sutured. If the defect is too large for primary closure, a skin graft may be necessary.

Acknowledgements

The illustrations are redrawn with permission from Silver, C. E. (1981) *Surgery for Cancer of the Larynx,* Churchill Livingstone, New York.

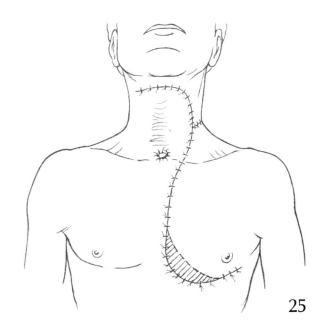

25

References

1. Billroth T, Gussenbauer C. Ulber die Erste durch T. Billroth am Menschen ausgefuhrte Kehlkopf-Extirpation und die Auswendung eines Kunstlichen Kehlkopfes. *Arch Klin Chir* 1874; 17: 343–56.

2. Stell PM. The first laryngectomy. *J Laryngol Otol* 1975; 89: 353–8.

3. Schwartz AW. Dr Theodore Billroth and the first laryngectomy. *Ann Plast Surg* 1978; 1: 513–16.

4. Alberti PW. The historical development of laryngectomy. II. The evolution of laryngology and laryngectomy in the mid-nineteenth century. *Laryngoscope* 1975; 85: 288–98.

5. Thomson StC. The history of cancer of the larynx. *J Laryngol Otol* 1939; 54: 61–87.

6. Holinger PH. The historical development of laryngectomy. V. A century of progress of laryngectomies in the northern hemisphere. *Laryngoscope* 1975; 85: 322–32.

7. MacComb WS, Fletcher GH. *Cancer of the Head and Neck.* Baltimore: Williams & Wilkins, 1967.

8. Gluck T, Soerensen J. Die Resektion und Extirpation des Larynx, Pharynx und Esophagus. In: Katz L, Presing H, Bumenfeld F, eds. *Handbuch der Spez. Chir. Ohres und der Obereu. Luftwege,* Vol. IV. Wurzburg: C. Kabitzch, 1931.

9. Ingals EF. Direct laryngoscopy. *Trans Am Laryngol Rhinol Otol Soc* 1911; 17: 26–9.

10. Lederman MB. The historical development of laryngectomy. VI. History of radiotherapy in the treatment of cancer of the larynx, 1896–1939. *Laryngoscope* 1975; 85: 333.

11. Martin H. *Surgery of Head and Neck Tumors.* New York: Harper & Bros, 1957.

12. Jackson C, Babcock W. Laryngectomy for carcinoma of the larynx. *Surg Clin North Am* 1931; 11: 1207–27.

13. UICC. *TNM Classification of Malignant Tumours,* 4th ed. Hermanek P, Sobin LH, eds. Berlin, Heidelberg, New York, London, Paris, Tokyo: Springer, 1987.

Vertical partial laryngectomy

Hugh F. Biller MD
Professor and Chairman, Department of Otolaryngology, The Mount Sinai Center, New York, USA

David J. Howard FRCS, FRCS(Ed)
Institute of Laryngology and Otology, Royal National Throat, Nose and Ear Hospital, London, UK

Introduction

Indications

The procedure of vertical partial laryngectomy is used to resect vocal fold cancers which extend to involve one or more of the following sites: (1) anterior commissure and opposite fold; (2) subglottic extension of 1 cm or less; (3) posterior extension to involve the vocal process or anterior face of the arytenoid.

The procedure is also used for tumours limited to the membranous vocal fold in young patients where irradiation may be contraindicated.

The procedure is used in select cases of recurrent tumour after treatment with radiotherapy. Three criteria must apply: the original lesion, before treatment with radiotherapy, is amenable to a vertical partial laryngectomy; the recurrence is in the same area as the original tumour; and subglottic involvement is less than 0.5 cm.

Contraindications to hemilaryngectomy

Cartilage invasion. This is always a contraindication to vertical partial laryngectomy.

Vocal fold fixation. When this is secondary to subglottic involvement or cricoarytenoid joint involvement it is a contraindication to partial laryngectomy. Vocal fold fixation from vocalis muscle invasion or tumour bulk is not necessarily a contraindication. Transglottic tumours should not be treated by a vertical partial laryngectomy because of the significant incidence of recurrence which is most probably a result of tumour in the pre-epiglottic space.

Preoperative assessment

In order to perform vertical partial laryngectomy and to be able to remove the tumour with adequate margins, it is essential that the exact extent of the lesion is recognized preoperatively. This may be determined by indirect laryngoscopy and direct laryngoscopy. In lesions which extend subglottically, it is necessary to be able to assess the exact distance from the free margin of the vocal fold. Additional information may be obtained by a computed tomographic scan or magnetic resonance imaging.

Operation

Anaesthesia and preparation of patient

The operation may be initiated with the patient under local or general anaesthesia. If local anaesthesia is decided upon then a tracheostomy is performed under local anaesthesia through a transverse incision two fingers'-breadth above the sternal notch. The trachea is opened and an endotracheal tube is inserted into the trachea. The opposite end of the tube is slipped under the drapes for the anaesthetist to connect to the anaesthetic machine. The patient is then anaesthetized. This procedure is performed under sterile conditions so there is no need to reprepare and drape the patient.

If general anaesthesia is used the patient is induced and anaesthesia maintained through a 7.5 mm oral endo-tracheal tube. The patient is positioned, with a small roll placed under the shoulders to allow maximum extension of the neck and is prepared and draped in the routine manner. The endotracheal tube is brought superiorly from the oral cavity and taped to the forehead over four or five sponges. The draping should be such that the anaesthetist can extract the endotracheal tube without contaminating the field. This will occur when the tracheostomy is completed and an endotracheal tube is inserted into the tracheostomy site. The distal end of this tube is then passed under the drapes for the anaesthetist to connect to the anaesthetic machine. The drapes are sutured in place.

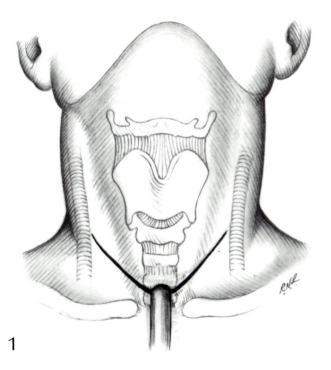

1

Incision

1

After completion of the tracheostomy and administration of the anaesthetic through the tracheostomy site, the transverse incision from the tracheostomy is extended bilaterally from the midline to the external jugular vein. This flap is elevated deep to platysma muscle and superior to the level of the hyoid bone. The flap is then sutured to the upper drapes.

Thyrotomy

2

The sternohyoid and sternothyroid muscles are separated in the midline. The anterior aspect of the thyroid cartilage, cricoid cartilage and first two tracheal rings are exposed. This may or may not require dividing the isthmus of the thyroid gland. An incision is made in the thyroid perichondrium in the midline, extending from the thyroid notch to the lower border of the thyroid cartilage. The perichondrium is elevated. The elevation is first performed with a 'peanut' swab and then completed with an elevator. The perichondrium on the side of the lesion is elevated posteriorly to approximately 1 cm from the posterior border of the thyroid cartilage.

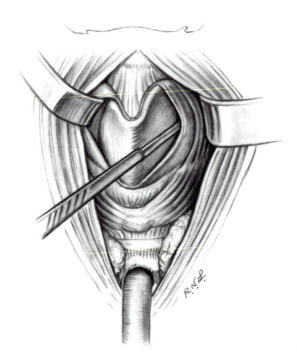

2

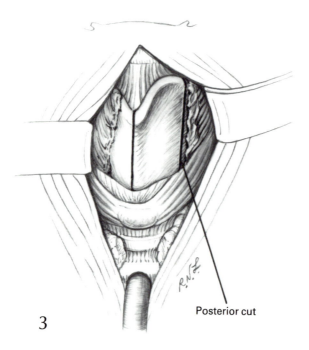

Posterior cut

3

3

On the contralateral side the perichondrium is elevated 1–2 cm. The posterior cut in the thyroid cartilage is placed 1.5 cm anterior to the posterior border of the thyroid cartilage. This cut runs in an inferosuperior direction. The anterior cut varies depending upon the anterior extent of the tumour. If the tumour of the vocal fold does not extend to the anterior commissure then the anterior cartilage cut is in the midline and extends from the base of the thyroid notch to the lower border of the thyroid cartilage.

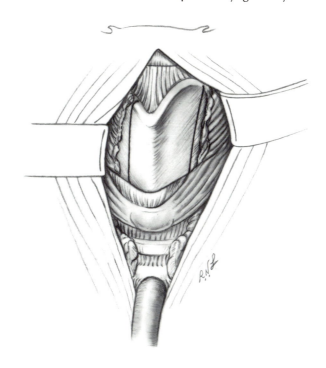

4

If, on the other hand, the tumour involves the anterior commissure, the anterior cut is placed approximately 1–1.5 cm from the midline on the side of lesser involvement and extends from the superior aspect of the thyroid cartilage to the inferior aspect.

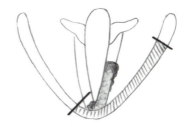

4

5

Following completion of the thyroid cartilage cuts, the cricothyroid membrane is incised transversely just above the cricoid cartilage. This transverse cut begins in the midline and extends along the upper border of the cricoid cartilage.

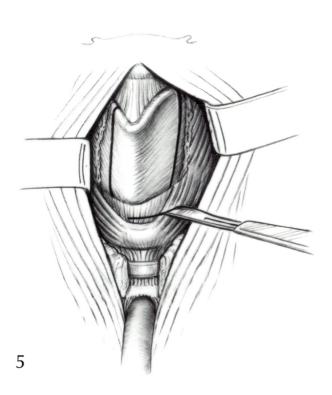

5

6

Through this incision, by the use of a hook, the subglottic mucosa is visualized on the side of greater involvement of the tumour. If the area is clear an incision is made following the upper border of the cricoid cartilage from the anterior midline laterally and posteriorly. This will allow sufficient exposure of the undersurfaces of the folds, but it will be difficult to see the undersurface of the anterior commissure.

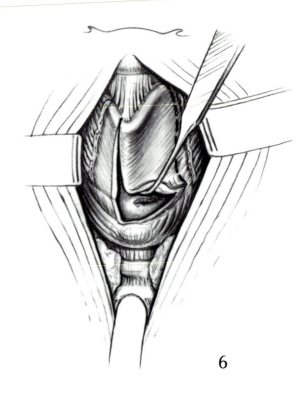

6

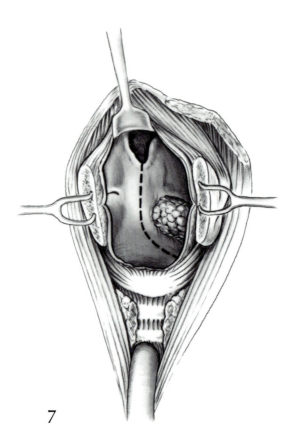

7

7

In order to visualize this area it is necessary to place the patient in the Trendelenburg position and to retract the cricothyroid membrane superiorly. An elevator is then introduced from below, between the vocal folds, and the normal vocal fold is abducted. The margins of the involved fold and the anterior commissure are then visualized. In order to perform this the patient must be paralysed. Only after the anterior commissure is visualized is the thyrotomy completed. A decision is then made whether to perform the thyrotomy through the anterior commissure or more laterally to include a portion of the opposite fold. Depending on this decision a scalpel is used to continue the superior extent of the thyrotomy either at the commissure or through a portion of the opposite vocal fold. The thyrotomy continues to the superior border of the thyroid cartilage. The two thyroid alae are then retracted with hooks.

Resection of tumour

8

The tumour is visualized. Normal vocal fold is retracted using a right-angle retractor and a tenaculum is placed at the false fold level of the hemilarynx to be resected. Scissors are then used to cut the soft tissue above the false fold at the level of the superior border of the thyroid ala which is being resected. As this incision progresses branches of the superior laryngeal artery will be encountered. These should be clamped and suture-ligated. After mobilization of the superior aspect of the hemilarynx, the inferior subglottic area is incised along the superior border of the cricoid cartilage. This incision continues posteriorly to the area of the cricoarytenoid joint. The posterior cut may either be through the vocal process, through the body of the arytenoid or posteriorly so the entire arytenoid is removed with the specimen, depending upon the extent of the lesion. After removal of the hemilarynx, bleeding vessels are cauterized. The cut margin of the opposite true vocal fold is sutured anteriorly to the perichondrium with interrupted 4/0 chromic sutures.

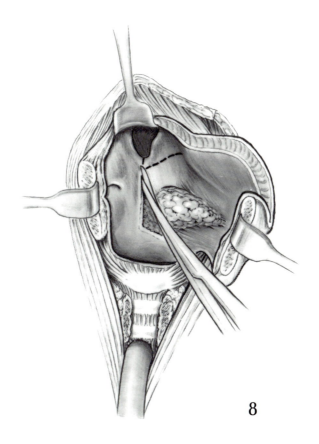

8

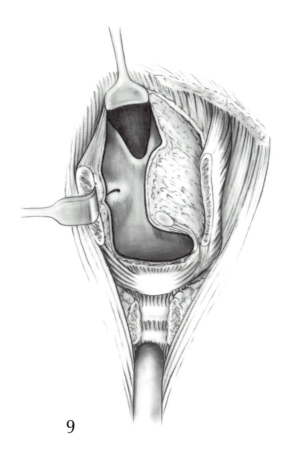

9

Closure when arytenoid present

9

The epiglottis is fixed anteriorly with a mattress suture of 0 chromic which extends from the perihyoid tissue through the petiole of the epiglottis and then through the perihyoid tissue where it is tied.

The reconstruction of the resected hemilarynx depends upon whether or not the arytenoid has been removed. If the arytenoid has not been removed then no reconstruction is performed and the laryngostome is closed by approximating the perichondrium on each side with interrupted absorbable sutures. The strap muscles are then reapproximated as the second layer.

Arytenoid reconstruction

10

If the arytenoid has been removed, it is essential to replace it to avoid a deficient posterior glottic chink, which results in significant aspiration. The closure of this posterior defect may be accomplished by the use of muscle fat, fascia, tendon or cartilage. The author prefers the use of free or pedicled cartilage.

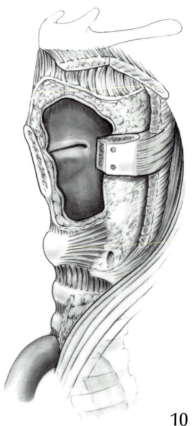

10

11

A piece of cartilage from the posterior border of the thyroid ala, tailored to measure approximately 1 cm × 5 mm, is wired to the arytenoid facet of the cricoid. The cartilage may be pedicled on the inferior constrictor muscle or may be used as a free graft.

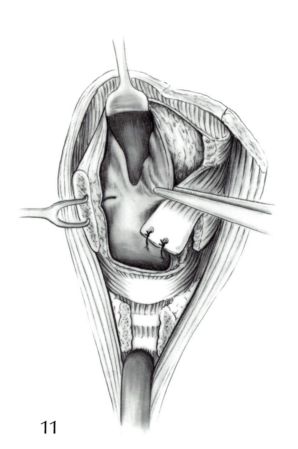

11

12

The mucosa from the postarytenoid, postcricoid and medial wall of the piriform sinus is mobilized, thinned and used to resurface the cartilage reconstruction as well as the area of the resected true and false fold. This mucosal flap is sutured with interrupted 4/0 chromic sutures along the subglottic area.

Closure

Closure of the laryngostome is accomplished by approximating the perichondrium from one side to the other with interrupted absorbable sutures. The strap muscles are approximated as a second layer. If in the resection the opposite vocal fold has been resected to such a degree that the anterior margin cannot be sutured to the anterior cartilage cut, then postoperative webbing of the anterior larynx may occur, leading to a decrease in the anteroposterior diameter and possibly stenosis. In view of this, a Silastic keel (Dow Corning, Reading, UK) is inserted anteriorly within the larynx in an attempt to avoid the webbing.

Closure is the same except that the keel extends anterior to the approximated strap muscles. This portion of the Silastic is pierced with a 2/0 nylon suture which is then fixed on either side of the neck with a button. The skin flap is reapproximated in layers. A Penrose drain is inserted and the endotracheal tube is replaced with a No. 7 or No. 8 tracheostomy tube with a cuff. A nasogastric tube is inserted and a light dressing is applied.

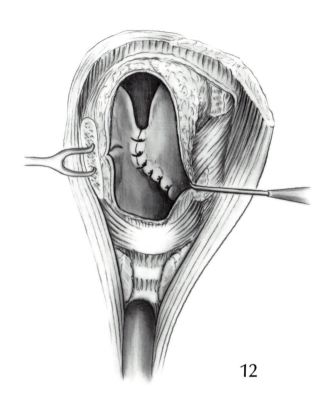

12

Postoperative care

Routine tracheostomy care is performed: humidified air via a collar mask, frequent tracheal suction, and adequate hydration. Prophylactic antibiotics are used routinely, beginning preoperatively and continuing until 12 hours postoperatively. Nasogastric tube feeding is instituted at approximately 48 hours after demonstration of adequate bowel sounds. Gentle walking is begun the morning after operation. The laryngeal airway is usually adequate for corking of the tracheostomy tube at approximately 6–7 days, except in patients who have had arytenoid removal and replacement, when corking can usually be done at 14 days. If the tracheostomy tube can be corked for 48 hours, it is then removed along with the nasogastric tube. The tracheostomy opening is taped and the patient is started on oral feeds. In general, aspiration is minimal or does not occur. Semisolids are preferable to liquids in the early stages of swallowing. The patient is usually discharged 2–3 days after removal of the tracheostomy tube.

In those patients with a keel in place, the tracheostomy tube is not removed. The nasogastric tube is removed at 7 days and the patient is discharged to be readmitted in 6 weeks for a laryngoscopy and removal of the keel. The tracheostomy tube is removed the next day.

Complications

There are only two significant complications: inadequate airway resulting in inability to decannulate the patient; and persistent aspiration.

The first is unusual but may occur in those patients who, after arytenoid removal and reconstruction, have a flap which becomes bulky and oedematous. This bulky flap may prevent decannulation because of an inadequate airway. In this case, a laryngoscopy is performed at 8 weeks and the flap is removed with a biting cup forceps or with the laser. Decannulation can usually be accomplished 1–2 weeks later.

Late stenosis from scarring may occur, thereby producing an inadequate airway requiring a tracheostomy. This complication usually requires corrective surgery of the larynx using thyrotomy and skin grafting with a stent. Occasionally, the stenosis may be corrected by using the laser perorally through the laryngoscope.

In patients with persistent aspiration the specific causative factor or factors must be determined. The larynx is visualized to assess whether there is glottic closure or incompetence. If glottic closure is adequate then it is necessary to evaluate whether there is oesophageal or cricopharyngeal obstruction. Videofluoroscopy is a useful investigation in these cases. If glottic closure is inadequate then correction is necessary. This may require Teflon injection or reoperation to correct the incompetence by muscle or cartilage implants.

Horizontal partial laryngectomy

Hugh F. Biller MD
Professor and Chairman, Department of Otolaryngology, The Mount Sinai Center, New York, USA

David J. Howard FRCS, FRCS(Ed)
Institute of Laryngology and Otology, Royal National Throat, Nose and Ear Hospital, London, UK

Introduction

Indications

This procedure is used to treat tumours which involve the epiglottis and/or the false cords. In selected cases it may be used to resect tumours involving the medial or anterior wall of the piriform sinus.

Contraindications

1. Tumour which crosses the ventricle to involve the true vocal fold.
2. Involvement of the interarytenoid space.
3. Significant involvement of the arytenoid which would prevent an adequate margin with disarticulation of the cricoarytenoid joint.
4. Limitation or fixation of the vocal fold.
5. Computed tomographic evidence of paraglottic involvement.
6. A 2 mm margin at the inferior extent of all supraglottic tumours.

Operation

Position of patient

1

The patient is placed supine with a pillow under the shoulders and the neck extended.

Anaesthesia

Anaesthesia is initiated and maintained by endotracheal intubation. After preparation and draping a tracheostomy is performed and anaesthesia is·then maintained through the tracheostomy site. This procedure is performed under sterile conditions and repeat preparation and draping is not necessary. An alternative method is to perform the tracheostomy under local anaesthesia after preparation and draping.

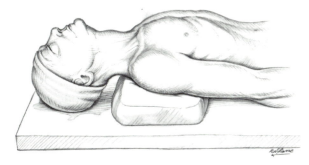

1

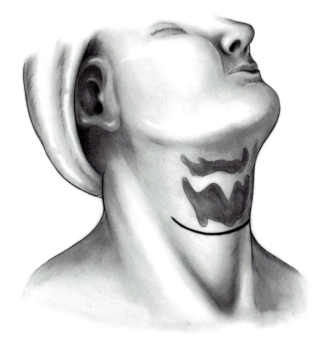

Incision

2

A transverse incision is made at the level of the cricoid cartilage if a neck dissection is not performed. If a neck dissection is being performed with the primary section, a modified H-type of incision is used. The neck dissection is completed before the primary tumour is resected and the block of tissue is left attached at the thyrohyoid membrane.

2

Thyrotomy

3

The strap muscles are cut at the superior border of the thyroid cartilage. On the side of the lesion these muscles are severed from the thyroid notch to the posterior border of the thyroid cartilage. On the side of lesser involvement they are sectioned only approximately midway to the posterior border. Perichondrium along the superior border of the thyroid cartilage is then incised and reflected inferiorly to the lower border of the thyroid cartilage. The superior cornu of the thyroid cartilage on the side of the lesion is mobilized.

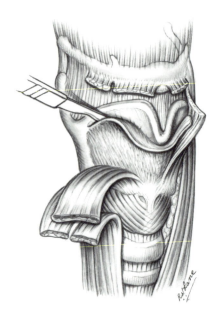

3

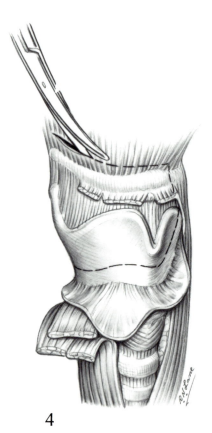

4

4

The cartilage is then marked before sectioning with a saw.

5

The anterior cut is at the junction of the lower two-thirds with the upper one-third of the thyroid ala. From this point, on the side of the lesion, the cut extends posteriorly to the mid-portion of the posterior border of the thyroid ala. On the contralateral side the cut extends superiorly to the mid-portion of the superior aspect of the thyroid ala. The hyoid bone is mobilized and the suprahyoid muscles are sectioned from the hyoid bone. The hyoid bone is cut at the lesser cornu on the side of least involvement. The pharynx is opened through the vallecula and the epiglottis grasped with a tenaculum.

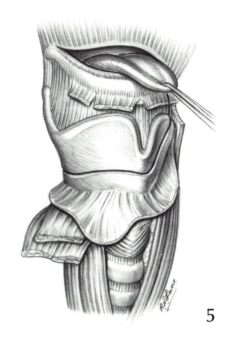

5

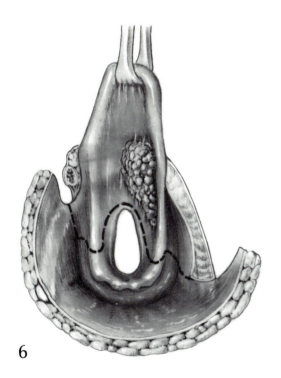

6

Resection

6

The resection begins on the side of least involvement by incising the margin of the epiglottis. The aryepiglottic fold is sectioned just above the arytenoid cartilage. All cuts are made after the tumour is adequately visualized. The ventricle and true vocal fold are observed. In order to improve visibility the patient is paralysed and the severed aryepiglottic fold is retracted laterally with a hook. The incision crosses the posterior aspect of the false fold to the ventricle and extends anteriorly to the anterior commissure. The entire supraglottis is then rotated to the side of greater movement.

7

The ventricle is incised with the epiglottis retracted and a similar resection is performed on the side of greater involvement. If necessary, a portion of the arytenoid or the entire arytenoid can be resected.

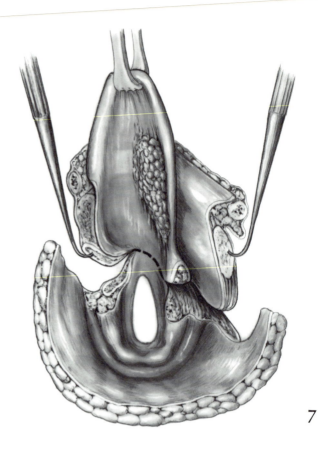

7

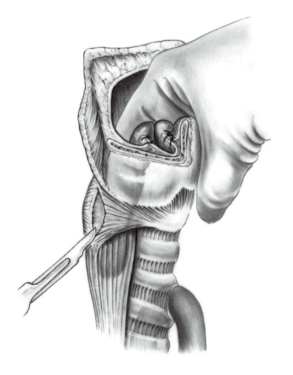

8

Reconstruction

8

A cricopharyngeal myotomy is performed posterior to the recurrent laryngeal nerve by incising the cricopharyngeal muscle over a finger placed in the upper oesophagus. The recurrent laryngeal nerve is not identified.

If the arytenoid has been resected it must be reconstructed in order to prevent a postoperative posterior glottic defect, which will result in aspiration. A free piece of cartilage is taken from the superior aspect of the thyroid ala and wired into place at the cricoarytenoid joint. The vocal process is then wired to the graft or the cricoid. The entire reconstruction area is covered by a flap from the adjacent mucosa.

Closure

9

The pharyngostome is closed by approximating the perichondrium and cut margin of the strap muscles to the base of tongue. This is a single-layer closure; the suture material used is 0 silk. All sutures are inserted and then they are tied, beginning at the site of least resection. The suture in front of the one to be tied is crossed so that the tension is removed from the suture being tied. The head is also flexed to relieve tension on the suture line. Closure on the side where the pharyngostome is largest is performed by a specially placed suture. En route from the base of the tongue to the perichondrium this suture passes from outside-to-in and inside-to-out at one or more areas of the cut margin of the lateral pharyngeal wall. This inverts the cut margin, thereby strengthening the closure. After the closure of the pharyngostome the flaps are reapproximated by suturing the platysma muscle and then the skin. If a neck dissection has been performed, vacuum drainage is used. If a neck dissection has not been performed two Penrose drains are used.

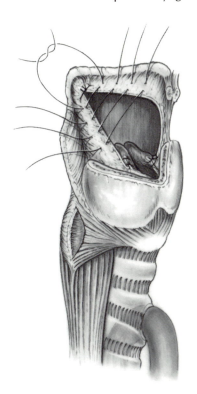

9

Postoperative care

The patient is fed by nasogastric tube. Routine tracheostomy care is instituted. Gentle walking is begun the day after operation. At 7 days the skin sutures are removed. At 14 days the tracheostomy tube is occluded for 24 hours, and if the airway is adequate the tracheostomy tube is removed. The tracheostomy site is allowed to close. Feedings are not begun until the tracheostomy site is closed. The nasogastric tube is removed at 18–21 days and peroral feedings are begun which initially consist of only solid foods, with intravenous supplementation given as required for the first 3–4 days. After feeding with solids is accomplished, liquids in the form of cold carbonated beverages can then be introduced.

Illustrations by Robert Lane

Surgery for the prevention and treatment of stomal recurrence

David J. Howard FRCS, FRCS(Ed)
Institute of Laryngology and Otology, Royal National Throat, Nose and Ear Hospital, London, UK

Introduction

This chapter deals with the principles and techniques of manubrial resection and mediastinal dissection in the prevention and treatment of stomal recurrence.

Pathology

The major problem is recurrent squamous carcinoma following treatment for laryngeal, hypopharyngeal or cervical oesophageal tumours. Occasionally, advanced malignancy of the tongue base or thyroid requiring laryngectomy may give rise to subsequent stomal recurrence. This is a highly lethal complication and even when treated aggressively carries a 5-year survival rate of approximately 20 per cent. Emphasis must therefore be placed on its prevention by all possible methods. Reports in the literature over the last 30 years have shown that stomal recurrence is associated with the following:

1. Primary subglottic carcinoma.
2. Transglottic carcinoma with subglottic extension.
3. Large bulky obstructive laryngeal carcinoma requiring emergency tracheostomy.
4. Advanced piriform fossa carcinoma.
5. Postcricoid carcinoma.
6. Cervical oesophageal carcinoma.

The overall incidence of stomal recurrence following laryngeal and pharyngeal surgery varies between 2 and 15 per cent in the larger reported series. The higher incidence of stomal recurrence in laryngeal carcinomas requiring initial tracheostomy is not necessarily due to tumour implantation into the tracheostomy wound. Indeed, the bulk of evidence is against this. The term 'stomal recurrence', although widely used, is often inaccurate; the disease in the stomal area often arises from paratracheal, pharyngeal and residual thyroid tissue rather than from the tracheal wall itself. Its appearance reflects inadequate resection of the primary diseases listed above.

Paratracheal nodes

Primary subglottic tumours and transglottic tumours with more than 5 mm of subglottic extension frequently spread to pre- and para-tracheal nodes. At initial surgery at least half of primary subglottic cancers have been shown to have microscopic paratracheal nodal metastases.

Thyroid gland involvement

Advanced piriform fossa, postcricoid and cervical oesophageal carcinomas also have an increased incidence of paratracheal nodal spread and additional involvement of the thyroid gland. This latter spread is often impossible to detect clinically.

Local spread into upper trachea

While the mucosal spread of the laryngeal lesions into the upper trachea may be obvious, the submucosal extent is impossible to assess clinically. Hypopharyngeal and cervical oesophageal lesions may involve the posterior and lateral walls of the trachea in a similarly undetectable way.

Bearing these in mind, the surgeon undertaking the initial laryngeal and/or pharyngeal excision must obtain:

1. An adequate low sectioning of the trachea.
2. A thorough resection of pre- and para-tracheal lymph nodes and the accompanying soft tissue of the paratracheal gutters.
3. At least an ipsilateral hemithyroidectomy and isthmectomy in piriform fossa and laryngeal disease.
4. A total thyroidectomy in postcricoid and cervical oesophageal disease.

Reliance on postoperative radiotherapy to control positive tracheal resection margins, paratracheal nodal or thyroid disease leads to frequent disappointment. In established stomal recurrence radiotherapy is very rarely curative and frequently fails to produce palliation. Chemotherapy has virtually no role to play.

Indications

It is difficult to give any absolute indications for the use of manubrial resection and mediastinal dissection at primary surgery, but they should be carefully considered in the laryngeal, pharyngeal and oesophageal lesions outlined above. In addition to the variety of size and location of the primary tumour, paratracheal and thyroid involvement, the shape and length of the patient's neck varies considerably. Modern radiological CT and MRI scanning cannot always be relied on to give accurate assessment of the extent of the tumour, and final judgement of the need for manubrial resection may have to be made at the time of surgery.

However, considering the overall poor results of treating established stomal stenosis, primary manubrial resection and mediastinal dissection are strongly advocated for the following conditions:

1. Most primary subglottic tumours.
2. Most cervical oesophageal tumours.
3. Laryngopharyngeal tumours where there is obvious paratracheal nodal involvement, with or without thyroid invasion, and where at least 2 cm of normal trachea cannot be obtained in the neck without tension.

The morbidity of the primary procedure is considerably less than that of the similar procedure undertaken for the treatment of stomal recurrence. Prevention is far better than attempted cure.

Surgical anatomy

Before undertaking this resection the head and neck surgeon should be familiar with the anatomy of the thoracic inlet, superior mediastinum and manubrium but should not be daunted by the procedure although large vessels abound in the area and are somewhat asymmetrically distributed and variable, the excision can be accomplished safely and within a relatively short time. It does not greatly extend the time of total laryngectomy, and in hypopharyngeal and cervical oesophageal procedures the improved access through the thoracic inlet facilitates reconstruction and may actually decrease the overall operating time.

1

The sternum is in two parts: manubrium and body. The manubrium is a flat, four-sided bone, broader above than below, and is connected to the body by a secondary cartilaginous joint. It is made of cancellous bone with a thin, compact cortex and haemopoietic marrow. The upper margin of the manubrium is concave (the suprasternal notch) and is traversed by the interclavicular ligament. The investing layer of deep cervical fascia attaches to the anterior and posterior borders of the suprasternal notch.

The medial ends of the clavicles articulate with each upper angle of the manubrium; the sternoclavicular joint has a strong fibrous capsule and disc. The costoclavicular ligament attaches the medial end of the clavicle to the first rib and its costal cartilage. The lateral border of the manubrium receives the first costal cartilage, forming a primary cartilaginous joint.

The anterior surface of the manubrium gives rise to pectoralis major along its lateral border and the tendon of sternomastoid is attached superomedially. Sternohyoid and sternothyroid originate posteriorly, but most of the posterior surface of the manubrium is bare.

The trachea, passing downwards and posteriorly, lies close to the suprasternal notch but is separated from the posterior surface of the bone by the left brachiocephalic vein and the lung margins in their pleural sacs. The left brachiocephalic vein is usually separated from the posterior surface of the bone by thymic remnants and/or fatty tissue.

The internal thoracic arteries are important posterolateral relations arising from the first part of the subclavian artery and descending behind the sternoclavicular joints to run close to the lateral borders of the manubrium. These vessels are at substantial risk if complete resection of the manubrium is attempted.

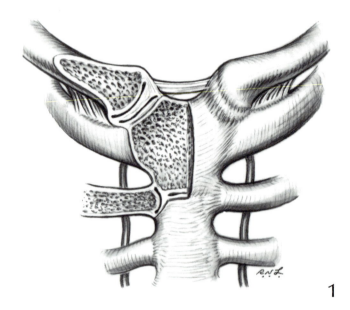

1

Superior mediastinum

The superior mediastinum lies between the thoracic inlet and a line passing horizontally backwards from the joint between the manubrium and body of the sternum to the lower border of the fourth thoracic vertebra. This horizontal plane is purely descriptive, not anatomical, as the anterior and posterior mediastinum are in direct continuity with the superior mediastinum.

The superior mediastinum is wedge-shaped, with the manubrium as its anterior boundary and the bodies of the first four thoracic vertebrae lying posteriorly.

Major arteries and veins

2

The concavity of the arch of the aorta lies behind the inferior aspect of the manubrium in the superior mediastinum passing, not from right to left, but backwards from the manubrium to the fourth thoracic vertebra. Thus the three major arterial branches of the arch (the brachiocephalic, left common carotid and left subclavian) pass upwards on the left side of the trachea. The brachiocephalic artery crosses gradually to the right so that the thoracic part of the trachea is enclosed by this asymmetrical V. The left vagus nerve and lung apex are separated from the trachea by the vessels, but the right vagus and lung apex are close to the trachea.

The major veins entering the superior mediastinum are the right and left brachiocephalic formed from their respective internal jugular and subclavian veins. The right brachiocephalic vein runs vertically downwards but the left vein passes almost horizontally across the superior mediastinum, to join the right vein at the lower border of the first right costal cartilage. The commencement of the left vein receives the thoracic duct and, in addition to the vertebral and internal thoracic veins, it also receives most of the blood from the inferior thyroid veins. The left superior intercostal vein and any thymic veins may also enter its mid portion.

Anatomical variations

These are relatively common and can be considerable in the root of the neck and superior mediastinum, but with care and good operative technique they rarely present significant problems at primary resection.

Trachea

The overall tracheal length averages 11 cm. It does not vary significantly with the overall height of the individual. However, the average distance from the cricoid to the suprasternal notch, 6 cm, has a wide range of variation (3.5–8 cm) and is a factor in assessing the initial operability and need for manubrial resection. Commonly a gain of at least 3 cm in length of tracheal resection can be gained after removal of manubrium.

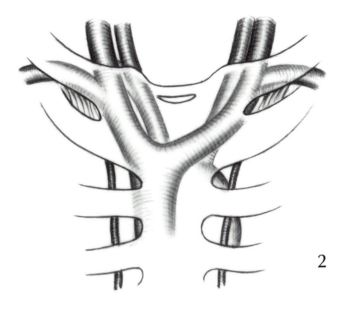

2

Brachiocephalic artery

Detailed anatomical cadaver dissections often report this artery as arising above the suprasternal notch in as many as 25 per cent of dissections. However, in over 40 cases to date, the author has experienced difficulty in establishing the tracheal stoma in relation to this artery in only one: in the live subject the elasticity and mobility of the vessels and soft tissues is far greater.

Left brachiocephalic vein

Running horizontally behind the body of the manubrium and enclosed in varying amounts of loose connective tissue, fat and thymic remnant, this vein is the most at risk. The smaller veins (mainly the inferior thyroid) draining into it require careful ligation but as with the artery its mobility is considerable, and even when it lies adjacent to the upper manubrium and suprasternal notch it rarely presents major problems during primary surgery.

Operations

PRIMARY EXCISION OF TUMOUR WITH MANUBRIAL RESECTION AND MEDIASTINAL DISSECTION FOR PREVENTION OF STOMAL RECURRENCE

Incision

3

A Gluck–Soerensen incision, as used for standard laryngeal and pharyngeal excisional surgery, is complemented by an additional vertical limb passing downwards to the level of the angle of Louis palpable at the manubriosternal joint.

If preoperative endoscopic and radiological studies have indicated extensive subglottic, postcricoid or cervical oesphageal tumour, it is important to assess the thoracic inlet early by division of the strap muscles and inspection and palpation of the thyroid, paratracheal nodes and major vessels. Occasionally gross disease fixed to the carotid arteries in the thoracic inlet will contraindicate further dissection. Unexpected extension and paratracheal involvement may indicate a change to include a manubrial and mediastinal procedure.

The vertical limb of the incision is deepened in the midline to the manubrial periosteum. Inferolateral skin and subcutaneous tissue flaps are then raised to expose the lower third of both sternomastoids, the medial third of clavicles and body of the manubrium. A deeper combined muscle and periosteal flap, comprising the medial portion of pectoralis major from the clavicles and manubrium with the associated periosteum, is then raised in the same direction. A combination of a wide curved periosteal elevator and some sharp dissection or needle diathermy is required to raise this flap from the anterior manubrium. The sternal and medial clavicular attachments of sternomastoid are divided to expose the sternoclavicular joints further.

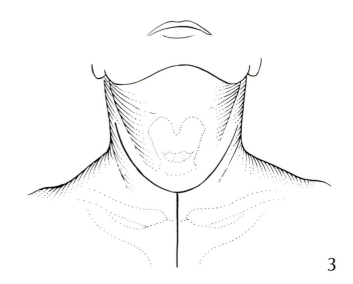

3

Excision of clavicular heads

4

The aim is to excise the medial clavicular heads and a significant proportion of the manubrial body as outlined. This allows an excellent view of the mediastinal contents and does not endanger the internal thoracic vessels; the absence of this part of the clavicles and the manubrium causes patients little difficulty. If enough bone is removed the cut ends of the clavicle do not obstruct the stoma on flexing of the shoulder joints and the costoclavicular ligament prevents 'floating' of the clavicles.

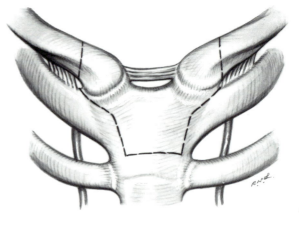

4

Manubrial resection

5

Division of the interclavicular ligament allows blunt finger dissection of the soft tissue from the posterior face of the manubrium. It is essential to ensure that the major vessels within this soft tissue are well clear of the bone before removal. The blunt dissection continues behind the clavicular heads, aided by occasional division of soft tissues using the tips of curved scissors placed directly onto periosteum.

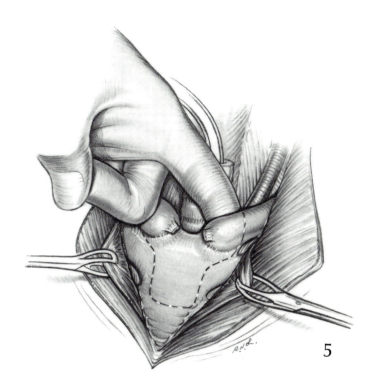

5

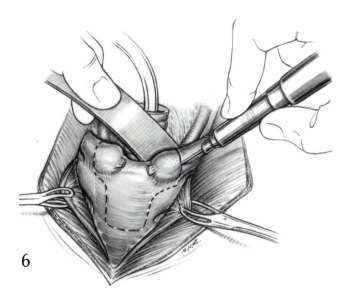

6

6

It is now possible to introduce a wide (2 cm) malleable copper strip behind all portions of the excisional area in order to protect the vessels and to allow safe division of the clavicle and manubrium by a high-speed fissure burr or oscillating saw (the author prefers the fine control and accuracy of the fissure burr). Minor soft tissue attachments, particularly joint capsule and posterior periosteum, may require scissor division as the bone segment is removed. Bone wax may be used to control any bleeding from the marrow spaces. Any sharp bone edges are reduced with a nasal rasp before commencing the mediastinal dissection.

Mediastinal dissection

The anterior wall of the trachea and left brachiocephalic vein are defined and the former is cleared down to the separation of the brachiocephalic and left common carotid arteries. The dissection of the paratracheal nodes and surrounding fat, first started in the neck, is carried down into the mediastinum, removing all tissue medial to the major arteries.

7

By bringing the mobilized larynx and cervical trachea forward it is possible to determine the level at which the trachea may be divided without exerting unacceptable pressure on related vessels and allowing good approximation to the skin edges of the vertical limb. If the disease allows oblique division of the trachea, this aids the stoma formation and lessens the tension on the mobilized trachea.

Dead space around the manubrial site can be a problem and is combated by covering the exposed manubrial edges by the periosteum/pectoralis major, approximating this to the posterior manubrial periosteum with catgut sutures. If the procedure is elective the sternohyoid musculature may be preserved and turned down to fill the space. After laryngectomy with subglottic extension the resection leaves only limited dead space which can be dealt with by the above procedure. After laryngopharyngectomy or laryngopharyngo-oesophagectomy with repair by myocutaneous flaps, free jejunum, transposed stomach or colon, the reconstructive tissues can be utilized to fill the dead space.

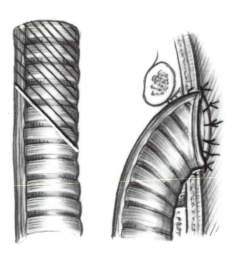

7

Closure

8

Primary wound closure is in two layers, using interrupted catgut sutures to the deep layer and Prolene (Ethicon Ltd, Edinburgh, UK) to the skin. If the stoma is deeply placed in the vertical skin incision, 3/0 Vicryl sutures (Ethicon Ltd, Edinburgh, UK) are recommended as they are not difficult to remove postoperatively. While suction drainage to dead space is preferable, leakage of air around the stoma site can be troublesome and the author uses a small corrugated drain in the inferior aspect of the vertical limb. Because the trachea is acutely angled to the stoma, standard indwelling tubes are best avoided. The author's preference is for no tube, but should peristomal oedema require it, a soft silicone tube or button is safe and effective. In all cases perioperative prophylactic antibiotic therapy with metronidazole and a cephalosporin is administered.

Postoperative management

With this preventive procedure carried out at primary excision the postoperative complications are minimal. The author has not experienced severe intraoperative or postoperative haemorrhage. In addition to preventing internal thoracic artery bleeding, this form of manubrial resection lessens the likelihood of pleural tear and pneumothorax. The author routinely uses bilateral chest drains in all laryngopharyngo-oesophagectomy cases.

Discharge from the drainage area lasting up to 3 weeks after surgery is related to the persisting dead space, but no cases of mediastinitis have been seen by the author.

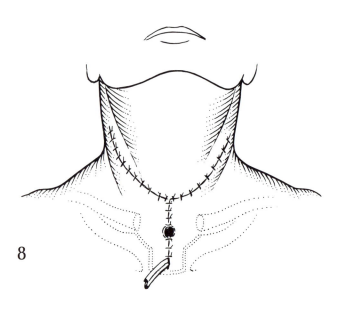

8

MANUBRIAL RESECTION AND MEDIASTINAL DISSECTION FOR THE TREATMENT OF ESTABLISHED STOMAL RECURRENCE

Stomal recurrence is an unpleasant and lethal complication, for which radical surgery offers almost the only hope of cure. Radiotherapy is very rarely curative and may have been given already as part of the primary treatment, so that a full course is not possible. It frequently fails to palliate. Chemotherapy at present has no role to play.

The low cure rate (5-year survival of 20 per cent) and previously documented high rate of complications continue to deter surgeons (and patients) from undertaking wide excisional surgery with manubrial resection and mediastinal dissection. However, in the last decade the use of the myocutaneous flap has markedly decreased the complication rate because it brings a new blood supply to the area and provides pharyngeal repair and protection for the great vessels. The author believes that the procedure can now be safely undertaken.

Likewise, if stomal recurrence necessitates resection of the residual pharynx then reconstruction by well-vascularized gastric transposition or free jejunal transfer provides healthy tissue to cover the great vessels and to obliterate dead space. The author's preference in this circumstance is for gastric transposition as the single orogastric anastomosis high in the neck and generous amounts of gastric tissue (and often omentum) to cover the vessels both help to decrease the local complication rate.

Patients with stomal recurrence are often elderly, with concomitant medical problems, and have compromised wound healing capabilities from previous surgery and irradiation. They must be informed of the serious consequences of the disease and the low cure rates for surgery, but in suitable patients the procedure is the only viable option for cure or worthwhile palliation.

Preoperative assessment of the limits of stomal recurrence is fraught with difficulty and techniques such as tracheal polytomography, barium swallow, CT and MRI scanning cannot be relied upon to ensure resectability and details of the degree of involvement of major vasculature. It is therefore of utmost importance that the patient and operating team understand that the initial part of the operation is an exploration to determine resectability. The initial dissection is directed laterally to assess involvement of the carotid arteries and it is common to have to dissect tumour from the carotid sheath.

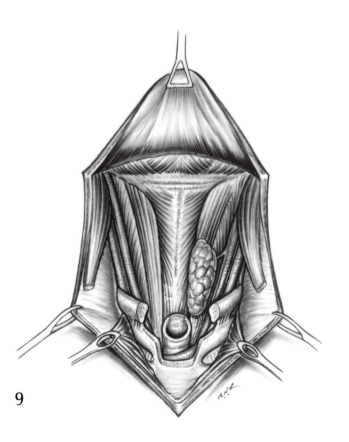

9

Resection and dissection

9

The operative procedure is similar to that already outlined, utilizing the previous Gluck–Soerensen incision and adding the vertical limb downwards in the midline over the manubrium. A 3 cm margin of skin, subcutaneous tissue and sternomastoid around the recurrence is included in the resection. After assessment of carotid involvement and resectability the manubrium is resected as previously described.

Dissection of the tissues involved then proceeds from superior to inferior and may necessitate removal of pharynx, residual thyroid, trachea, cervical oesphagus and all associated paratracheal areolar and lymphoid tissue. The brachiocephalic and left common carotid arteries should be identified and cleared and the left innominate vein may be retracted downwards or resected. Finally the trachea is divided as low down as necessary to release the specimen. *Illustration 9* shows the defect after excision in a case where pharynx and contralateral thyroid did not require resection. These early localized stomal recurrences are unfortunately in the minority.

Reconstruction and repair

Following excision of pharynx/oesophagus

The author's preference is for gastric transposition with its single high anastomosis and generous amounts of new tissue. Free jejunum, transposed colon and pectoralis major reconstruction of the pharynx all involve less reliable anastomoses. It is the anastomotic leak, with its effects on the adjacent vessels, and mediastinitis that causes the morbidity and mortality in this group. Whatever the surgeon's choice of pharyngeal reconstruction it should be of the highest standard and is definitely not for the occasional operator.

Inability to form a new tracheal stoma in the skin of the vertical incision over the resected manubrium is very rare. The anterior stomach wall occupying the stomal excision site can be skin grafted directly with good results; it does not require cover with a further deltopectoral or pectoralis major flap.

Following excision of stomal recurrence without pharyngeal or oesophageal resection

Initially, the author used to rotate a complete pectoralis major myocutaneous flap into the stomal defect and form the new tracheal stoma in the centre of the myocutaneous flap. However, necrosis of the surrounding flap and subsequent problems of stomal stenosis have meant that the stoma is now formed, as before, in the vertical limb of the initial incision and pectoralis major simply rotated into the defect above the new stoma. Pectoralis major is left attached to the clavicle in the region of the thoraco-acromial vessels but its insertion onto the humerus is divided so that the muscle flap can be mobilized in the standard way and easily rotated into the defect.

The muscle flap is considerably less bulky than the complete myocutaneous flap and is easily approximated to the edges of the skin defect. It then readily accepts a split thickness skin graft. The decreased bulk allows the inferiorly placed stoma to be far less affected and the muscle flap conforms to the surrounding tissues with less tension and impairment of its vascularity. This has been found to be an excellent method with few complications and better overall results.

Postoperative management

There are few postoperative complications with both of the above techniques provided that anastomotic leakage does not occur. Dedicated nursing and medical staff are required, with meticulous attention being paid to all factors affecting healing and the conditions of the new stoma and flaps. Many patients undergoing resection for stomal recurrence will have had total thyroidectomy and parathyroidectomy and will require appropriate replacement therapy.

Further reading

Mast WR, Jafek BW. Mediastinal anatomy for the mediastinoscopist. *Arch Otolaryngol* 1975; 101: 596–9.

Sisson GA, Bytell DE, Becker SP. Mediastinal dissection – 1976: indications and newer techniques. *Laryngoscope* 1976; 87: 751–9.

Harrison DFN. Resection of the manubrium. *Br J Surg* 1977; 64: 374–7.

Schuller DE, Hamaker RC, Gluckman JL. Mediastinal dissection: a multi-institutional assessment. *Arch Otolaryngol* 1981; 107: 715–20.

Surgical methods to aid vocal rehabilitation after laryngectomy

A. D. Cheesman FRCS
Royal National Throat, Nose and Ear Hospital and Head and Neck Unit, Charing Cross Hospital, London, UK

David J. Howard FRCS, FRCS(Ed)
Institute of Laryngology and Otology, Royal National Throat, Nose and Ear Hospital, London, UK

Introduction

The literature dealing with voice restoration after laryngeal surgery is vast. In no other area of laryngology has the ingenuity of surgeons, patients, speech therapists, nurses, scientists and prosthetic manufacturers been more apparent. The history of these efforts is a fascinating one and began even before the Edinburgh surgeon, T. H. Watson, removed a syphilitic larynx in 1866. The history is beyond the scope of this chapter, but the authors recommend that all surgeons dealing with significant numbers of laryngectomy patients should study this literature carefully for there is much in the past which is still of relevance. An understanding of the basic physiology of voice and speech is also vital.

Physiology

Voice is the vibrating column of air that results from phonation at the vocal folds and is driven by the expiratory air flow from the lungs. Speech results when voice is resonated and articulated by the upper vocal tract.

Speech thus has four components: (1) the initiating expiratory air flow from the lungs; (2) the phonatory vibration from the vocal folds; (3) enhancement by the resonators of the upper vocal tract; and (4) articulation by the articulators of the upper vocal tract.

1 & 2

Following laryngectomy there is a loss of voice due to the surgical removal of the folds (the vibrator) and redirection of the expiratory air flow (the initiator) out through the stoma. The resonators and articulators are generally unaffected. Successful rehabilitation of the voice requires the restoration of an initiator and a new vibrator. Fortunately the muscular walls of the reconstructed pharynx can function as a remarkably effective vibrator which is known as the pharyngo-oesophageal (P–E) segment. To initiate a vibrating column of air or voice, air must be introduced into the oesophagus below the P–E segment. This can be achieved by the transoral injection of air as seen in conventional oesophageal speech, or by rediversion from the respiratory tract by a surgically created tracheo-oesophageal fistula. This latter type of initiator obviously has the greatest potential for the restoration of near normal voice, allowing loud and sustained speech.

Consequently most surgical interest is currently concerned with fistula techniques with or without prostheses. The main alternative method of speech rehabilitation is some form of electromechanical device to create a vibrating column of air directly in the upper vocal tract where it can be articulated.

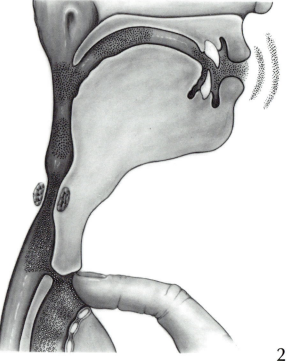

1

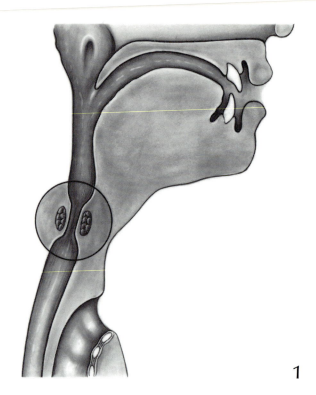

2

Selection of a vocal rehabilitation technique

The incidence, distribution and management of laryngeal cancer varies considerably around the world and management plans proposed by American and European authors may not be appropriate in many parts of the world. Many of the currently recommended prostheses are not readily available and their expense may be an important factor. It is also very important for the surgeon to realize that prosthetic speech rehabilitation is an on-going method of treatment requiring both time and expertise for success, consequently cooperation with a speech therapist is recommended.

The choice of the best mode of communication postoperatively in any given setting requires consideration of the medical, social, psychological and educational aspects of each patient and should involve discussion between the surgeon, speech therapist and the patient and his relatives, preferably before laryngectomy.

Medical factors

The age, dexterity and general medical condition of the patient are important considerations. For example, those patients with significant arthritis, poor vision, tremors, stomal stenosis, copious tracheal mucus, tracheal hypersensitivity, chronic alcoholism or severe depression may be poor candidates for many of the modern tracheo-oesophageal fistula techniques requiring prostheses. These patients sadly often fail to develop adequate oesophageal speech and an electronic neck vibrator device may be their only possible means of communication.

The effect of radiation on vocal rehabilitation techniques remains a highly controversial area. The sore throat, oedema, loss of saliva and reduced compliance of the residual pharyngo-oesophageal tissue seen during radiotherapy undoubtedly impairs the acquisition of voice. However, an individual's reaction to radiation treatment is extremely variable, and while some are able to continue with speech therapy and actually develop oesophageal speech during the treatment, others have such marked reactions that they find it impossible to use even a simple electronic neck vibrator because of pain and oedema.

There are conflicting views when considering the long-term effects of radiotherapy. In the authors' practice prior irradiation has not been found to be a contraindication to any methods of voice restoration, except for the Staffieri procedure (see p. 520).

Surgical factors

While still subject to debate, there is no good evidence that the type of neck incision, method of total laryngectomy, or use of concomitant neck dissection, have any appreciable effect on vocal rehabilitation. However, most surgeons involved in surgical speech rehabilitation feel that the method of pharyngeal reconstruction is of vital importance and generally will make some attempt to adjust its post-laryngectomy tonus. Similarly, those patients with advanced disease who undergo laryngectomy and multiple surgery such as fistula repair, myocutaneous flaps and further neck dissections do undoubtedly have a significantly reduced chance of effective communication.

Other surgical factors which affect the outcome of vocal rehabilitation are problems with the articulators, tongue, floor of mouth and oropharynx – most notably the accidental division of one or other hypoglossal nerves during routine total laryngectomy.

The debate regarding the importance of inferior constrictor repair continues. In the past, preservation and repair of these muscles was thought a necessity for the production of a good oesophageal voice. More recently Singer et al.[1] and others have reported cricopharyngeal muscle spasm as being a major factor in preventing acquisition of voice and recommend a posterior myotomy of the pharynx at the time of laryngectomy, or as a later secondary procedure in those cases of failed oesophageal voice. Our own experience shows that a low short myotomy of the reconstructed pharynx is important for the easy production of both oesophageal and fistula voice.

Social and psychological factors

While most surgeons and speech therapists feel that motivation plays an important role in the development of speech following laryngectomy, it is something that has proved elusive to define and the literature contains conflicting studies. The individual's sex, level of intelligence, employment and income have not been found consistently to correlate with the outcome. However, in common with other colleagues, the authors feel that patients from large active families, particularly those with supportive partners, develop better communication skills. There is no doubt that those patients who achieve good vocal rehabilitation have a considerably improved quality of life compared with those who are unsuccessful and this is the basis of our current study.

Surgical techniques

Prior to 1980 there were a variety of different surgical procedures designed to create a fistula but they were all complicated by either a tendency to stenosis or aspiration.

3

The most commonly used procedure is that described by Staffieri and in unirradiated patients it can have very gratifying results. However, in the authors' practice most cases have had primary radiotherapy and our experience of the Staffieri neoglottic procedure has been unsatisfactory. In the developing world this procedure may have much to offer where prostheses are not freely available and the quality of radiotherapy is questionable.

Primary total laryngectomy with speech rehabilitation will probably produce the best cure rate with minimal functional mutilation.

The demonstration of an effective simple tracheo-oesophageal puncture procedure by Singer and Blom[2] in 1980 started the current enormous enthusiasm for surgical speech rehabilitation. They used a simple one-way valve that allows air diversion into the oesophagus on occluding the stoma with a finger, and prevents aspiration into the trachea during swallowing. Similar prostheses were rapidly introduced, such as those by Panje and the Gronigen group. There was a period of considerable competition between the various prostheses in the early 1980s and several significant improvements have been made.

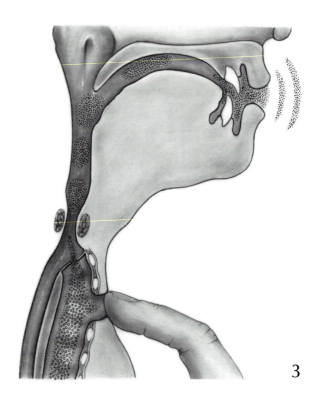

3

4

Most of the current available prostheses have their proponents but the authors have mainly used the Blom–Singer group of prostheses which they find give the most consistent results. However it is true to say that the fitting of these particular valves needs both care and experience. Currently we use both the standard duck-bill prosthesis and the low pressure prosthesis, particularly in those patients with either increased pharyngeal tone or a narrow oesophageal segment.

The use of this method of speech rehabilitation by an experienced team is generally very successful, over 90 per cent of patients initially acquiring voice. With time the continued use of fistula voice as the primary mode of communication by patients declines, reaching about 70 per cent by 12 months. The success rate is higher in those patients with primary puncture performed at the time of laryngectomy. In such cases the surgeon can control the method of pharyngeal reconstruction and voice production can virtually be guaranteed.

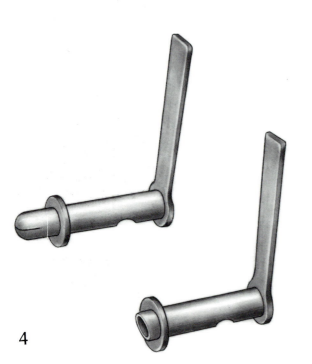

4

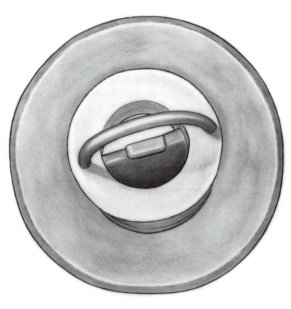

5 & 6

Blom and Singer have also developed a stomal valve which allows the patient to phonate without the need to occlude the stoma by a finger.

5

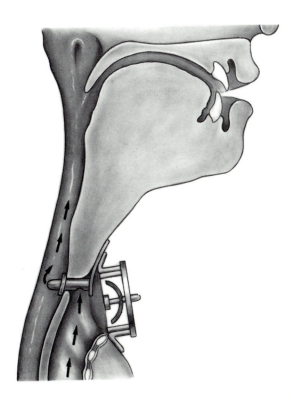

6

Preoperative

Primary puncture

Those patients undergoing primary puncture at the time of total laryngectomy should receive full preoperative counselling from both the surgeon and speech therapist. They are given an explanation of the timescale of events postoperatively and some simple initial details with regard to the valve, the likely acquisition of speech, and some realistic expectation of what it will be like. Further counselling by an experienced laryngectomee is of considerable value.

Those established laryngectomees who seek secondary speech rehabilitation require particularly careful assessment to ensure satisfactory results. This is especially true of those who have failed to acquire oesophageal voice.

Secondary puncture

An assessment of the function of the P–E segment is essential and the air insufflation test described by Taub and Bergner[3] has been advocated as the best method. It consists of inserting a 14 Fr gauge red rubber catheter transnasally into the upper oesophagus. The examiner blows air into the oesophagus via the catheter, thus eliminating any problems the patient may have with air injection into the oesophageal reservoir. The patient opens his/her mouth and as the catheter is gently manipulated up and down the vocal tract, passive oesophageal voice may be heard. This allows the examiner to assess the presence or absence of a vibrating segment, the air pressure required to produce voice, and the resistance to air flow through the P–E segment. Used without videofluoroscopy this test is not entirely reliable as there is uncertainty of the position of the end of the catheter and a qualitative assessment of the P–E segment is not possible. Consequently, videofluoroscopy is an important part of our detailed work-up of patients requesting secondary puncture or, perhaps more appro-

priately, analysis of why they fail to achieve oesophageal voice.

We undertake a detailed assessment which includes a questionnaire covering the patient's previous surgery, the amount of speech therapy and the present status of their voice and swallowing. Videofluoroscopy is performed at a combined clinic involving an ENT surgeon, radiologist, speech therapist, and audiovisual recording technician. The radiological appearances of the reconstructed pharynx and upper oesophagus are recorded during the events of swallowing, attempted oesophageal phonation, and phonation with air insufflation. It is only by viewing the dynamic aspects of the whole vocal tract that problems can be defined and categorized.

The first part of videofluoroscopy is a straightforward barium swallow study and this is used to detect the presence of a stricture which will not dilate during the swallow. The presence of a stricture, if short, may be corrected by local pharyngeal surgery, but if the stricture is long then correction with a distant skin flap or free jejunal graft with microvascular anastomosis is essential for good voice rehabilitation as well as improving the swallow.

The next two steps in videofluoroscopy study the dynamic changes of the pharynx during phonation, the changes being demonstrated by initially coating the pharyngeal wall with barium. The patient is first asked to attempt phonation which tests both the injection and vocal phases of oesophageal speech. Subsequently the injection phase is bypassed by using air insufflation to inflate the oesophageal reservoir and then phonation is again attempted. Experience in over 250 videofluoroscopies with pressure recordings has allowed us to classify our patients according to variations in muscular tone of the reconstructed pharynx. There is a spectrum of tonicity from hypotonicity through normal tonicity (as seen in good oesophageal speakers) to those with increased pharyngeal tone which we have classified at two levels – hypertonicity with increased tone, and spasm with a very high muscular tone.

Hypotonic pharyngeal musculature

7

These patients demonstrate the rapid passage of barium through the pharynx during barium swallow and with both attempted phonation and insufflation very little narrowing is seen in the region of the P–E segment. The voice is weak and whispery. A P–E segment can be created by digital pressure on the front of the neck and this is rewarded by an increase in vocal strength.

Normal tone of the pharyngeal musculature

The correct tonicity is demonstrated in good oesophageal speakers who generally have a single well-defined P–E segment and an easy production of voice. Further studies of the P–E segment in those patients where the method of pharyngeal repair was controlled at the time of laryngectomy, with a view to enhancing voice rehabilitation, show a smooth entry from the oesophagus into the P–E segment to be an important factor.

Increased pharyngeal tone

1. *Hypertonicity.* With hypertonic patients there is often some narrowing of the pharynx during barium swallow but this generally can be seen to dilate up on some swallows. With attempted phonation and air insufflation often two or three P–E segments are seen, and the speech is often strained and erratic. On insufflation, voice production is achieved if air blowing is applied gently. These patients will benefit from secondary myotomy but can often be managed with a low pressure prosthesis.
2. *Pharyngeal spasm.* Pharyngeal spasm is a severe degree of hypertonicity and there is complete obstruction to air flow through the P–E segment. On attempted phonation, air fails to pass through the P–E segment to charge the oesophageal reservoir. When the oesophageal reservoir is inflated by insufflation, the P–E segment again closes tightly and no air passes through it to produce voice. These patients occasionally have voice following laryngectomy, but it is typically of short duration with a high-pitched tone and has been described as having a 'Donald Duck' quality. This is classified as pharyngeal voice, with the vibrating

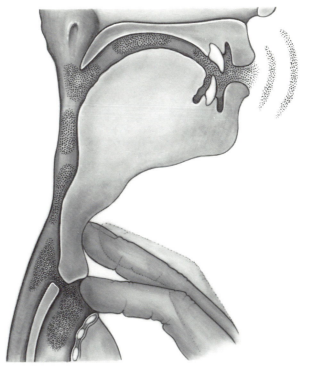

7

segment located between the base of tongue and posterior pharyngeal wall and a small air reservoir in the upper pharynx.

Patients with frank pharyngeal spasm require a myotomy for vocal rehabilitation and often obtain dramatic results both for oesophageal and fistula speech. The patient's speech is videotaped before and after surgery. This allows independent assessment of the success of voice production and more complex measures of vocal function can be made. An ENT assessment is made of the stoma size and contours. The patient is then counselled about his failure to acquire oesophageal voice and informed of the rehabilitative surgery necessary to achieve satisfactory speech. An assessment is also made of the patient's intelligence, motivation and any relevant problems such as alcoholism, visual deficiencies, locomotor difficulties and adverse social circumstances.

Operations

VOICE RESTORATION AS A PRIMARY PROCEDURE

The authors have been assessing the results of tracheo-oesophageal puncture performed at the time of laryngectomy as a primary procedure since 1983. To date over 100 patients have had primary voice restoration undertaken. The main consideration in performing total laryngectomy for carcinoma must be to achieve a radical excision of tumour giving the best chance of cure.

The tracheo-oesophageal puncture is performed once the larynx is removed and prior to repair of the pharynx. Correct siting, shape and size of the tracheostome are important, and the trachea is cut at an oblique angle leaving a high posterior wall. A small disc of skin is excised, and the stoma is included in a Gluck–Soerensen incision or placed in a separate incision below. It is essential to ensure an adequate diameter of 15–18 mm depending on the size of the patient's fingers and good skin-to-mucosal apposition is obtained by careful suturing, the tension of the trachea being borne by subcutaneous sutures through the peritracheal fascia.

A flat anterior aspect of the neck adjacent to the stoma allows a more comfortable fitting of the tracheo-oesophageal prosthesis and in some patients the stomal valve. This is achieved by performing a bilateral sternomastoid tenotomy.

Horizontal closure of the pharyngeal defect is preferable and ensures a pharynx with a large lumen. This involves mucosal closure by suturing vallecular mucosa to the upper edge of the hypopharynx or postcricoid mucosa. Flexion of the head is sometimes required at this stage. The mucosal repair is reinforced by suturing together the two inferior constrictors loosely in front of the pharynx. These are also sutured to the suprahyoid muscles. Prior to pharyngeal closure a 2–3 cm posterior myotomy is performed in the region of the cricopharyngeus muscle and upper oesophageal sphincter to avoid hypertonicity or subsequent problems with spasm.

The residual thyroid gland is sutured laterally so that it is clear of the proposed tracheo-oesophageal puncture site. The upper end of the posterior wall of the trachea is sutured to the oesophagus in preparation for the tracheo-oesophageal puncture which is performed through the posterior tracheal–anterior oesophageal wall 5 mm from the future mucocutaneous junction of the tracheostome. A 14 Fr Ryle's tube is passed through the puncture and then distally down the oesophagus into the stomach and serves as the feeding tube in the postoperative period. Following its removal at 10–14 days after the operation, an appropriately sized Blom–Singer valve is inserted prior to postoperative speech therapy.

VOICE RESTORATION AS A SECONDARY PROCEDURE

Secondary puncture may be performed either as a planned procedure after laryngectomy or for failure to acquire oesophageal voice. Although in the hands of an experienced surgeon primary puncture is generally successful, many surgeons are unhappy with the idea of primary puncture, preferring to get full and satisfactory healing after laryngectomy before contemplating a fistula technique. Even with meticulous technique at total laryngectomy, subsequent fistula formation could in theory be attributed to the valve prosthesis. It is not always possible at laryngectomy to predict the ultimate intratracheal angle at the stoma, and it is common to have oedema around the tracheostome so that occasionally the airway is compromised if a prosthesis is in place. Finally, in the immediate postoperative period there may be significant oedema of the hypopharynx, particularly in those patients who have received recent radiotherapy, to cause difficulty with both swallowing and vibration of the pharyngo-oesophageal segment mucosa, and this may result in initial patient discouragement. A planned secondary procedure is still most commonly employed and is usually undertaken 4–6 weeks after total laryngectomy. In the intervening period an electro-larynx is used to improve communication and minimize post-laryngectomy depression, but the speech quality is mechanical and often difficult to understand so not all patients find it beneficial.

As mentioned already, the preoperative assessment before secondary puncture, particularly in failed oesophageal speakers of long standing, may reveal factors such as a small stoma, pharyngeal stricture or hypertonicity which will require additional surgery to overcome these factors prior to insertion of the valve.

Operative technique

Many variations of this simple procedure have been described. It is usually done under general anaesthesia using a small 4.5 mm or 5 mm cuffed endotracheal tube inserted in the tracheostoma. This can be removed for short periods if necessary to allow better access during the procedure.

While a wide variety of modified oesophagoscopes and bronchoscopes have been described for this technique, the authors use a standard adult Negus (distally-lit) bronchoscope which is passed under direct vision into the pharynx approximately 5 cm past the level of the stoma. It is then rotated 180° and slowly withdrawn until the light can be seen clearly through the posterior wall of the upper trachea in the midline. The puncture is then made through the transilluminated party wall into the lumen of the bronchoscope.

One method uses a custom-made flexible sharpened trocar to which is attached a 14 Fr catheter. The trocar and catheter pass safely through the upper pharynx within the lumen of the bronchoscope and are brought out through the mouth. The catheter is then repassed back down the oesophagus towards the stomach and could be used as a feeding tube, but it is our custom to resume feeding after 24 h.

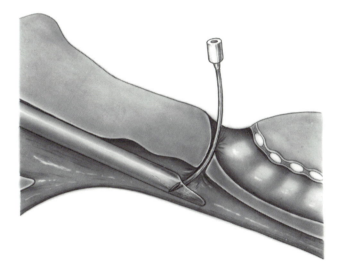

8

8

Blom and Singer in their initial report described a technique using a trocar fashioned from a disposable 14 Fr gauge intravenous catheter set, bent to form a C-shaped curve and introduced through the tracheo-oesophageal party wall into the tip of the bronchoscope. The needle is then removed and the disposable intravenous catheter remains positioned in the bronchoscope.

9

The distal end of this catheter is then attached to a 14 Fr urethral catheter and following dilatation of the tracheal puncture with a right-angled haemostat, the catheter can be drawn into the bronchoscope for a distance of 3–4 cm.

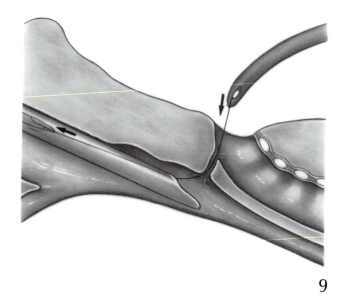

9

10

10

The intravenous catheter is then released from the catheter which is pulled back a little until there is only 1 or 2 cm inside the bronchoscope. An alligator forceps is then used to tip the end of the catheter down into the oesophagus where it is pushed for a distance of 5–6 cm. After making sure that the catheter is positioned correctly in the oesophagus pointing downwards, the broncho-scope is withdrawn.

A 2/0 silk suture is used to sew the catheter to the skin immediately above the mucocutaneous junction. The catheter is additionally bent and taped to the chest and, if necessary, the patient may be fed through this catheter for the next 2 days, minimizing the risk of leakage around the catheter into the mediastinum.

10

Postoperative management

Valve fitting

On the second postoperative day the catheter is removed and the length of the fistula tract is measured with the gauge to determine the correct size of Blom–Singer prosthesis. With the catheter out, open-tract voicing is attempted by exhaling against an occluded stoma. If good voice is obtained then we can be sure that the vocal tract is satisfactory for speech rehabilitation. Normally a correctly sized duck-bill prosthesis is used as these are easier for the patient to manage; however, if voice production is poor, a low-pressure prosthesis is more appropriate. It is very important to ensure that the prosthesis is correctly placed with the inner retention flange in the oesophageal lumen. During the following month the oedema around the puncture often decreases and the prosthesis can be sized down one or even two lengths. The patient then receives instructions with regard to stoma occlusion, proper breath control, articulation, muscle relaxation and removal, cleaning, and replacement of the Blom–Singer valve. The diet remains unrestricted and patients are released from hospital 4–7 days later.

Outcome

As stated previously, initial voice acquisition should be possible in around 90 per cent of patients, but these impressive figures reduce to approximately 70 per cent at 1 year for both primary and secondary puncture patients. Unfortunately, preoperative expectations from both patient and surgeon may be unrealistic and there is no doubt that with the primary patients some may dislike the sound of their tracheo-oesophageal voice when comparing it with their normal voice. The secondary patients, who have had time to realize how difficult life is without a voice, have a better acceptance of the change in voice quality and are generally more enthusiastic for the procedure. This is, perhaps, fortunate as secondary patients often have an increased incidence of problems, but significant complication is rare. While the majority of patients are trouble-free once the valves have been fitted, a number of minor problems are encountered – particularly when patients are initially fitted with the voice prosthesis. These difficulties require the combined efforts of the otolaryngologist, speech therapist and patient and it is necessary to maintain a constant level of enthusiasm to ensure the continued success of the technique.

Complications

Apart from the personal enthusiasm already mentioned, patients need general support in the environment to which they are returning, and initial help to deal with the cleaning and manipulation of the voice prosthesis. Adequate manual dexterity is required for this and it is important that the patient can visualize the fistula site. While some patients remove and clean their prosthesis daily, others will leave them in place for many months without removal. The average life of the prosthesis is about 3 months but varies from weeks to many months.

Extrusion

It is now rare for voice prostheses to extrude spontaneously if they have been correctly sized initially. The majority are accidentally pulled out by patients during prosthesis cleaning and manipulation. In patients who use a tracheostoma valve to allow hand-free voicing, the flange of the underlying prosthesis may become adherent to the edge of the tracheostoma valve and is dislodged when the housing is removed.

Cases have been reported where the prosthesis has been inhaled and required removal via a bronchoscope. It is important that the patient carries a 14 Fr whistle-tip red rubber catheter at all times and is therefore able to insert this into the fistula site. If they have difficulties they must attend an ENT department within 1–2 h as, without the placement of this catheter, the fistula closes rapidly in some patients. Attending an ENT unit unfamiliar with tracheo-oesophageal fistula techniques is often unsatisfactory and may lead to confusion, as many patients have learnt to their cost. Fistulae which have begun to stenose may be dilated with urethral dilators and catheters of increasing size until the voice prosthesis can be reintroduced. In expert hands this can be undertaken many hours later and avoids the necessity of repuncture. In most large series, 10–20 per cent of cases have required repuncture at some time.

Aspiration and dysphagia

Leakage through the lumen of the voice prosthesis is generally a sign that the prosthesis needs replacing; it may also occur when the prosthesis is over-fitted and the excess length causes the duck-bill to touch the posterior oesophageal wall and results in incompetence of the valve. This sometimes occurs with correctly sized valves and can be overcome by using the low-pressure prosthesis which has a shorter intraoesophageal length. Videofluoroscopy is advised in such cases to confirm the diagnosis and to exclude the presence of any concomitant pathophysiology.

Tissue reaction at fistula site

Granulations may form around the tracheal opening of the fistula and these may be associated with crusting and bleeding. They are usually managed by silver nitrate cautery or cryocautery on an outpatient basis, but occasionally they may be so prominent as to require removal of the voice prosthesis and insertion of a catheter for 48 h. In severe cases a trunk of tissue may grow around the lumen of the fistula, pouting out into both the trachea and the oesophagus at each end of the fistula and eventually rendering the use of the prosthesis difficult owing to occlusion of the airway and leakage. Surgical removal of these outgrowths may be occasionally required and it may be necessary to close the fistula and repuncture at a later date. Histological examination of these tracts in the authors' series have demonstrated chronic inflammation and fibrosis, the cause of which remains unknown. Silicone prostheses may stimulate a foreign body reaction which may be exacerbated by secondary bacterial infection or fungus.

Fungal contamination

Silicone and other medical plastics are prone to fungal infestation in some patients. *Candida* eats into the silicone rendering the valves incompetent and is also probably a factor in causing stoma granulations. It is easily recognizable by the pink staining of the prosthesis on removal. Such problems are treated by soaking the prosthesis each day in hydrogen peroxide solution and the patient needs to use two prostheses on alternate days. The pharynx and fistula tract should also be periodically disinfected by sucking a amphotericin lozenge daily for 14 days.

Conclusion

Most complications with Blom–Singer prostheses can be overcome by simple voice prosthesis re-selection or minor surgery. When the prosthesis has extruded it is often possible to salvage the situation by prompt catheter re-insertion and/or dilatation. All procedures of this nature are dependent upon careful patient selection and regular follow-up and this will obviate many of the complications. The constant enthusiasm and support of the medical team encouraging patients to seek expert advice promptly is paramount to success in this rewarding area of speech rehabilitation.

References

1. Singer MI, Blom ED, Hamaker RC. Further experience with voice restoration after total laryngectomy. *Ann Otol Rhinol Laryngol* 1981; 90: 498–502.

2. Singer MI, Blom ED. An endoscopic technique for restoration of voice after laryngectomy. *Ann Otol Rhinol Laryngol* 1980; 89: 529–33.

3. Taub S, Bergner LH. Air bypass voice prosthesis for vocal rehabilitation of laryngectomees. *Am J Surg* 1973; 125: 748–56.

Further reading

Cheesman AD, Knight J, McIvor J, Perry A. Tracheo-oesophageal 'puncture speech'. An assessment technique for failed oesophageal speakers. *J Laryngol Otol* 1986; 100: 191–9.

Lund VJ, Perry A, Cheesman AD. Blom–Singer puncture. Practicalities in everyday management. *J Laryngol Otol* 1987; 101: 164–8.

Milford CA, Perry A, Mugliston TA, Cheesman AD. A British experience of surgical voice restoration as a primary procedure. *Arch Otolaryngol Head Neck Surg* 1988; 114: 1419–21.

Bleach N, Perry AR, Cheesman AD. Surgical voice restoration with the Blom–Singer prosthesis following laryngopharyngo-oesophagectomy and pharyngogastric anastomosis. *Ann Otol Rhinol Laryngol* 1991; 100: 142–7

Illustrations by Gillian Lee

Surgical management of vocal fold paralysis

Patrick J. Bradley FRCS
Consultant Otolaryngologist and Head and Neck Oncologist, University Hospital, Nottingham, UK

Introduction

The human larynx has three major functions which are the maintenance of the airway, protection of the airway and phonation. Interference with any of these functions will make the patient symptomatic and cause him to seek medical advice. The most frequent symptom at the time of presentation is hoarseness of voice. Clinical examination of the larynx is mandatory in the evaluation of every patient who presents with alteration of voice. Not infrequently, a unilateral immobile vocal fold (vocal fold paralysis) is seen either by indirect laryngoscopy or nasoendoscopy. Further investigations to elucidate the cause are required, as the finding of an immobile vocal fold is only the effect of some pathological event. Radiological evaluation may include a chest radiograph, skull base series and more commonly a computed tomography (CT) scan or magnetic resonance imaging (MRI) from the skull base to the mediastinum. Evaluation of the swallow mechanism and the oesophagus by contrast radiology may be required. After these investigations have been completed the patients are frequently subjected to endoscopy (laryngoscopy/bronchoscopy/oesophagoscopy) to evaluate the larynx and to confirm the histological nature of any abnormality found clinically or demonstrated by radiology. At the time of endoscopy it is mandatory to test the fixity, laxity or dislocation of the cricoarytenoid joint and also to evaluate whether the fold is fixed because the laryngeal musculature is invaded by tumour or involved by fibrosing or muscular disorders.

The selection of patients for surgical treatment in unilateral vocal fold paralysis cannot be made without determining the prognosis of the paralysis. The following factors influence the prognosis:

1. Aetiology of paralysis. Trauma or neuronitis may have a favourable outcome. Prognosis is poor if the nerve has been sectioned at surgery, invaded by tumour or involved by progressive neural disease.
2. Duration of paralysis. Spontaneous recovery usually takes place within 1 year of onset, in most cases 6 months. Recovery after 1 year is extremely rare.
3. Position of the paralysis. The more medially the paralysed fold is located the better the prognosis.
4. Electromyographic (EMG) findings. The presence of action potentials induced by voluntary activity, including phonation, heralds a likely recovery.
5. Stroboscopic findings. The presence of complete glottic closure and mucosal wave on the paralytic fold indicates a favourable outlook.

When the prognosis of spontaneous recovery of vocal fold function is determined to be poor, surgical intervention is indicated. Patients with a favourable prognosis should be treated expectantly, including speech therapy. If the prognosis cannot be determined, surgery is usually reserved until 6–12 months have elapsed. When the patient has a concomitant disordered protective mechanism causing aspiration and/or a weak cough, surgical intervention is indicated, for example a patient with terminal disease who is not expected to live for a long time.

Aims of management

Treatment is directed to correcting the functional disturbance, creating an airway, and improving the voice or swallow. Correction of one disturbance should not jeopardize any of the other laryngeal functions.

UNILATERAL VOCAL FOLD PARALYSIS

The surgical methods available are intracordal injection, medialization by thyroplasty, nerve–muscle pedicle re-innervation, laryngeal nerve reinnervation and a combination of the above.

INTRACORDAL INJECTION

Indications

The most frequent indication is glottic incompetence caused by unilateral vocal fold paralysis. Treatment is seldom indicated to aid with the management of aspiration when both vocal folds are positioned in abduction. Excellent results can be anticipated when it is used to restore a satisfactory cough.

Contraindications

Surgery or injection should not be used in the treatment of non-organic or functional disorders, or for vocal paralysis in which recovery is anticipated.

Injection materials

Polytetrafluoroethylene (Teflon)

Teflon (E. I. du Pont de Nemours and Company, UK) is the most frequently used substance. Its use indicated when a permanent result is required. Removal is difficult but can be performed endoscopically using a carbon dioxide laser.

After Teflon injection the fold may become red and oedematous and the patient may develop a fever, transient hoarseness and a mild to moderate stiff neck with swollen cervical lymph nodes. The acute postinjection reaction may require a tracheostomy. Foreign body granulomas have been recorded. In acute fulminant reactions, usually associated with upper respiratory tract infections, steroids and antibiotic therapy may be indicated.

Collagen (Phonogel)

Phonogel is bovine dermal collagen which has been solubilized, purified and reconstituted in phosphate buffered physiological saline. The proprietary manufacturing process removes the most highly species-specific segments of the collagen molecules, reducing the potential for the animal collagen to cause an untoward reaction in humans. Following injection the collagen implant forms a cohesive mass which is colonized by loose connective tissue cells. The implant gradually resorbs and is replaced to some extent by the loose connective tissue. Adverse reactions are predominantly local, with a self-limiting hypersensitivity response.

Gelfoam

This is indicated for patients who have a presumed temporary paralysis, such as lower cervical nerve injury following posterior fossa or skull base surgery. Trauma to the recurrent laryngeal nerve during thyroid surgery or cardiac surgery is ideally treated by Gelfoam injection (Upjohn, Kalamazoo, Michigan, USA).

Gelfoam paste injection may be used as a trial before the injection of Teflon to determine possible vocal quality. The Gelfoam paste injection may be repeated if its effect is not adequate and may have a physiological effect for up to 3 months. The Gelfoam paste is made up at the time of the injection. A 1 g jar of sterile Gelfoam powder is mixed in a small basin with 4–4.5 ml sterile saline. A firm paste is developed by vigorous mixing and stirring. This paste is rolled into a cylinder and placed in the chamber of a 5 ml disposable syringe. The chamber of the Arnold–Brunning gun is filled from the 5 ml syringe. Care must be taken to ensure that air bubbles are not trapped within the injection material to avoid underinjection of the paste. Resorption of the Gelfoam is gradual, occurring almost imperceptibly between 6 and 12 weeks after injection. Since the resorption is gradual, the patients may well develop compensation by overclosure of the other mobile fold.

Other materials

These include silicone, paraffin, diced collagen, bone paste, tantalum powder, glycerine and autologous fat.

Basic techniques

Injection can be undertaken transorally using a direct or indirect laryngeal method or by the transcutaneous method through the cricothyroid space. Injection performed by direct laryngoscopy is the easiest and the most popular method. Using the Dedo–Pilling laryngoscope with the Lewy suspension apparatus, it is possible to perform the procedure with the operating microscope. If performed by indirect laryngoscopy, local anaesthesia is to be recommended to aid with the correct placement and evaluation of the vocal function during the procedure. Topical mucosal anaesthesia using lignocaine to the oral cavity and oropharynx helps with the introduction and placement of the endoscope and blocking of the superior laryngeal nerves. Used at the level of the greater horn of the hyoid it aids patient tolerance of the endoscopy. When using the transcutaneous technique the use of the nasoendoscope with video monitoring is essential. When employing any technique under general anaesthesia, caution needs to be used so that correct placement of the paste is achieved and that 'too little' rather than 'too much' is employed. Injection is performed with microscopic visualization using a specially designed injection apparatus such as the Arnold–Brunning Intralaryngeal Teflon set, the McKelvie Teflon Gun, the Nagashima silicone injection set, or the Collagen Xomed Corporation set. Injection is conducted slowly and carefully with visual and if possible auditory monitoring.

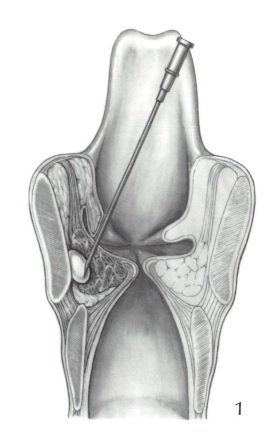

1

Injection under direct vision

The aims are to move the vocal fold towards the mid-sagittal plane and to increase the bulk of the atrophic vocal fold.

1 & 2

The site of injection varies somewhat with the type of the material being used. Teflon or silicone is injected in the lateral portion of the thyroarytenoideus muscle and/or in the space between the thyroarytenoideus muscle and the thyroid cartilage. Injection is first placed laterally and slightly anterior to the tip of the vocal process of the arytenoid cartilage. If this procedure does not bring about a satisfactory result, an additional injection is made lateral to the midpoint of the membranous vocal fold.

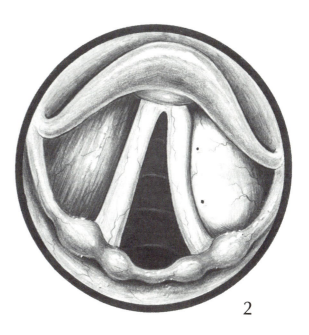

2

3

Collagen can be injected more superficially because its consistency is close to that of human tissue.

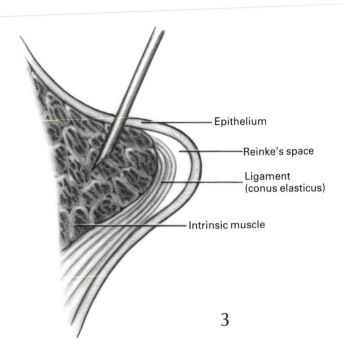

Epithelium

Reinke's space

Ligament (conus elasticus)

Intrinsic muscle

3

Transcutaneous injection

The nasal, pharyngeal and laryngeal mucosa is anaesthetized with topical 4 per cent lignocaine. The patient is placed in the supine position. The fibrescope connected to the video camera is inserted through the nose to just above the vocal folds. The fibrescope image is viewed on the television monitor throughout the procedure. Injection is made through the anterior cervical skin. The needle is inserted at the level of the upper edge of the cricoid cartilage 5–6 mm from the midline on the affected side. The needle is directed laterally, superiorly and posteriorly through the cricothyroid space. To monitor its movement the needle is moved medially back and forth as it proceeds. When small movements are observed in the area laterally and slightly anterior to the tip of the vocal process, the injection is begun. Injection is conducted gradually and carefully with visual and auditory monitoring.

The injection of Teflon or silicone should be placed lateral to the fold and at a depth of 5–6 mm. This moves the vocal fold towards the midline without affecting its free mucosal margin. The most critical area for injection is the midportion of the membranous vocal fold. The second most important area is the junction of the posterior and the middle thirds. Successful glottic closure of the anterior two-thirds of the fold will result in an excellent voice, even though a small cleft remains posteriorly.

Patients with a unilateral vocal fold paralysis are all assessed and advised by the speech therapist. In patients who achieve reasonable to good voice, therapy should be continued. Patients who do not show any improvement within a few sessions, or who have a poor cough with aspiration, are potential candidates for Teflon injection.

Patients are told that the procedure will be carried out under a general or local anaesthetic. They will need to be admitted to hospital the day before and will need to remain in hospital for the night after the procedure. All are told that there is a risk that the airway may be narrowed and that in approximately 1 per cent of cases there is a need for tracheostomy. This tracheostomy will be closed within a few days when the swelling subsides. Should the swelling not reduce it may be necessary to perform another operation to remove some of the Teflon. The patients are also told that they may need a second injection if their symptoms are not improved. The greatest improvement is usually in the patients' ability to cough, followed by voice and, possibly, improvement in swallowing. The patients are told that the voice improvement has a tendency to fade with usage as the day progresses. The majority of patients are delighted with the symptom improvement produced by a single injection. Some surgeons recommend the regular use of antibiotic and steroid cover to reduce the risk of infection and to minimize the possibility of reactive oedema. I do not recommend this as a routine and each case should be treated on its own merits. All patients are kept in hospital overnight following injection and initial voice rest is essential to prevent oedema.

Injection into the anterior half of the membranous vocal fold should be avoided as this causes localized protrusion of the vocal fold edge and results in inadequate glottic closure. Similarly, injection into the mucosa should also be avoided, as this reduces mucosal pliability and interferes with the mucosal vibratory wave and may subsequently lead to dysphonia. The needles used should be bevelled and the route of the injected substance should be lateral.

Advantages

The technique is reasonably safe and reliable provided the defect to be overcome does not exceed 2–4 mm at the posterior glottic area. The bolus of the injected substance, Teflon or silicone, should be sufficient to restore a good cough and improve the volume of the voice.

Disadvantages

The technique will not overcome a greater than 4 mm posterior glottic chink and although it will medialize the vocal fold it will not restore the ability of the vocal fold to tense. While volume is improved, pitch may not alter, and approximately 1 per cent of patients are at risk of a tracheostomy.

Limitations of Teflon intracordal injection

Patients must be informed of the possible need for tracheostomy and should not be injected when the airway is compromised. It is preferable to wait for up to 12 months after the onset of paralysis. Diplophonia or other forms of dysphonia may persist following injection, resulting from underinjection, extrusion or displacement of the material. It may not be possible to visualize the larynx by the usual laryngoscopic methods required for injection, e.g. in patients with trismus or cervical arthritis. In approximately 15 per cent of patients there is no improvement in voice quality following injection.

MEDIALIZATION SURGERY

The following techniques are most frequently used to treat unilateral vocal fold paralysis but are also occasionally used for glottic insufficiency caused by surgery or trauma. The techniques available are surgical augmentation, medialization laryngoplasty and arytenoid rotation.

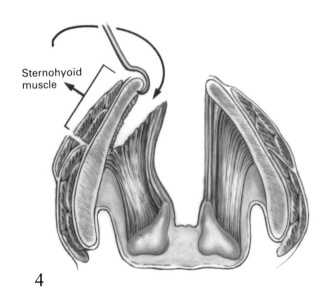

Sternohyoid muscle

4

Surgical augmentation

4

The aim is to place augmentation material (autograft cartilage, silicone or muscle) immediately inside the thyroid cartilage at the level of the vocal fold, and thus move the vocal fold medially.

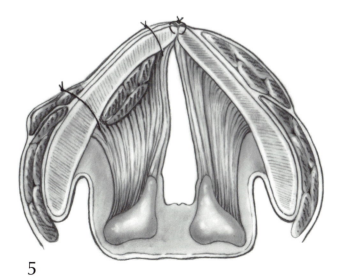

5

5

The surgery may be conducted under local anaesthesia, with nasoendoscopy and video monitor control. A horizontal skin incision is made along the lower edge of the thyroid cartilage on the paralysed side. Following elevation of the skin anterior to the thyroid cartilage, the sternohyoid muscles are retracted laterally, exposing the thyroid cartilage. A superior, anterior, anteroinferior or window approach can be used to gain entry to the inner aspect of the thyroid ala.

Following any of these approaches the augmentation material should be placed lateral to the vocal fold.

Medialization laryngoplasty

The aim is to move part of the thyroid ala medially at the level of the vocal fold, pushing the vocal fold edge towards the midline.

6

Under local anaesthesia, the thyroid ala is exposed. The rectangular section of cartilage which is to be medialized is outlined. The upper edge is positioned horizontally at the mid-level of the anterior angle of the thyroid ala. The lower edge is placed parallel to the upper edge. The distance between the two edges is approximately the same as one quarter of the height of the anterior angle of the thyroid ala. The anterior edge of the rectangle is located approximately 5 mm from the midline, whereas the posterior edge is located slightly posterior to the anteroposterior midpoint of the thyroid ala, where the tip of the vocal process of the arytenoid cartilage is located. A knife or an oscillating saw is used to cut through the cartilage. The inner perichondrium should not be sectioned.

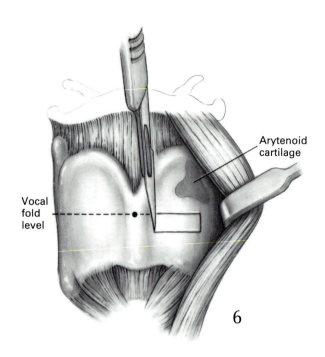

Arytenoid cartilage

Vocal fold level

6

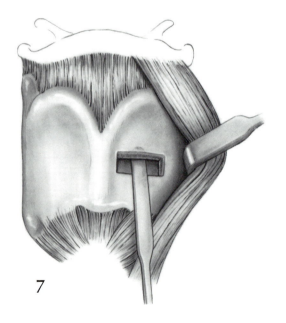

7

7

The mobile quadrangle is then displaced medially while the patient phonates.

8

When the best location of the displaced segment is determined, it is held in place by inserting a silicone flange through the window. The size of the flange should be adjusted depending on the location of the segment to be held. Besides the auditory monitoring, visual monitoring by means of a fibrescope may be employed to aid with selecting the best displacement. The wound is closed in a standard fashion.

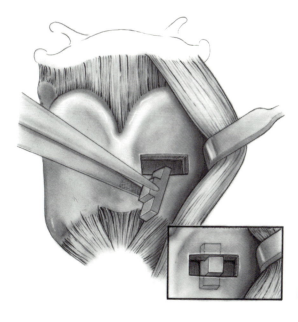

8

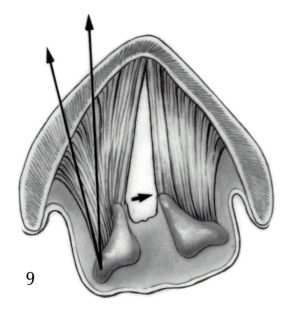

9

Rotation of the arytenoid cartilage

9

This procedure rotates the arytenoid cartilage by pulling the muscular process in the direction of the force of the adductor muscle, bringing the tip of the vocal process towards the midline.

The surgery is performed under local anaesthetic. A horizontal skin incision is made at the mid-thyroid cartilage level from the middle of the anterior neck to the anterior border of the sternocleidomastoid muscle on the affected side. The thyropharyngeal muscle of the inferior constrictor muscle is exposed and vertically sectioned along the posterior edge of the thyroid cartilage. The cricothyroid joint is dislocated and the posterior edge of the thyroid ala is reflected anteromedially. The mucosa of the piriform sinus is elevated upwards. The location of the muscular process is identified by palpation of the upper rim of the cricoid cartilage anteroposteriorly. The crico-arytenoid joint is opened laterally. The muscular process is pulled anteromedioinferiorly with a 3/0 nylon suture. The nylon suture is then fixed to the thyroid ala through two small drilled holes. The holes are made near the junction of the anterior third and the lower fourth of the thyroid ala. The necessary extent of the pull is determined by auditory and visual monitoring. Excessive pull causes overadduction of the vocal fold, resulting in difficulty with phonation if not with respiration. The wound is closed in layers in a standard fashion. The operation has the advantage that it can be used when the posterior glottic chink is greater than 4 mm.

NERVE–MUSCLE PEDICLE REINNERVATION

This procedure aims to provide restoration of adduction of the paralysed fold but also has the potential for restoring the tensing capability of the vocal fold with the resultant possibility of a superior voice. It is indicated in those patients who are considered to have a 'valuable voice', such as lawyers, clergymen, actors, singers and others who depend upon their voices for a living.

10

An incision is made at the lower border of the thyroid cartilage on the paralysed side to expose the sternocleido-mastoid muscle. This muscle is retracted and the branch of the ansa hypoglossi to the anterior belly of the omohyoid is identified. The nerve–muscle pedicle is produced, care being taken to identify the actual point of entry of the nerve into the muscle

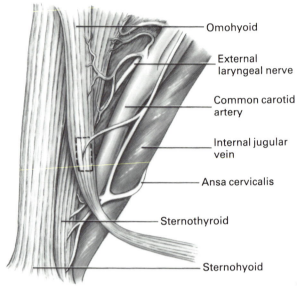

— Omohyoid

— External laryngeal nerve

— Common carotid artery

— Internal jugular vein

— Ansa cervicalis

— Sternothyroid

— Sternohyoid

10

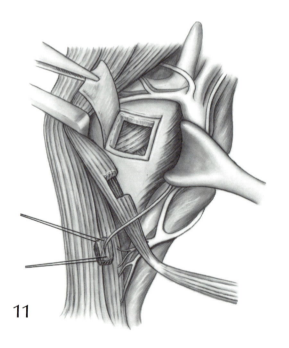

11

11

The strap muscles are retracted to expose the perichon-drium of the thyroid cartilage. A posteriorly based flap of perichondrium is incised and mobilized from the inferior half of the thyroid cartilage, a window is then produced in the lower half of the thyroid ala with the oscillating saw, leaving an intact strut along the inferior and posterior aspects of the thyroid cartilage. The underlying muscle thus exposed is the lateral thyroarytenoideus muscle, the major tensor and adductor of the vocal fold.

12

The nerve–muscle pedicle is sutured to it using two or three sutures of 5/0 nylon. The perichondrial flap is returned and sutured lightly in place and the neck wound is closed in the usual fashion.

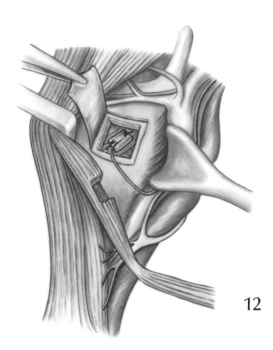

12

Results

The principle of nerve–muscle pedicle reinnervation has been reconfirmed by several authors, but the clinical success has not been widespread. It should be emphasized that, while this technique may not give universally good results, it should be considered in patients who require a voice that is more than just 'adequate'. Teflon injection remains the procedure of choice for most patients because it is inexpensive, gives almost immediate improvement and its results are generally good. Possible additional explanations for the voice improvement after reinnervation include the use of postoperative speech therapy, postoperative oedema due to the trauma, the possibility that implanted muscle may add bulk to the paralysed vocal fold and that muscle fibrosis following surgery may affect the final position of the arytenoid or vocal fold. Some patients have improved voice without any demonstrable movement of the fold; this may be due to increased tone or perhaps a slight change in the level of the vocal fold, allowing the normal side to oppose the paralysed side for vibration.

RECURRENT LARYNGEAL NERVE REINNERVATION

This procedure aims to restore innervation to the intrinsic muscles of the larynx and is particularly indicated following known surgical trauma to the vagus or recurrent laryngeal nerves in the neck. It is contraindicated if there is no distal stump of the recurrent laryngeal nerve.

13

Under general anaesthesia, an oblique incision is made to gain access to the paratracheal region near the second and third tracheal rings and the ansa hypoglossi, immediately superficial to the internal jugular vein. The fascia between the strap muscles and the sternomastoid muscle is opened and the internal jugular vein is exposed. Using a nerve stimulator, the ansa hypoglossi with the branch to the sternothyroid muscle is identified. It is then dissected towards its muscular termination inferiorly. The recurrent laryngeal nerve is identified in the tracheo-oesophageal groove or sulcus. The nerve must be intact from this site superiorly into the larynx.

The ansa and the recurrent laryngeal nerve should be divided far enough inferiorly to allow sufficient length for a tension-free anastomosis. This is most critical in those patients in whom the contralateral ansa is used. The anastomosis is performed under the operating microscope, using three 10/0 nylon sutures. The wound is closed in the usual manner and drained.

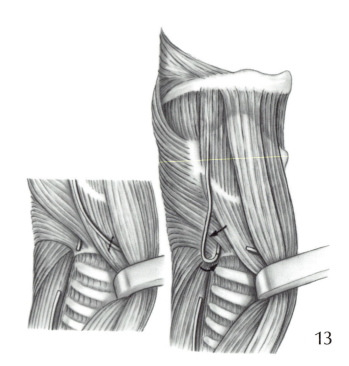

13

This reinnervation procedure may produce a voice superior to that following intracordal injection and is a simple procedure with no serious side effects. The larynx is not invaded, manipulated or injected. Nerve transfer has two increments of voice improvement. The first is usually immediate and is thought to be secondary to sternothyroid muscle denervation that results from the ansa hypoglossi transection. The main phonatory improvements, however, take 2–3 months following the procedure, during which time the axons grow through the nerve anastomosis and traverse the distal stump of the recurrent laryngeal nerve to reach the paralysed muscles.

Many explanations have been suggested for the excellent phonatory quality achieved by this technique. Severance of the sternothyroid muscle branch results in medialization of the ipsilateral thyroid cartilage lamina, which in turn medializes the entire vocal fold. Reinnervation of the laryngeal muscles by the ansa cervicalis produces resting tone in the thyroarytenoid, lateral cricoarytenoid, posterior cricoarytenoid and interarytenoid muscles. This tends to stabilize the arytenoid cartilage, and the nerve transfer reproduces normal vocal fold muscle tone and hence normal vocal fold compliance.

Frequently an injection of Gelfoam paste in the ipsilateral fold provides the patient with the advantages of immediate improvement during the early portion of the 2–3 month interval during which the innervation is taking place.

BILATERAL VOCAL FOLD PARALYSIS

Lesions of the vagus or recurrent laryngeal nerve in the neck or mediastinum below the origin of the superior laryngeal nerve leave the innervation of the cricothyroid muscle intact. Bilateral involvement of the nerves will result in the folds being in the paramedian or median position, thus allowing the patient a good voice but little airway. However, the symptoms and physical findings of bilateral vocal fold palsy may vary for several reasons. The first reason is that the injury may involve only a portion of a recurrent laryngeal nerve or one of its extralaryngeal branches. Forty per cent of patients have two or more extralaryngeal subdivisions of the recurrent laryngeal nerves. Secondly, the superior laryngeal nerve, which innervates the cricothyroid muscle, may continue to function unless the injury is in the high vagal region, and the extent of this adductor activity varies in different people. Thirdly, when a recurrent laryngeal nerve is severed, a typical lower motor neurone paralysis develops. The initial muscular flaccidity produces a cadaveric or paramedian cordal position, but in time, as atrophy and fibrosis develops, the muscular contracture draws the cord back to the midline.

Numerous surgical procedures have been described to improve the airway in patients with bilateral vocal fold paralysis in the paramedian position, and include tracheostomy, arytenoidectomy, vocal fold lateralization and reinnervation procedures. Whatever procedure is undertaken the voice is usually made worse to a greater or lesser extent as a consequence of improvement of the airway.

TRACHEOSTOMY

(*See* also chapter on 'Emergency and elective airway procedures: tracheostomy, cricothyroidotomy and their variants', pp. 27–44.)

The most direct approach to the problem of airway distress caused by bilateral vocal fold paralysis is to bypass the obstruction. Hence, a tracheostomy is often part of the management of patients with this disorder. Tracheostomy has the advantage of being simple and direct and provides an immediate solution to the problem of airway obstruction. It can be performed under local anaesthesia, even in patients who are otherwise very poor surgical risks. Tracheostomy may be well tolerated for prolonged periods of time, sometimes for years, and has been considerably improved by the introduction of the newer types of lightweight, relatively inert, plastic tubes.

The voice is not impaired, provided that the tracheostomy tube is significantly smaller than the circumference of the trachea itself so as to permit the passage of air around the tube when it is occluded with the finger. Alternatively, a fenestrated tracheostomy tube incorporating a speaking valve may be used.

The use of the 'button' type tracheostomy has the advantage that virtually none of the tube is within the tracheal lumen itself and it usually does not require neck tapes for support. Many patients with bilateral vocal fold paralysis have a resting airway that is sufficient for quiet activity, or at least for conversational activity while the patient is sitting. Thus it may be possible to keep the tracheostomy corked except during times of exertion, and perhaps at night while asleep. This will permit use of the voice without a valved tube and without digital occlusion of the tube. The cork can be removed at will, providing an effective bypass for those times when the airway proves inadequate.

Permanent tracheostomy is a less than satisfactory means of rehabilitation. Most patients do not find wearing a tube for the rest of their lives a pleasant prospect. The tubes need modification if clothing is to be worn; at least two-thirds of the patients are women because of their higher incidence of thyroid disease, and the cosmetic problem produced by a tracheostomy is a significant one.

The potential complications of long-term tracheostomy use must be considered. These include:

1. Formation of granulation tissue, with subsequent bleeding and infection at the tracheostomy site.
2. Tracheal stenosis either at the tracheostomy site or at the distal point where the tip of the tube may traumatize the trachea.
3. Possible tracheal erosion with secondary haemorrhage from the innominate artery or other vessels.
4. Diminished cough efficiency with a subsequent increase in the incidence of pneumonitis and upper respiratory tract infections.
5. The presence of the tracheostomy tube may interfere with swallowing, adding a further difficulty for these patients.

Arytenoidectomy and vocal fold lateralization procedures

These procedures should ideally preserve a 1–2 mm space between the membranous folds, maintaining the voice, and a 5–6 mm gap in the arytenoid bed to provide airway improvement. Every millimetre is critical in these procedures – 'the better the technique, the better the result'. Tissue resection may be undertaken either endoscopically or by an open approach.

Initial attempts at surgical improvement of the airway in such patients were through a laryngofissure. Excision of one or even both vocal folds and ventricles were employed. These procedures generally failed because of intraluminal cicatrization. The technique of submucous resection of the vocal fold was advocated. Variations of this approach included submucous resection of the arytenoid. Extralaryngeal methods were then developed, such as disarticulation of the arytenoid, but the results were not uniformly successful. Nowadays effective and safer endoscopic microsurgical methods are available. All of the methods described involve surgery to the arytenoid or the posterior end of the membranous vocal fold.

ARYTENOIDECTOMY

This may be carried out endoscopically or by a laryngofissure or lateral approach. Endoscopic excision of the arytenoid by microdissection under magnification can be difficult and bloody, thus making it impossible to position sutures. With the advent of the carbon dioxide laser, endoscopic laser arytenoidectomy can be performed efficiently with little bleeding and allows endoscopic suturing if this is desired.

The operation is performed using general anaesthesia and the usual precautions taken with laser endoscopy. Suspension microlaryngoscopy and a 400 mm objective lens coupled to the carbon dioxide laser are required. The laser is set at 10 W with a 0.1 second repeat mode focused spot size 0.8 mm. Moistened neurosurgical pledgets are placed in the subglottic space to protect the trachea and endotracheal tube if the latter is used.

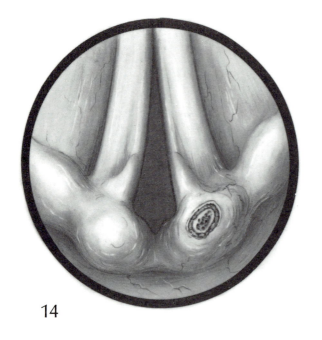

14

14

After exposure of the arytenoid cartilages and the posterior commissure, the mucoperichondrium overlying the accessory cartilages and the apex of one arytenoid are vaporized to expose the underlying cartilage. The corniculate cartilage and the apex of the arytenoid cartilage are vaporized with the laser in continuous mode, then the mucoperichondrium overlying the upper border of the arytenoid cartilage is ablated with the laser back in repeat mode.

15

The upper body of the arytenoid cartilage is vaporized.

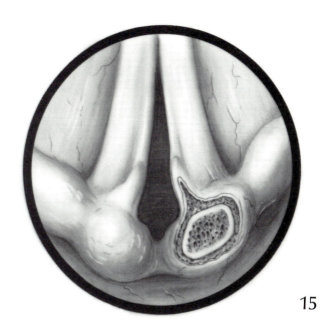

15

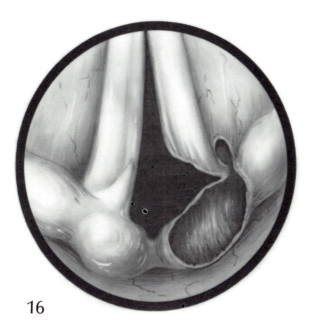

16

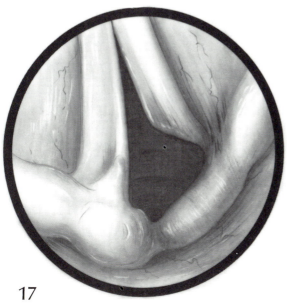

17

16 & 17

By altering the laser between interrupted mode to destroy the mucoperichondrium and continuous mode for evaporation of the cartilage, the arytenoid can be ablated. Great care is needed to prevent vaporization of the interarytenoid mucosa. Postoperatively the patient should be covered by broad-spectrum antibiotics and an intraoperative dose of dexamethasone.

This procedure results in good preservation of voice and is rapid and atraumatic. However, it requires a laryngologist experienced with the laser and familiar with the three-dimensional anatomy of the arytenoid via the endoscope. There is a possibility of postoperative oedema, granuloma formation, posterior glottic scarring and cricoid perichondritis. Revision surgery may be indicated if resection or subsequent fibrosis produce inadequate airway improvement.

VOCAL FOLD LATERALIZATION

The following procedure may be used as primary treatment in bilateral vocal fold paralysis but is particularly useful in patients whose airway remains impaired following arytenoidectomy.

18

Segmental removal of the thyroarytenoid muscles adjacent to the vocal ligament is undertaken towards the conus elasticus and thyroid cartilage. This can be done by using microcautery or a carbon dioxide laser.

19 & 20

Vocal fold lateralization and closure of the defect is achieved by sutures introduced via the lumen of two hypodermic needles, under endoscopic visualization and control.

The resulting voice in these patients may be more coarse and breathy but most patients prefer this to the alternatives of chronic glottic obstruction or a permanent tracheostomy.

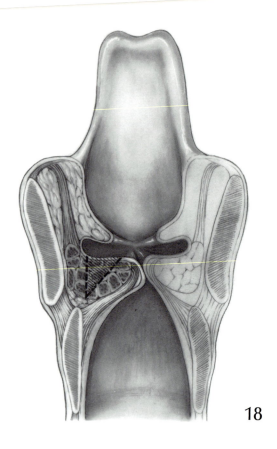

18

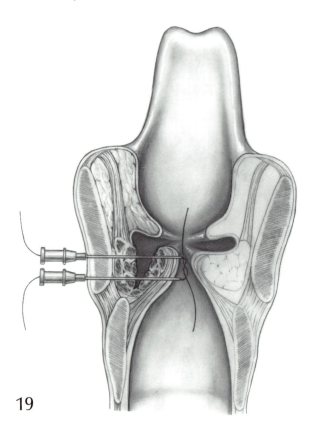

19

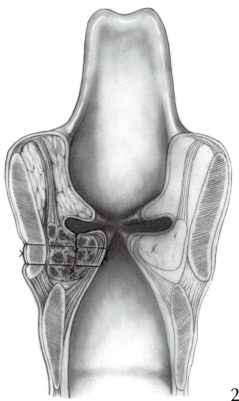

20

LARYNGOFISSURE AND ARYTENOIDECTOMY

The procedure is performed under general anaesthesia with a tracheostomy. The tracheostomy and thyrotomy incisions should be kept separate. A 4–5 cm horizontal incision is made at the cricothyroid level. The strap muscles are retracted, exposing the cricothyroid membrane and the thyroid cartilage. A precise vertical midline incision is made in the cricothyroid membrane. The thyroid cartilage is split with a knife or a cutting saw. A haemostat is inserted into the anterior commissure and the commissure is incised precisely in the midline. A self-retaining retractor is used to retract the thyroid alae, taking care not to traumatize the severed anterior ends of the vocal folds.

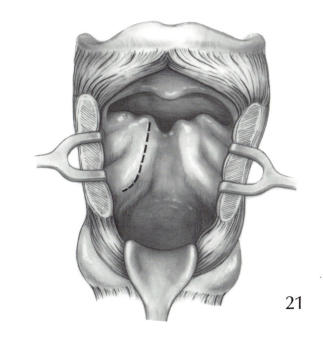

21

21

Local anaesthetic with adrenaline is injected around the arytenoid to be removed. A hockey stick incision is made vertically down the arytenoid with a horizontal limb along the vocal process.

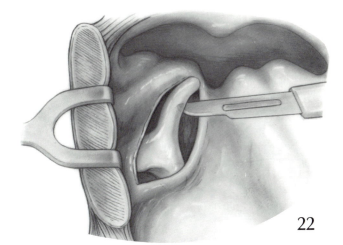

22

22

A Frears elevator and No. 15 blade knife are used to mobilize the perichondrium of the cartilage. Skin hooks help to stabilize the tissues and minimize the local tissue trauma. Bleeding is controlled by bipolar coagulation.

23

The incision is sutured with interrupted plain 5/0 catgut. No stents or lateralization sutures are usually necessary. The thyrotomy incision is closed over a drain to prevent surgical emphysema or haematoma. Postoperative antibiotics and routine tracheostomy care are required. The patients are usually hospitalized for a few days and allowed home with a non-cuffed tracheostomy tube. Decannulation can proceed when the arytenoid bed area has settled sufficiently and this may take from a few days to many weeks.

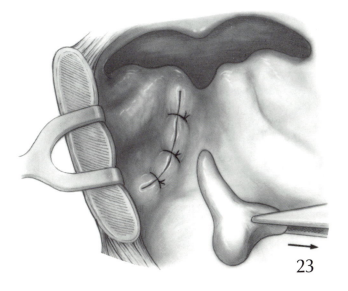

23

LATERAL EXTERNAL ARYTENOIDECTOMY (WOODMAN PROCEDURE)

24

Following an incision along the anterior border of sternomastoid muscle, it is retracted posteriorly and the strap muscles anteriorly. The inferior constrictor muscle is dissected from the posterior margin of the thyroid ala and the cricothyroid joint incised and dislocated. The thyroid ala is retracted anterolaterally so that the arytenoid anatomy can be palpated. The posterior and lateral cricoarytenoid muscles are incised beneath the arytenoid cartilage.

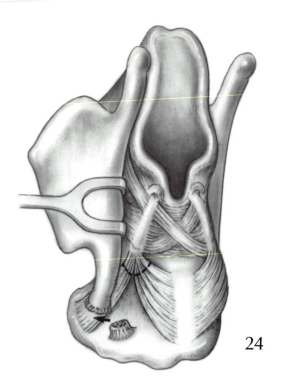

24

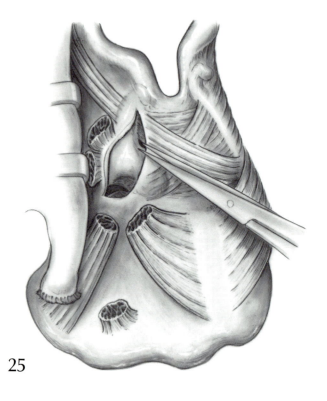

25

25

The cricoarytenoid joint is separated by spreading fine-point scissors in the joint space and the arytenoid cartilage is removed by traction and dissection through a vertical incision. The tip of the vocal process is preserved.

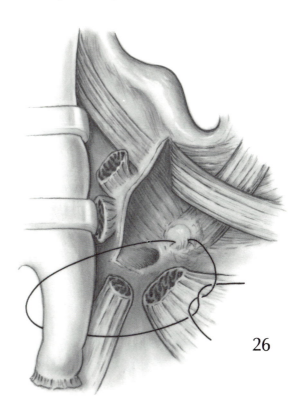

26

26 & 27

A 2/0 monofilament suture is then placed either around the inferior cornu of the thyroid cartilage or through its substance, fixing the vocal fold to the lateral wall of the larynx in abduction. The suture is tightened while the vocal fold is visualized by direct laryngoscopy to obtain the appropriate vertical position and lateral displacement. The inferior constrictor muscle is reapproximated with 4/0 chromic catgut and the wound drained before skin closure.

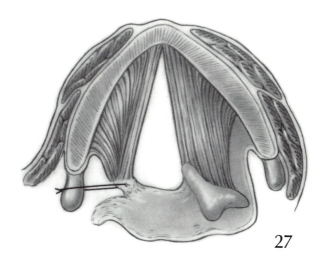

27

Reinnervation procedures

NERVE–MUSCLE TECHNIQUE

This technique aims to return vocal fold function to near normal at no further expense to the voice. It is contraindicated in patients who have had previous surgery or radiotherapy that has violated the necessary nerve pedicle.

The technique is similar to that of the unilateral vocal fold reinnervation. The lateral margin of the thyroid ala is palpated, and a double hook is used to rotate the larynx towards the opposite side. The jugular vein is retracted and the diagonal fibres of the inferior constrictor muscle are exposed. These fibres may be carefully separated to expose the reflection of the piriform sinus. Careful dissection will expose the fibres of the posterior crico-arytenoid muscle, which are easily identified by the fact that they run at right angles to the fibres of the inferior constrictor. When in doubt, the surgeon may simply continue carefully spreading the muscle fibres until the cricoid lamina is reached. In such circumstances the posterior cricoarytenoid muscle will be identified by 'backing out' one layer, and no harm will result from this manoeuvre. Once located, the surface fibres of the posterior cricoarytenoid may be lightly scarified with a scalpel blade if previous dissection has not roughened the muscle somewhat. The prepared nerve–muscle pedicle is then brought into position and sutured in place by two or three 5/0 nylon sutures. The wound is closed in the standard fashion.

DENERVATION OF THE LARYNX

Denervation of the larynx with gross disturbance of its protective function produces laryngeal incompetence. Lesions involving the vagus nerve above the origin of the superior laryngeal nerve usually result in a lateral position of the paralysed vocal fold due to abolition of the adductor action of the cricothyroid muscle. Severe intractable aspiration due to laryngeal incompetence is invariably associated with a combination of motor and sensory defects affecting all the neural pathways. Many neurological conditions, including traumatic, infective and neoplastic lesions, may involve the lower cranial nerves at the level of the medulla, the brainstem or the skull base.

Management of such patients is dependent on the aetiology and likely natural history of the neural defect, particularly with regard to possible recovery. The age of the patient and the associated disease status must be considered and whether the patient is seen in the acute or chronic phase of the clinical state.

The aims of management are the maintenance of an adequate airway, prevention of aspiration and preservation of voice. Evaluation of such patients includes endoscopy, videofluoroscopy and electromyography to aid with planning rehabilitation.

The methods of management available in these patients include tracheostomy, augmentation of the vocal folds, epiglottopexy, laryngeal closure procedures, laryngo-tracheal separation and diversion, and total laryngectomy.

TRACHEOSTOMY

The establishment of a tracheostomy with an inflatable cuffed tube may provide some protection of the airway in these patients during swallowing and give a portal for suction clearance of the chest. However, the presence of the tracheostomy may in itself increase the swallowing difficulties and aspiration making nasogastric, gastrostomy or jejunostomy feeding mandatory. In the long term this may be an unsatisfactory combination.

AUGMENTATION

Severe aspiration following denervation of the larynx is rarely helped significantly by augmentation of either the supraglottis or vocal folds and as a consequence a wide variety of laryngeal closure procedures have been advocated.

LARYNGEAL CLOSURE

The operation allows restoration of respiration and swallowing without aspiration, but sacrifices phonatory function. Many techniques have been described including vocal fold suturing, supraglottic closure, high tracheal closure, submucosal posterior cricoid cartilage resection and subglottic laryngeal closure. Such procedures may be offered to patients with severe aspiration in whom there is neither a protective nor a phonatory function to the larynx. This type of surgery may in theory be reversed should the patient's condition improve and the need for phonation be anticipated. One of the advantages of subglottic or high tracheal closure is that the mobility of the vocal folds can be evaluated at frequent intervals. All of these procedures listed above have their enthusiasts, and meticulous care and multiple-layered suturing are required, otherwise the closure will dehisce.

EPIGLOTTOPEXY

This procedure prevents aspiration and is relatively easy to reverse. It may allow some vocal function in the short term and preserves the voice for the long term. The patient must have the mental stature and manual dexterity to perform closure of the tracheostomy as a prerequisite to phonation.

Endoscopic assessment of the epiglottic anatomy is helpful in patient selection. Assessment of the length and width of the epiglottis in relation to the laryngeal inlet are necessary.

28

Under general anaesthesia a suprahyoid pharyngostomy is performed via the suprahyoid incision shown.

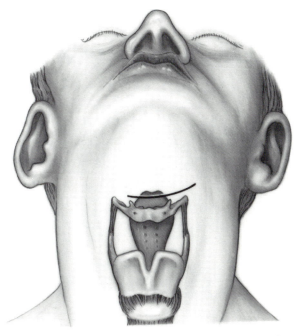

28

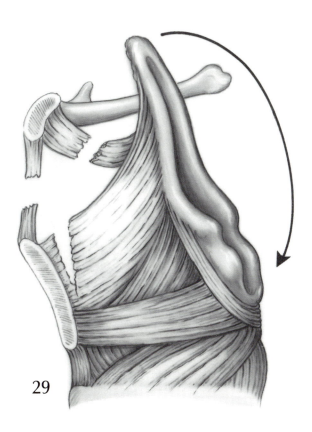

29

The hyoepiglottic and the thyroepiglottic ligaments are severed and the tensile strength of the cartilage is diminished by two or three linear cuts into the upper surface of the cartilage. After this procedure, the epiglottis will assume a posterior position.

29

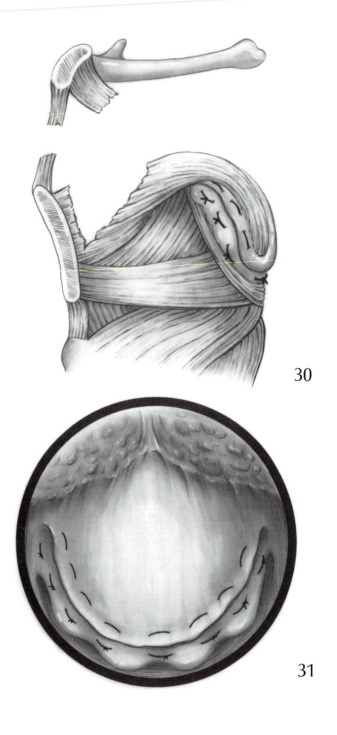

30 & 31

The mucosal surfaces of the epiglottis, aryepiglottic folds and arytenoids are denuded. 2/0 silk horizontal mattress sutures are all individually placed prior to tying. After surgery, a small area can frequently be detected that has opened and which can be used as a one-way valve for phonation, yet prevent aspiration. Should this opening not appear some time after surgery, then depending on the neurological recovery and the desire for phonation, a reversal procedure may be performed endoscopically.

30

31

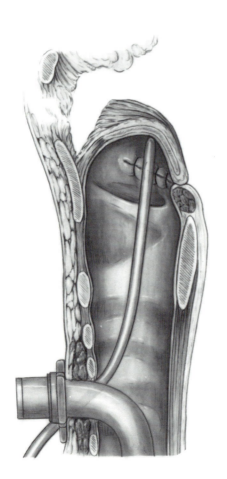

32

32

A probe can be introduced through the tracheostomy site and passed through the vocal folds tenting the epiglottis. With the laser or conventional microlaryngeal instrumentation, any size of opening can be created. As the size of the window increases the effort required for phonation decreases.

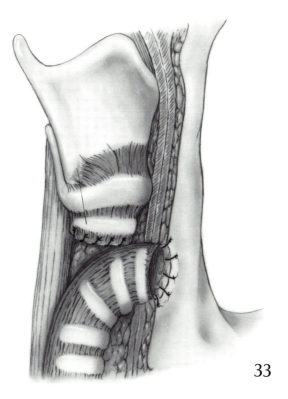

33

LARYNGOTRACHEAL SEPARATION/TRACHEO-OESOPHAGEAL DIVERSION

33 & 34

These are dependable techniques which completely divide the respiratory tract and protect from aspiration for an indefinite period of time, while preserving the malfunctioning larynx and its neural input. They are potentially reversible and the neurological status of the residual larynx can be periodically assessed. The separation procedure has the disadvantage that swallowed food may pool in the larynx and a tracheocutaneous fistula may form in the subglottic pouch.

TOTAL LARYNGECTOMY

Ultimately a total laryngectomy may be the surgical procedure of choice in some patients with an incompetent larynx, and may be indicated when other procedures have been performed without any improvement of the patient's condition. It may be indicated in patients for whom the prognosis for rehabilitation or long-term survival is poor, in those who have other associated medical problems, or in patients who are likely to have poor wound healing. Limited pharyngeal excision facilitates pharyngeal closure without undue tension on the suture lines. The strap muscles are not removed and are utilized to reinforce the pharyngeal closure. This approach removes the source of the aspiration and prevents further soiling of the respiratory tract. While there is an obvious finality associated with the operation, the patient may be spared numerous surgical procedures and the danger of continued aspiration. With the current neoglottic reconstructive techniques the patient's voice may be restored in the future if the condition warrants it.

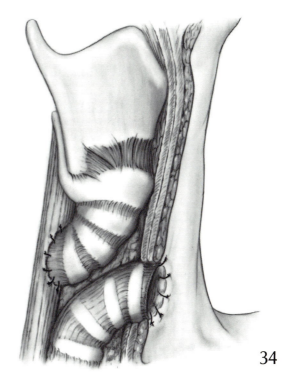

34

VOCAL FOLD PARALYSIS IN CHILDREN

In the small child or the newborn an abnormal cry should suggest that there may be an abnormality affecting the larynx, and appropriate investigations including endoscopy may be indicated. Vocal fold paralysis/paresis is the second most common diagnostic category after laryngomalacia in the aetiology of stridor presenting during early infancy. The incidence of vocal fold paralysis is higher in patients with central nervous system disease and may be unilateral or bilateral. Increased diagnosis of this condition may be attributed to the use of nasoendoscopic evaluation of the upper airways of problem children. Many children may be misdiagnosed as having laryngomalacia. As they subsequently grow and develop no further symptoms may present, but later in life, even into adulthood, the abnormality of the vocal fold may be first detected.

Management

Mmanagement of vocal fold palsy in children may be different from that in adults. The vocal fold paralysis may be transient and the paralysis may resolve once the congenital abnormality is corrected or treated properly. Vocal fold paralysis should be looked for in children who have had cardiac surgery, patent ductus arteriosus correction, repair of tracheo-oesophageal fistula or in children with dysmorphic features with a hoarse cry (Moebius syndrome or Klippel–Feil syndrome). Management of the child usually requires no surgical intervention, although occasionally speech therapy is effective. In children over the age of 5 years who have a persistent abnormal voice, evaluation should be undertaken in the same manner as in an adult.

In children with bilateral vocal fold palsy the relative urgency of surgical intervention is dependent on the severity of the patient's condition, particularly with regard to respiratory difficulties, with or without stridor. Management plans may have to be reviewed frequently to evaluate the changes in the status of laryngeal functions. In severe cases endotracheal intubation or a tracheostomy may be necessary. By correcting the neurological status, e.g. hydrocephalus, the paralysis may be expected to improve. Progress can be observed by frequent use of the nasopharyngoscope.

Surgical procedures available to treat bilateral vocal fold paralysis have been described previously.

Further reading

Crumley RL. Teflon versus thyroplasty versus nerve transfer: a comparison. *Ann Otol Rhinol Laryngol* 1990; 99: 759–63.

Dedo HH. Avoidance and treatment of complications of Teflon injection of the vocal cord. *J Voice* 1988; 2: 90–2.

Isshiki N, Taira T, Kojima H, Shoji K. Recent modifications of thyroplasty type 1. *Ann Otol Rhinol Laryngol* 1989; 98: 777–9.

Isshiki N. Arytenoid adduction for unilateral vocal cord paralysis. *Arch Otolaryngol* 1978; 104: 555–8.

Kaufman JA. Laryngoplasty for vocal cord medialisation: an alternative to Teflon. *Laryngoscope* 1986; 96: 726–31.

Ossoff RH, Duncavage JA, Shapshay S, Krepsi YP, Sisson GA. Endoscopic laser arytenoidectomy revisited. *Ann Otol Rhinol Laryngol* 1990; 99: 764–71.

Singer MI, Hamaker RC, Miller S. Restoration of the airway following bilateral recurrent laryngeal nerve paralysis. *Laryngoscope* 1985; 95: 1204–7.

Tucker HM. Vocal cord paralysis in small children: principles in management. *Ann Otol Rhinol Laryngol* 1986; 95: 618–21.

Tucker HM. Combined laryngeal framework medialisation and reinnervation for unilateral vocal fold paralysis. *Ann Otol Rhinol Laryngol* 1990; 99: 778–81.

Lateral rhinotomy

V. J. Lund MS, FRCS
Institute of Laryngology and Otology, Royal National Throat, Nose and Ear Hospital, London, UK

Introduction

This technique, which was for many years unaccountably neglected, affords excellent access to the nasal cavity and lateral nasal wall. Strictly speaking lateral rhinotomy refers only to the actual approach but through it removal of the entire lateral wall and septum can be effected. It thus combines excellent access and minimal postoperative morbidity, both functional and cosmetic.

The operation is generally attributed to E. J. Moure from Bordeaux, who described it in 1902 for the removal of frontoethmoidal tumours[1]. However, references to a similar procedure were made by Michaux and Bruns in 1848 and 1872 respectively[2,3].

Surgical anatomy

See chapter on 'External operations on the frontoethmoid sinuses', pp. 555–564.

Indications

This approach was originally intended for removal of frontoethmoidal tumours which might then be followed by radiotherapy if disease had compromised the cribriform plate or roof of the ethmoids. This has been completely supplanted by craniofacial resection, which nevertheless continues to utilize the lateral rhinotomy approach inferiorly.

The procedure is still valuable for the following:

1. Malignancy confined to the nasal cavity, e.g. malignant melanoma[4].
2. Benign neoplasms arising within the nasal cavity, medial maxilla, ethmoids, pterygomaxillary region and nasopharynx, e.g. angiofibroma, inverted papilloma, osteoma, ossifying fibroma and neurofibroma[5].

Haemostasis can be effected in the more vascular lesions by ligation of the sphenopalatine artery in the lateral nasal wall or of the internal maxillary artery via the antrum.

The procedure can be performed at virtually any age but size of the individual will limit the access provided.

Contraindications

Any lesion in this region which appears to have compromised the cribriform plate or roof of the ethmoids, or where the orbital apex is affected, is more safely and effectively treated by a formal craniofacial resection.

Preoperative

If careful examination of the nasal cavity (preferably with fibreoptic endoscopy) reveals a lesion confined to septum or inferior turbinate, little investigation is required other than histological confirmation. Any potentially more extensive lesion on the lateral wall or in the superior nasal cavity should be investigated by computed tomography with direct coronal images and in selected cases by magnetic resonance imaging, with gadolinium-DPTA enhancement to establish that this approach is appropriate.

Anaesthesia and preparation

The procedure is performed under general anaesthesia, with the patient 15° head up in the reverse Trendelenburg position. The incisional area is injected with a small amount of local anaesthetic, such as 1 per cent lignocaine with 1:200 000 adrenaline, and a temporary tarsorrhaphy is performed on the operative side with 5/0 silk.

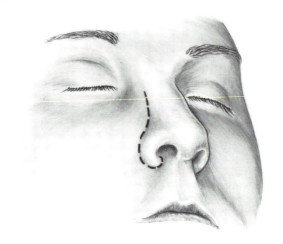

1

Operation

Incision

1 & 2

For the best cosmetic results the incision should run from the level of the medial canthal ligament, equidistant from medial canthus and dorsum of the nose. It travels down the nasomaxillary groove and accurately follows the ala round to finish in the nasal cavity. All layers are divided, and cutting superiorly towards the pyriform aperture mobilizes the inferior lateral wall, allowing it to be swung back and retracted with a stay suture. Branches of the superior labial artery to the vestibule usually require ligation.

Procedure

Depending upon the access required, the skin and periosteum is elevated over the nasal bone and frontonasal process medially and laterally to the orbital rim, and on to the face of the maxilla as far as the infraorbital foramen. Similarly, the medial canthal ligament can be detached from the anterior and posterior lacrimal crests (although complete detachment is rarely required), the lacrimal sac displaced laterally and the orbital periosteum widely freed from the lamina papyracea, which can readily be achieved using ribbon gauze and a malleable copper retractor. The anterior ethmoidal vessels can be cauterized and divided to improve access.

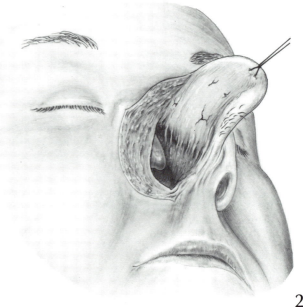

2

3

The bone can then be removed piecemeal with nibblers or Hayek forceps. Superiorly, while removing the inferior part of the frontonasal process of the maxilla, it is often possible to preserve the orbital rim. To facilitate bone removal from the lateral wall of the nasal cavity, soft tissue is dissected with a Freer elevator. In extensive mucosal lesions, the inferior nasal mucosa can be completely 'sleeved', allowing an en bloc removal including the inferior turbinate, which can be freed with sharp dissection and scissors posteriorly.

Further bone is removed at the anteromedial corner of the maxilla until the antral cavity is approached and the anterior and medial walls diverge. A straight osteotome is used to fracture and remove the medial bony wall and the antral lining is completely removed if necessary. The ethmoid sinuses can then be cleared under direct vision via the nasal cavity and orbit. The need for further resection, such as removal of the septum or posterior antral wall, will be determined by the individual case.

En bloc resection of the lateral nasal wall and ethmoid has been termed 'medial maxillectomy'[6].

Closure and postoperative management

The cavity thus created is packed with 2-inch gauze soaked in Whitehead's varnish (compound iodoform paint) which is removed at a week to 10 days depending on the circumstances, under local or occasionally general anaesthesia. Use of this antiseptic preparation achieves haemostasis and allows re-epithelialization of the cavity without recourse to split-skin grafting. The patient is kept on broad spectrum antibiotics, such as cefuroxime and metronidazole or amoxycillin/clavulanate, until the pack is removed.

The incision is closed with 4/0 chromic catgut and 5/0 silk or Prolene (Ethicon Ltd., Edinburgh, UK). Considerable care must be taken to approximate the alar region to prevent subsequent contracture and 'lift' of the margin. A small pressure dressing is applied overnight.

Most patients experience some degree of crusting following surgery, for which an alkaline nasal douche is helpful until the condition naturally resolves, usually within 6 months.

Variations

It is possible to limit or extend the incision and resection.

1. Limitation of the incision in very localized disease will obviate cosmetic problems at the alar margin.
2. Extension of the incision:
   (a) Superiorly under the medial eyebrow as in a Lynch–Howarth approach and as originally described by Moure[1].
   (b) Superiorly onto the glabella in a midline forehead crease to the hairline for craniofacial resection[7].
   (c) Inferiorly round the alar margin and through the medial philtrum and upper lip[8].

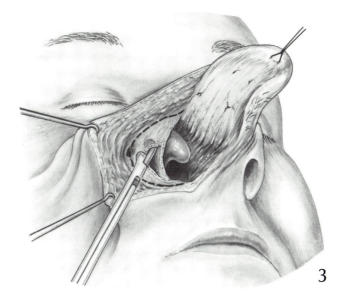

3

Complications

Early

Early complications include haemorrhage, blepharitis and oedema of the lids, paraesthesia due to infraorbital nerve damage, wound infection, cerebrospinal fluid leak and meningitis.

All of these are rare if good surgical technique is employed.

Late

1. *Epiphora.* This can occasionally occur if the nasolacrimal duct is transected and then stenoses. In these circumstances the sac can be marsupialized[8] or the duct stented[9].
2. *Cosmetic.* Alar lift, vestibular stenosis and webbing of the incision in the medial canthal region can usually be avoided by surgical technique. Columellar retraction and saddling can be a consequence of the surgical excision or result from unintentional septal perforation.
3. *Diplopia.* This rarely occurs unless the incision is extended superiorly to affect the trochlea.
4. *Telecanthus.* This has been said to occur if the medial canthal ligament is not reapproximated. In practice it rarely occurs[10].
5. *Obstruction of the frontonasal recess* leading to subsequent *mucocele formation.* This complication is exceptionally rare as the area is either undisturbed or completely cleared. Similarly, sinusitis is a rare theoretical consequence.
6. *Nasocutaneous fistula.* This is said to occur occasionally in patients who receive radiotherapy, but this has not been our personal experience.

References

1. Moure EJ. Traitement des tumeurs malignes primitives de l'ethmoide. *Rev Hebd Laryngol* 1902; 2: 401–12.

2. Mertz JS, Pearson BW, Kern EB. Lateral rhinotomy: indications, technique and review of 226 patients. *Arch Otolaryngol* 1983; 109: 235–9.

3. Lawson W, Biller HF. Lateral rhinotomy. In: Blitzer A, Friedman W, Lawson W, eds. *Surgery of the Paranasal Sinuses*. Philadelphia: WB Saunders, 1985: 197–203.

4. Lund VJ. Malignant melanoma of the nasal cavity and paranasal sinuses. *J Laryngol Otol* 1982; 96: 347–55.

5. Harrison DFN. Lateral rhinotomy: a neglected operation. *Ann Otol Rhinol Laryngol* 1977; 86: 756–9.

6. Sessions RB, Larson DL. En bloc ethmoidectomy and medial maxillectomy. *Arch Otolaryngol* 1977; 103: 195–202.

7. Cheesman AD, Lund VJ, Howard DJ. Craniofacial resection for tumours of the nasal cavity and paranasal sinuses. *Head Neck Surg* 1986; 8: 429–35.

8. Schramm VL, Myers EN. 'How I do it' – head and neck. A targeted problem and its solution. Lateral rhinotomy. *Laryngoscope* 1978; 88: 1042–5.

9. Sessions RB, Humphreys DH. Technical modifications of the medial maxillectomy. *Arch Otolaryngol* 1983; 109: 575–7.

10. Bernard PJ, Lawson W, Biller HF, Lebenger J. Complications following rhinotomy: review of 148 patients. *Ann Otol Rhinol Laryngol* 1989; 98: 684–92.

Illustrations by Robert Lane and Gillian Lee

External operations on the frontoethmoid sinuses

V. J. Lund MS, FRCS
Institute of Laryngology and Otology, Royal National Throat, Nose and Ear Hospital, London, UK

Introduction

History

The development of surgery in the frontoethmoid region resulted in two main approaches, that designed to enhance drainage while preserving facial contour and that aiming to eradicate irreversibly diseased mucosa at the expense of cosmesis. The former has obviously achieved ascendancy over the latter in the post-antibiotic era and there is fortunately no longer a place for the radical and inevitably disfiguring sinusectomy described in 1898 by Reidel[1].

Exenteration of the ethmosphenoid system was modified and popularized by Howarth[2] in the UK and Lynch[3] in the USA. They both emphasized the importance of removing all diseased frontal sinus mucosa and creating adequate drainage. Failure to maintain long-term patency of the frontonasal recess was the chief cause of failure and resulted in the emergence of the osteoplastic flap. A variety of exogenous and endogenous materials have been used to promote obliteration of the sinuses; abdominal fat has proved the most popular.

The decreasing incidence of chronic frontal sinusitis, the over-estimation of recurrence associated with the Lynch–Howarth technique, and undoubted cosmetic and infection problems of the osteoplastic flap has led to a swing back to the Lynch–Howarth operation in the UK. The osteoplastic flap continues to be popular in North America[4]. However, the objectives of these procedures can now be achieved in many instances by intranasal endoscopic surgery. Addressing the underlying pathophysiology offers a 'functional' approach which often obviates more radical surgery[5].

Surgical anatomy

The cruciate ethmoid bone forms the central support for the anterior cranial fossa. Above the horizontal bar protrudes the crista galli; below the perpendicular plate and at either end of the horizontal bar are lateral air cell labyrinths. In an adult, the whole bone is 2.5 × 2.5 × 2 cm, pyramidal in shape, with the apex pointing anteriorly and the base abutting the sphenoid.

The anterior and posterior ethmoidal vessels are important landmarks to the level of the cribriform plate. The rule of 24–12–6 can be applied to the medial wall of the orbit representing, respectively, the average distance in millimetres from the anterior lacrimal crest to the anterior ethmoidal foramen, from anterior to posterior ethmoidal foramen and from posterior ethmoidal to optic canal[6]. This situation can be very variable with the last distance being between 3 and 8 mm, 16 per cent of the population having no anterior ethmoidal foramen and 30 per cent multiple ethmoidal foramina[7].

The frontal sinus is radiologically recognizable in 50 per cent of subjects by 6 years of age and is fully developed by 15 years of age though it may be undeveloped in 1–2 per cent[8]. It is extremely variable in shape, size and drainage and is often divided into a transverse and vertical part. Incomplete bony septa compartmentalize the sinus though a complete intersinus septum is usually present in 90 per cent of individuals[9]. Supernumerary sinuses and diverticula further complicate the situation. Drainage of the frontal sinus may be directly into the frontonasal recess in the anterior middle meatus or additionally through the ethmoidal cells, paths directly related to the embryological development of the sinus.

Operations

EXTERNAL FRONTOETHMOIDECTOMY
(Lynch–Howarth frontoethmoidectomy)

Indications

1. Frontoethmoidal mucoceles.
2. Chronic infection unresponsive to conservative medication.
3. Complications of acute ethmoiditis and frontal sinusitis, e.g. orbital cellulitis allowing drainage and decompression.
4. Recurrent polyposis, particularly when previous intranasal surgery may have destroyed surgical landmarks.
5. Access for ethmoidal artery ligation in the treatment of epistaxis, transethmoidal hypophysectomy, dacryocystorhinostomy, repair of cerebrospinal fluid leaks nasoseptal flaps and decompression of malignant exophthalmos.

Preoperative evaluation

Radiological examination may include plain sinus radiographs, hypocycloidal tomography and computed tomography, depending on availability. The role of magnetic resonance imaging has yet to be established, though in the absence of malignancy it will probably be superfluous.

Anaesthesia and preparation

A general anaesthetic is given via an oral tube with pharyngeal pack, with the additional application of topical vasoconstrictors.

The patient is placed in the reversed Trendelenburg position with 15° head flexion. Skin preparation of the forehead and upper face is performed taking care that nothing contaminates the eye. A temporary tarsorrhaphy is employed to avoid accidental damage to the cornea.

Incision

1

This is made slightly curved and extends down to the level of the medial canthus of the eye. It may be extended under the eyebrow to facilitate access to the frontal sinus, but division of the supratrochlear neurovascular bundle should be avoided if possible. The soft tissues are very vascular and significant bleeding from the angular vein is often encountered. A definite single cut down to bone will expose and facilitate clamping the bleeding vessels.

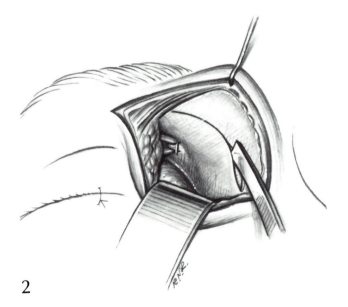

1

2

The periosteum is incised and elevated with a Freer elevator to expose the nasal process of the maxilla, frontal bone and medial wall of the orbit. Care is taken where the periosteum is adherent to the frontonasal and frontoethmoidal sutures, to avoid damage to the trochlea and prolapse of orbital fat. The trochlea is best displaced by sharp dissection. The lacrimal sac is elevated from its groove and displaced laterally.

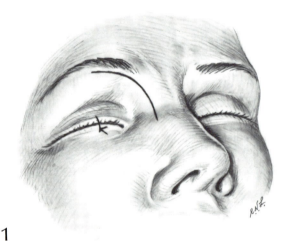

2

Ligation of ethmoidal vessels

3

Dissection continues posteriorly to reveal the anterior ethmoidal vessels, which are ligated with sutures or neurosurgical clips or, more often, coagulated with bipolar diathermy. The posterior ethmoidal vessels indicate the posterior limits of the ethmoidal cells and are also ligated or diathermy applied. One centimetre ribbon gauze soaked in topical adrenaline aids dissection, and while the use of a Ferris Smith retractor may be helpful, retraction of the orbital periosteum is best performed with a malleable copper retractor.

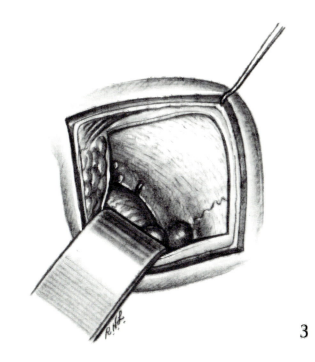

3

Exposure and exenteration of ethmoid sinuses

4

The thin medial wall of the orbit can now be penetrated using a Tilley Henkel forceps. Occasionally a hammer and gouge may be required. The ethmoidal cells can be exenterated under direct vision, up to and including the sphenoid.

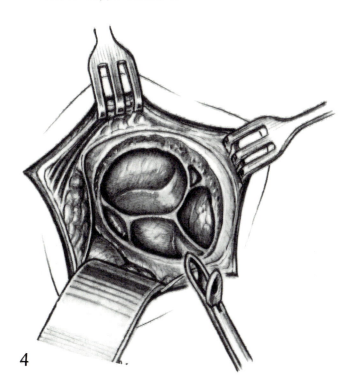

4

5

Similarly, the frontal sinus is entered via the medial floor through the anterior ethmoidal cells. The amount of floor removed will depend upon the access required to deal with the disease, but routinely it is advisable to remove at least the medial wall to open the frontonasal region.

The insertions of the middle and superior turbinates are thus exposed and the position of the cribriform plate defined superiorly. While not infallible, the middle turbinate represents an important landmark to the plate and should be retained at least until the end of the operation.

All diseased lining mucosa is removed except in areas of exposed dura, bearing in mind the variable anatomy of the sinuses. In the case of frontal sinus mucoceles, an attempt should be made to open the intersinus septum to provide an additional, albeit unphysiological, drainage route.

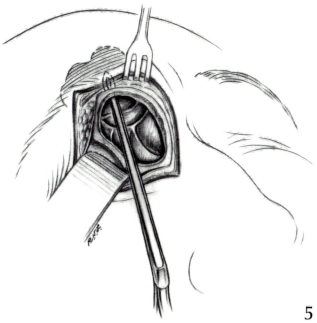

5

Frontal sinus drainage

6

Despite extensive removal of bone in the region of the frontonasal recess, subsequent fibrosis and new bone formation may lead to obstruction. To maintain patency, a fenestrated Silastic tube (Dow Corning, Reading, UK), 1 cm in diameter, is placed from the frontal sinus through the ethmoidal region to open in the nasal cavity, though it should not abut the septum too obliquely. The size of the tube ensures that it remains in place but the length of time that it is left has not been established. However, 3–5 months appears adequate in the majority of patients to maintain a permanent channel. Many other more complicated methods have been described using mucoperiosteal flaps and split-skin grafts. Alternatively, intranasal endoscopic visualization and clearance of the region during and after the operation can be used to maintain patency, obviating the use of foreign material.

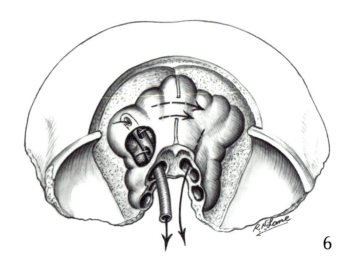

6

Closure

The periosteum, subcutaneous tissues and skin are sutured carefully with catgut and silk. The trochlea region should be formally reattached to the periosteum of the frontal bone with a Prolene stitch (Ethicon, Edinburgh, UK) to avoid damage to superior oblique function[10]. The eye should be washed at the end of the operation with saline to remove blood, and chloramphenicol ointment instilled to prevent conjunctivitis. A pressure dressing is applied for 24 hours. Skin sutures can be removed at 4–5 days.

It is advisable to apply gentle suction to the nasal cavity using a Silastic tube postoperatively.

Complications

Incision. Oedema, infection, paraesthesia, damage to the medial palpebral ligament and webbing of the wound may all result. Careful positioning of the incision and surgical technique will avoid most of these. Fistula formation is rare after accurate wound repair.

Failure to attach the trochlea may result in vertical diplopia due to underaction of the superior oblique muscle. If this persists, it can usually be corrected with a prism modification to spectacles or occasionally by eye muscle surgery.

Haemorrhage. This is usually due to retraction of ethmoidal vessels before adequate haemostasis is achieved.

Leak of cerebrospinal fluid. Dural exposure, either surgically or by the pathological process, is not uncommon and mucosa should not be disturbed in these regions. Damage to tubes of dura running on the olfactory nerve fibres to the superolateral wall may also produce this complication. If leakage results, it should be treated with appropriate antibiotics and closed primarily with fascia lata, tissue glue, gelatin (Gelfoam, Upjohn, USA) or a septal mucosal flap in conjunction with a fat/muscle graft.

Periorbital damage. This results in prolapse of fat into the surgical field and is best dealt with immediately. The pressure dressing minimizes swelling, and postoperative epiphora and diplopia are usually transient even when the latter results from decompression after long-term displacement.

Visual loss. This is unusual but can obviously result if the globe is injured and is a theoretical complication after long-term displacement, in which case prophylactic steroids are indicated, prior to decompression.

Frontonasal recess obstruction and recurrence of pathology. Failure to maintain frontonasal recess patency may result in subsequent mucocele formation and/or the original disease process may recur.

TRANSORBITAL ETHMOIDECTOMY
(Patterson's operation[11])

Indications

The indications given for the Lynch–Howarth procedure also apply to this operation. In addition, access to the orbital floor for trauma and decompression can be gained by this route.

Anaesthesia and preparation

These are the same as for the Lynch–Howarth operation.

Incision

7

After a temporary tarsorrhaphy, the incision, 2 cm long, is made in the natural crease of the nasojugal fold, one finger's-breadth below the inferior lash margin, extending not further than the midpoint of the orbital rim. Stay sutures can be used as retractors.

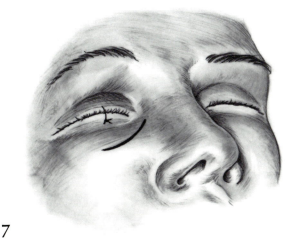

7

Dissection

8

The orbicularis muscle is split and the periosteum elevated at the orbital margin with meticulous care. Dissection reveals the origin of the inferior oblique muscle (except in 9 per cent of patients where the muscle is intraperiosteal)[7] and the lacrimal sac medially. The orbital floor is exposed and dissection continues postero-superiorly as far as the posterior ethmoidal vessels which are clipped or treated with diathermy. Malleable copper retractors are again useful. The lacrimal sac is mobilized and retracted laterally, allowing the ethmoidal cells to be entered via the lamina papyracea under direct vision, progressing posteriorly until the compact bone of the sphenoid, encompassing the optic canal, is reached. The height of the cribriform plate relative to the middle turbinate should always be borne in mind. The sphenoid sinus may be opened.

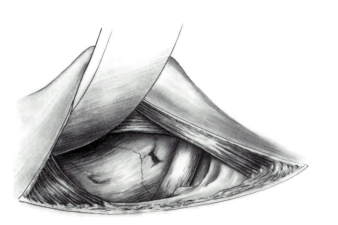

8

Decompression

9

Orbital decompression can be effected by removal of the medial wall inferior to the ethmoidal vessels, and the floor as far laterally as the infraorbital canal. If necessary, this can be combined with a lateral orbitotomy to remove bone on either side of the canal. In cases of trauma, repair of the orbital floor may be readily performed using Silastic sheeting or fascia lata. For greater visualization of the maxillary sinus it may be preferable to combine the Patterson's with a Caldwell–Luc approach.

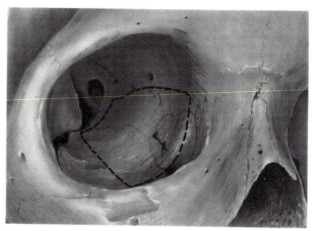

9

Closure

The wound is closed in layers with a separate layer of catgut to the split fibres of the orbicularis muscle. Occasionally temporary nasal packing is indicated. A pressure dressing should be applied for 24 hours and sutures removed after 4–5 days.

Complications

These are similar to those for the Lynch–Howarth procedure, with recurrence of disease and transient epiphora associated with oedema of the orbicularis muscle and lacrimal sac being the commonest. Previous intranasal ethmoidectomy may have led to fibrous adhesions between nasal mucosa and orbital periosteum, so considerable care is needed when dissecting orbital periosteum to avoid tears and prolapse of orbital fat.

OSTEOPLASTIC FLAP

Indications

1. Chronic suppuration which has failed to respond to all other means of treatment. The success of the external frontoethmoidectomy has limited its use.
2. Removal of osteomata through the craniofacial approach is preferable for extensive lesions (*see* chapter on 'Craniofacial approach for ethmoidal tumours' by Cheesman in the 4th edition of the 'Nose and Throat' volume of *Operative Surgery*).
3. Repair of trauma.

4. Treatment of frontoethmoidal mucoceles by this procedure has been advocated in the USA.

The use of this operation, originally advocated by Macbeth[12] and Goodale and Montgomery[13], with and without obliteration, has been largely superseded by the external frontoethmoidectomy and the craniofacial procedure.

Contraindications

If the ethmoids, sphenoid or maxilla are also extensively involved, it may be difficult to gain adequate access to these sinuses by this approach alone.

Preoperative evaluation and preparation

Radiographs of the frontal region are mandatory to determine the extent of the sinus and pathological changes. Hypocycloidal and computed tomography are usually indicated. From plain radiographs, a template can be made for use during the operation. The template is cut from Silastic sheeting which can be readily sterilized.

Prophylactic antibiotics are recommended with premedication. If the coronal incision is to be employed, the skin should be shaved 4 cm back from the hairline and prepared. If obliteration with abdominal fat is to be performed, the abdomen should be prepared with the intention of making the incision in the left iliac fossa.

The operation is performed under general anaesthesia, in the reversed Trendelenburg position, with the head positioned so that the plane of the forehead is horizontal. Temporary bilateral tarsorrhaphies are performed, and local infiltration of the proposed incision with lignocaine and adrenaline is helpful.

Incision

10

A coronal incision is made 2–3 cm behind the hairline, cutting through skin, subcutaneous tissue and frontalis muscle, but taking care not to incise the periosteum. The incision is extended inferolaterally to just anterior to the root of the helix. The flap is elevated inferiorly in the plane between frontalis muscle and periosteum to the supraorbital rims and glabella. Neurosurgical clips are useful for haemostasis.

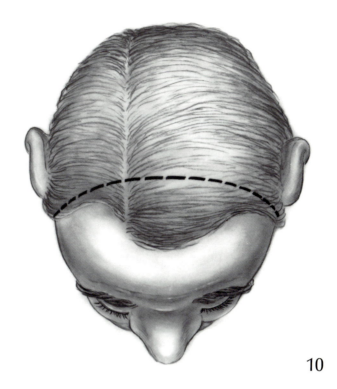

10

11

Alternatively, a 'spectacle' incision may be used and connected across the glabella. This is suitable when the sinus is small and on no account must the eyebrows be shaved.

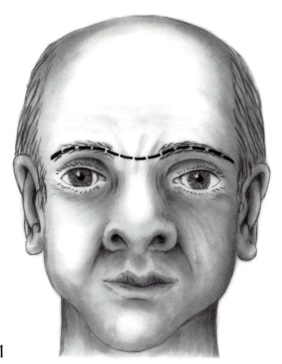

11

Removal of the anterior frontal sinus walls

12

The sterilized template is placed over the frontal sinuses, aligning supraorbital rims exactly and the superior and lateral margins are marked with methylene blue. Alternatively, wires or needles dipped in methylene blue, pushed through the skin to mark the periosteum, have been employed to define the sinus margin.

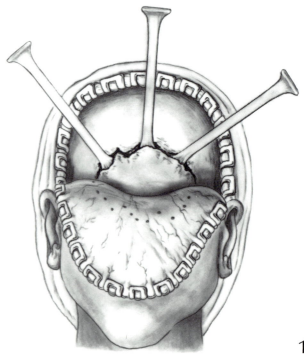

12

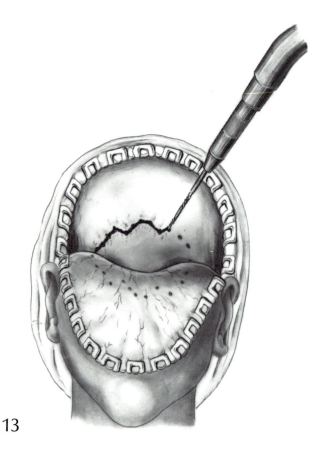

13

The periosteum is incised along this line down to bone and elevated 2–3 mm on each side of the incision to facilitate closure. A cut is made round this outline with a fissure burr or oscillating (Stryker) saw, cutting just inside the line to ensure the incision is within the limits of the sinus and bevelling it obliquely to prevent the bone falling in on replacement. The supraorbital and supratrochlear nerves should be preserved.

13

14

The intersinus septum is often thick enough to require breaking with a chisel or curved osteotome so that the flap can be prised down and forwards, hinged inferiorly along the floor of the frontal sinus. The supraorbital rims and glabella can be particularly thick in males so a separate cut may be helpful in the nasion.

14

Exenteration of the sinus mucosa

15

Except in areas of dural exposure, all diseased tissue can be removed, stripping the mucous membrane completely. It is particularly important to remember the complexity of frontal sinus anatomy with incomplete septa, supernumerary sinuses and diverticula. Finally, the bone should be burred to remove all traces of mucosa.

The frontonasal duct may be cleared if drainage is contemplated using a large Silastic tube, but more usually the last vestiges of mucosa are inverted to obliterate this region.

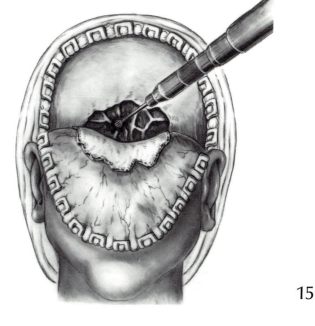

15

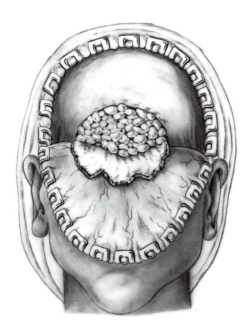

16

16

If fat is used in an attempt to obliterate the sinus, it is removed from the left lower quadrant of the anterior abdominal wall and must be handled with care to avoid trauma. (The right side is avoided to prevent confusion with an appendicectomy scar.) The fat should completely fill the sinus cavity. Bone chips or bone paté has also been used for this purpose.

Closure

17

The bony flap is replaced and the periosteal layer repaired meticulously. The skin is sutured in two layers, lateral drains inserted and a pressure dressing applied for 24 hours.

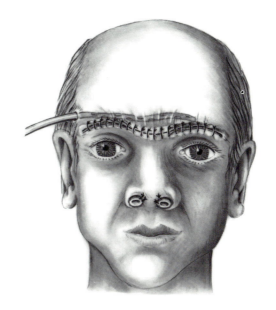

17

Variations

The operation is most often used for conditions affecting both frontal sinuses but it can be modified so only one sinus is opened. This is achieved by cutting parallel and lateral to the intersinus septum as shown on radiographs.

The approach can also be extended into a lateral craniotomy for large lesions arising in the lateral superior orbit.

Complications

Cosmesis.   Frontal bossing, bony depression and nasal skin necrosis have been reported, so meticulous care in repair is required. Subsequent cranioplasty and bone grafting may be necessary. The receding male hairline may make even the best scars visible with time.

Haemorrhage with haematoma formation under the flap.   This is avoided by careful haemostasis and an adequate pressure dressing postoperatively.

Infection of primary and abdominal donor site. Osteomyelitis of the frontal bone flap will have disastrous cosmetic results. It is therefore most important that prophylactic antibiotics should be used.

Cerebrospinal fluid leak.   Dural tears may result from inaccurate use of the template or as a result of pathological osteolysis and require primary repair with fascia lata or similar grafts.

Recurrence of original pathology.   This has been reported to be as high as 25 per cent[14].

References

1. Reidel BM. Schennke Inaugural Dissertation, Jena, 1898.

2. Howarth WG. A radical frontal sinus operation. *J Laryngol Otol* 1923; 38: 341–3.

3. Lynch RC. The technique of a radical frontal sinus operation which has given me the best results. *Laryngoscope* 1921; 31: 1–5.

4. Rubin JS, Lund VJ, Salmon B. Frontoethmoidectomy in the treatment of mucoceles: a neglected operation. *Arch Otolaryngol* 1986; 112: 434–6.

5. Stammberger H. Endoscopic endonasal surgery – concepts in treatment of recurring rhinosinusitis. Part I. Anatomic and pathophysiologic considerations. *Otolaryngol Head Neck Surg* 1986; 94: 143–56.

6. Rontal E, Rontal M, Guilford FT. Surgical anatomy of the orbit. *Ann Otol Rhinol Laryngol* 1979; 88: 382–6.

7. Harrison DFN. Surgical approach to the medial orbital wall. *Ann Otol Rhinol Laryngol* 1981; 90: 415–19.

8. Schaeffer JP. *The Nose, Paranasal Sinuses, Nasolacrimal Passageways and Olfactory Organ in Man: Agenetic, Developmental and Anatomic-Physiological Considerations.* Philadelphia: Blakiston, 1919.

9. Lund VJ. Anatomical considerations in the aetiology of fronto-ethmoidal mucoceles. *Rhinology* 1987; 25: 83–8.

10. Lund VJ, Rolfe ME. Ophthalmic considerations in fronto-ethmoidal mucoceles. *J Laryngol Otol* 1989; 103: 667–9.

11. Patterson N. External operations on the frontal and ethmoidal sinuses. *J Laryngol Otol* 1939; 54: 235–44.

12. Macbeth RG. The osteoplastic operation for chronic infection of the frontal sinus. *J Laryngol Otol* 1954; 68: 465–77.

13. Goodale RL, Montgomery WW. Experiences with osteoplastic anterior wall approach to the frontal sinus: case histories and recommendations. *Arch Otolaryngol* 1958; 68: 271–83.

14. Schenk NL. Frontal sinus disease: III. Experimental and clinical factors in failure of the frontal osteoplastic operation. *Laryngoscope* 1975; 85: 76–92.

Illustrations by Robert Lane

Radical maxillectomy

V. J. Lund MS, FRCS
Institute of Laryngology and Otology, Royal National Throat, Nose and Ear Hospital, London, UK

Introduction

The maxilla comprises a bony box or body with four processes – zygomatic, frontal, alveolar and palatine, which must be divided for its removal. The bone has four surfaces – nasal, orbital, infratemporal and anterior, any of which may have been breached by disease, this depending to a large extent on the thickness of the bone in these areas.

History

The first total maxillectomy was probably carried out by Gensoul in 1827[1]. Lizars described the first radical maxillectomy in the UK in 1829[2] though Syme also performed a similar procedure at virtually the same time[3]. In 1842 William Fergusson removed a large tumour from the maxilla of a 12-year-old girl without general anaesthesia in 16 minutes before an audience of 200 medical students[4].

Indications

1. Removal of malignancy arising within the maxilla, either within the sinus or from the bone itself. To satisfy oncological criteria, disease should be confined to within the sinus cavity which, due to late presentation, is rarely the case. Frequently orbital clearance is required and exenteration of the ethmoid labyrinth. Extensive ethmoidal involvement where there is any possibility of compromise of the cribriform plate is better managed by craniofacial resection, which can be combined with maxillectomy and orbital clearance.
2. Removal of extensive benign pathology affecting the maxilla. Fortunately these lesions are rarely encountered but after years of neglect significant disfigurement may have resulted from fibro-osseous conditions, though a total maxillectomy would only be performed in the last resort.
3. The Weber–Fergusson approach can be employed for extensive angiofibromas which have substantially eroded the maxilla, extending laterally into the infratemporal fossa and which cannot be encompassed by the lateral rhinotomy approach. This approach should be compared with the mid-facial degloving procedure (*see* chapter on 'Mid-facial degloving', pp. 571–575). Having achieved access, the residual maxilla is conserved.

Contraindications

In the past many patients with extensive antroethmoidal disease underwent total maxillectomy and orbital clearance which nowadays would be treated by craniofacial resection. An accurate radiological appraisal to determine intracranial spread is necessary in these patients.

Preoperative

Adequate histological and radiological assessment is mandatory. Computed tomography (in both direct axial and coronal planes with contrast) defines the extent of the pathology, the type of which will be confirmed by biopsy. Differentiation between tumour mass, inflammation and fluid can be difficult on computed tomography and may be resolved by magnetic resonance[3].

It is important that the patient is assessed by a prosthedontist before operation to take impressions of permanent dentition and existing dentures for modification. Broad spectrum antibiotics are given with the premedication.

The need for orbital clearance may be readily apparent on clinical and radiological grounds but equivocal cases may only be determined at operation and these possibilities must be discussed with the patient before the operation.

Anaesthesia and preparation

The operation is performed under general anaesthesia with the patient supine in the reversed Trendelenburg position. An oral cuffed endotracheal tube is used taped to the opposite side of the mouth and an additional pharyngeal pack is recommended. After routine preparation of the face, a temporary tarsorrhaphy is performed on the affected side.

Operation

Incision

1

The classic 'Weber–Fergusson' incision runs approximately 2–3 mm below the lower lash margin which allows skin to be detached from the orbicularis oculi. If the incision is placed too low, disfiguring oedema can result; if placed too close to the lash margin, ectropion may occur. The incision extends beyond the lateral canthus and is continued from the level of the medial canthus, down the side of the nose in the crease as for lateral rhinotomy, cutting straight through nasal mucosa. It then curves round the ala to the midline of the columella, and the upper lip is divided with Mayo scissors while holding firmly either side, to maintain haemostasis, until clips can be applied to the superior labial vessels. It is important to make the angle at the medial canthus as obtuse as possible as the blood supply to this corner may be jeopardized, particularly after radiation, and may subsequently break down.

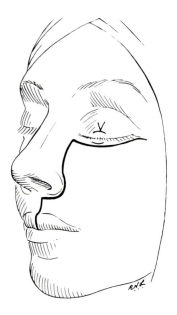

1

2

The upper lip skin edges can be held back with an Allis retractor or a stitch through subcutaneous tissue while the rest of the incision is completed. The cut continues in the alveolar buccal sulcus, passes round the maxillary tuberosity and crosses the palate at the junction of the soft and hard palates. A cutting diathermy is helpful to minimize bleeding. Finally the incision is completed from posterior to anterior through the mucous membrane of the hard palate just lateral to the midline and joins the alveolar buccal incision in the region of the first incisor which, if present, must be removed.

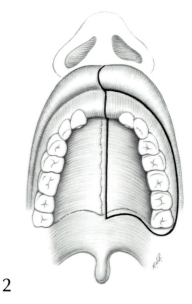

2

Elevation of skin and mucosa

3

The entire skin flap including buccinator can now be raised, revealing the maxillary bone and pyriform aperture back to the zygomatic arch and lateral margin of the malar bone, exposing the orbicularis intact around the eye. The orbital rim is defined and the orbital periosteum carefully dissected to reveal the orbital floor, traumatizing the orbicularis oculi as little as possible. Careful inspection of this region, particularly along the infraorbital canal, is important to ensure that no tumour invasion has occurred, in which case orbital clearance would be indicated. Similarly the lamina papyracea of the medial wall must be examined along its entire length as tumour may escape into the orbital apex by this route.

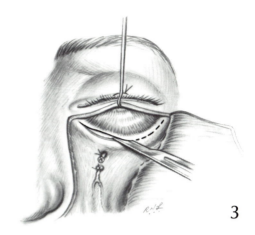

3

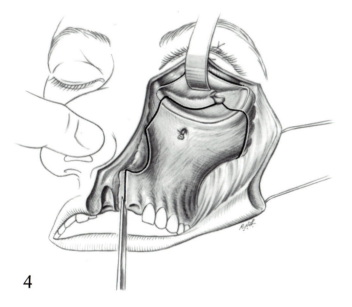

4

Division of bony attachments

4

The malar bone is divided by a Gigli saw passed into the lateral part of the infraorbital fissure with curved forceps. A Stryker saw may also be used, particularly when the bone has been weakened by tumour invasion. The zygoma is similarly divided after detachment of the masseter. The incision is carried across the floor of the orbit and through the frontal process to join the piriform aperture.

5

A Gigli saw, fissure burr or osteotome and chisel may be used to divide the hard palate, starting from the incisor socket and passing posteriorly, lateral to the attachment of the nasal septum. The hard and soft palates have already been divided leaving only the pterygoid process to be separated. This is best done with a large curved osteotome inserted behind the tuberosity in the groove between it and pterygoid process. A variable amount of force and leverage will detach the bone but the pterygoid muscle fibres must be cut with curved Mayo scissors before the specimen is free. The maxilla is grasped with Lions forceps and rocked while cutting the final attachments. After removal of the maxilla, a hot pack should be available to place in the cavity immediately to diminish bleeding from the internal maxillary artery.

After several minutes the cavity can be inspected and, if necessary, the artery ligated; sometimes a transfixion suture to the pterygoid muscles is needed. The detached pterygoid plates should be removed to contour the cavity and the ethmoid labyrinth exenterated, bearing in mind the level of the cribriform plate. The anterior wall of the sphenoid is opened and any roughened bony edges smoothed. The cavity may be washed with saline at this point.

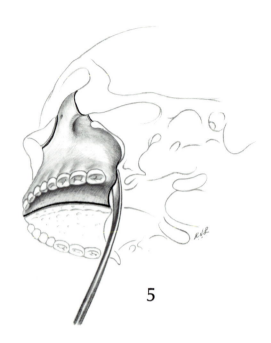

5

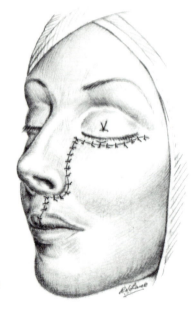

6

Closure of skin

6

The cavity is now checked for haemostasis and a 2-inch ribbon gauze soaked in Whitehead's varnish inserted, sufficient to line the cavity without obstructing the temporary prosthesis. The skin flap is laid back and closed with subcutaneous catgut and fine silk sutures, with particular care in the medial canthal region and at the vermilion border.

Insertion of the prosthesis

The prosthedontist now fashions a temporary obturator using gutta percha on the pre-formed denture which attaches to the existing dentition and fills the palatal defect, restoring facial contour. Use of the Whitehead's pack and obturator prevents contracture and obviates the need for skin grafting of the cavity. Normal speech and diet can thus be achieved in the immediate postoperative period. Similarly temporalis flaps to close the palatal defect are unnecessary and hamper subsequent cavity inspection. In the edentulous, the prosthesis may have to be temporarily wired in place.

Having removed the tarsorrhaphy suture, the eye is carefully rinsed of blood, some chloramphenicol (Chloromycetin) ointment introduced and an eye pad with tulle gras applied followed by a light pressure dressing for 24 h.

Postoperative management

7

The patient may commence on a soft diet on the first postoperative day but should continue on antibiotics until removal of the pack and stitches 5–7 days later. This is combined with minor modifications to the temporary prosthesis, after which a permanent light-weight obturator can be fashioned.

The cavity can be readily inspected and regular douching minimizes crusting which usually settles after a few months.

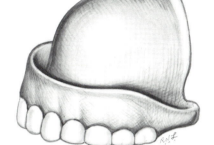

7

Complications

1. Haemorrhage from the internal maxillary or occasionally from ethmoidal vessels can occur but adequate haemostasis and the Whitehead's pack usually avoids this problem.
2. Cerebrospinal fluid leak can occur if over-enthusiastic exenteration of the ethmoids is performed.
3. Ophthalmic problems. The preservation of the suspensory ligament of Lockwood, medial palpebral ligament and posterior portion of the orbital floor provide adequate support for the eye, resulting in excellent function in most patients.

4. Cosmetic problems may result from poor placement of the lower lid incision resulting in lymphoedema or ectropion. This may require later surgical intervention. An acute angle below the medial canthus may result in a defect, especially in irradiated skin. Care must be taken at the ala to avoid contracture, which lifts the upper lip in an apparent 'sneer', and careful approximation of the vermilion border is important.

Variations

Orbital clearance

8

Many maxillary sinus malignancies may have invaded the orbit at presentation. This necessitates orbital clearance, as opposed to 'exenteration' where the eyelids are also removed, though to no oncological advantage. A modified Weber–Diffenbach incision is used which skirts both lash margins. Attention to the angle acuity as the nasofacial incision is extended inferiorly is again important. Using stay sutures the eyelid skin can be retracted and elevated from the underlying tarsal plates.

The clearance of the orbit is completed after elevation of the facial flap. There is no advantage in performing this in continuity with the maxillectomy, which is actually facilitated by the initial clearance of the orbital contents. The orbital periosteum is elevated and freed around the entire bony socket, bearing in mind its adherence to the suture lines and the trochlea. The medial and lateral suspensory ligaments are detached and a finger can be swept round the socket completing the dissection. Finally the orbital apex is divided with curved Mayo scissors and the eye removed. Care is taken not to traumatize unduly the globe, which can be sent for use in corneal grafting.

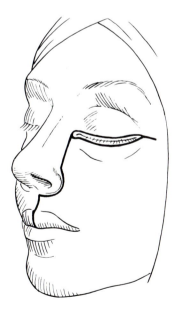

8

9

A hot pack is inserted in the orbit and the remaining contents inspected to define tumour invasion and complete haemostasis, usually with ligation of the ophthalmic artery. The maxillectomy is completed as before but with additional amounts of the bony orbit being removed as necessary. The orbit is lightly packed with Whitehead's varnish ribbon gauze but insufficient to affect the skin of the socket. The edges of the lids are carefully approximated so that the skin will eventually fall back to line the socket, although it will usually move with respiration in the first few weeks after the pack is removed. At 7–10 days after surgery a general anaesthetic is given to allow removal of the packing and any modification of the obturator which had been positioned at the end of the initial operation.

Once the skin of the orbital socket is well seated an orbital prosthesis can be fashioned based on preoperative photographs. This can be attached to spectacles or sometimes self-retaining in the cavity using 'glues', although these may traumatize the surrounding skin. Osseointegrated implants are playing an increasingly important role in the rehabilitation of these patients in our unit, but their use remains confined to specialist centres at present.

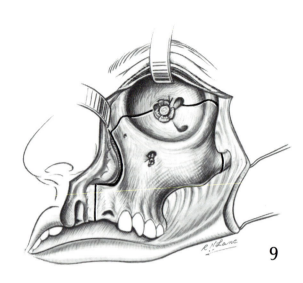

9

Extended radical maxillectomy

Involvement of anterior cheek skin will necessitate resection and reconstruction either with local flaps or more probably a pedicled or free myocutaneous flap.

Extension through the posterior wall into the pterygoid musculature will require further clearance of this region and the infratemporal fossa, although clearance of malignant tumour which has extended thus far must be regarded as principally palliative. Similarly, extension through the orbital apex into the middle cranial fossa is prognostically disastrous, although radioactive seeding of the area may be beneficial.

A craniofacial approach is indicated if ethmoidal extension with anterior cranial fossa involvement is suspected.

References

1. Gensoul PJ. *Lettre Chirurgicale sur Quelques Maladies Graves du Sinus Maxilliare avec Atlas de Huit Planches en Couleur*. Paris: Bailliere, 1833.

2. Lizars J. Removal of the superior maxillary bone. *London Med Gaz* 1829–30; V: 92–3.

3. Syme J. Excision of the upper jaw. *Edinb Med Surg J* 1829; xxxii: 238–9.

4. Fergusson W. Lecture 10. In: *Lectures on the Progress of Anatomy and Surgery During the Present Century*. London: Churchill & Sons, 1867.

5. Lund VJ, Howard DJ, Lloyd GAS, Cheesman AD. Magnetic resonance imaging of paranasal sinus tumours for craniofacial resection. *Head Neck Surg* 1989; 11: 279–83.

Mid-facial degloving technique (sublabial approach) for nasal and paranasal sinus resection

David J. Howard   FRCS, FRCS(Ed)
Institute of Laryngology and Otology, Royal National Throat, Nose and Ear Hospital, London, UK

Introduction

This technique allows exposure of the structures of the middle third of the face without external skin incisions. The first full description of this technique was published by Casson et al.[1] in 1974. It has not been commonly used but is slowly gaining its place in the repertoire of the head and neck surgeon. It must be stressed that it does not completely supersede the standard approaches of lateral rhinotomy and the Weber–Fergusson incision but it will provide an equally good exposure and operative result in many cases previously treated by these two approaches.

The mid-facial degloving procedure requires skill in both basic sinus and rhinoplastic surgery as the approach involves bilaterally extended sublabial Caldwell–Luc incisions, coupled with soft tissue elevation of the entire nasal dorsum.

1

This degloving allows good exposure of the nasal cavities and the bones of the middle third of the face, with considerable mobility of the upper lip. With appropriate dissection, retraction and bony removal, the nasal septum, nasopharynx, ethmoids, sphenoid sinus, pterygo-palatine area and infratemporal fossa can all be explored. Control of the internal maxillary artery is easily obtained. The steps may be duplicated bilaterally if necessary in the removal of extensive lesions.

The degloved area of skin is supplied by the facial and infraorbital arteries which remain intact so that other skin incisions may be added to provide additional exposure. Combination with transpalatal, temporal, orbital and frontal operations is possible for extensive lesions.

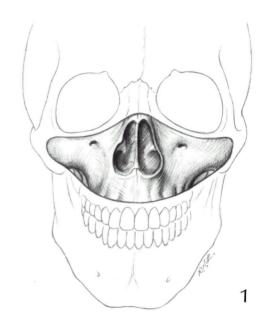

1

Indications

1. For the resection of benign nasal and sinus disease, particularly inverting papilloma, angiofibroma and fibro-osseus disease.
2. Septodermoplasty and repair of large septal perforations.
3. Mid-facial fractures.
4. Mid-facial osteotomies.
5. Mid-facial bone grafting for contour restoration.
6. Selected malignant tumours which can be adequately encompassed with the exposure.

All the above are ideally carried out in children and adolescents where external incisions may be particularly undesirable.

Advantages

1. Good exposure of the nasal cavities, mid-third of face and central skull base.
2. Allows additional modification and extension.
3. No external scarring.
4. Minimal postoperative complications.
5. Successful control of a wide variety of disease.
6. Good patient tolerance.

Disadvantage

The only disadvantage is the occasional occurrence of nasal vestibular stenosis.

Contraindications

The procedure is contraindicated in extensive lesions of the skull base involving the frontal sinuses, orbit and cribriform plate. These are more appropriately treated by external approaches or craniofacial surgery. A dividing line between the size of the lesion resectable by a mid-facial degloving approach and other more radical approaches will depend on the particular pathology, an individual patient's anatomy and the experience of the surgeon. It is therefore a dividing line that cannot be rigidly defined.

Preoperative procedures

The patient is warned before the operation about postoperative facial bruising and oedema. The likelihood of, and the timescale of resolution of, postoperative intranasal crusting is also discussed, particularly in those patients undergoing removal of the more extensive lesions. Advice is also given to the patient with regard to infraorbital numbness and paraesthesia which may be experienced after the operation.

Operation

The operation is performed under general anaesthesia; the endotracheal tube is positioned centrally in the mouth and fixed to the chin. The patient is supine in a reversed Trendelenburg position with approximately 15° of head-up tilt. The head rests on a ring to facilitate intraoperative positioning. Vasoconstriction of the nasal mucosa is produced using either Moffat's solution or 5 per cent cocaine solution on pledgets applied intranasally. Additional haemostasis is produced using xylocaine with adrenaline 1:200000 injected into the proposed incision sites in the soft tissue of the nose, buccogingival sulcus and anterior face of maxilla. Suture tarsorrhaphies or corneal protectors are placed bilaterally. Skin preparation may be used and head drapes applied. A head lamp is desirable, preferably with fibreoptic illumination.

2

A bilateral sublabial incision is carried out straight down to the level of bone and with a lateral extent out to the maxillary tuberosity on both sides.

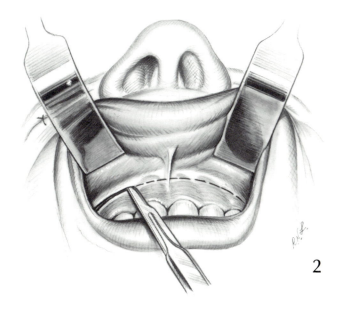

2

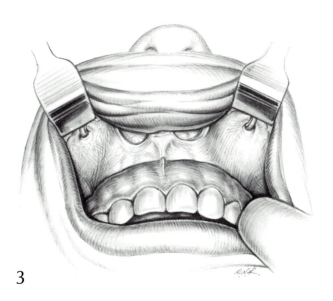

3

3

The periosteum over the anterior face of the maxilla is raised with the soft tissues bilaterally, taking care to identify and preserve the infraorbital nerves.

4a, b & c

Routine rhinoplasty-type intercartilaginous incisions are made. These enable separation of the soft tissues of the nose from the upper lateral cartilages. The periosteum overlying the nasal bones is elevated as far laterally as possible and superiorly to the root of the nose. A transfixion incision is then performed along the dorsal and caudal borders of the cartilaginous septum from the medial crura of the lower lateral cartilages. This incision is further extended across the floor of the nose to the lateral aspect of the pyriform fossa connecting with the intercartilaginous incision to complete circumvestibular release. Sharp dissection laterally then connects the skeletonized nose with the anterior maxillary areas already elevated.

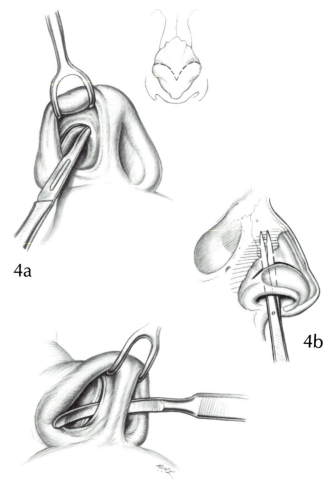

4a

4b

4c

5

The skin of the middle third of the face can now be degloved from the skull all the way superiorly to the frontonasal suture line, infraorbital rim and, laterally, the zygomatic process. The mouth can then be retracted laterally sufficiently to dissect behind the maxillary sinus into the infratemporal fossa where the internal maxillary artery can be ligated or clipped if necessary before commencing resection.

It is now possible to gain excellent access to the nasal cavities, nasal septum and enter the maxillary sinus anteriorly in the usual way. Excellent exposure of the nasopharynx can be obtained by the following steps:

1. Removal of the anterior wall of the maxilla.
2. Removal of the posterior wall of the maxilla.
3. Control of the internal maxillary artery.
4. Removal of the lateral wall of the nose, including the perpendicular process of the palatine bone.

Ethmoidectomy and sphenoidectomy may now be carried out under good visualization. The whole nasal septum is accessible and may be removed if necessary up to the level of the cribriform plate. The posterior wall of the sphenoid sinus, pterygoid muscles and plates, and the base of sphenoid are the posterior limits of resection. The cribriform plate and anterior cranial fossa are the superior limits and the lateral limit is the coronoid process of the mandible. The inferior boundary is the palate although obviously removal of the palate and inferior maxillectomy are easily undertaken with this approach.

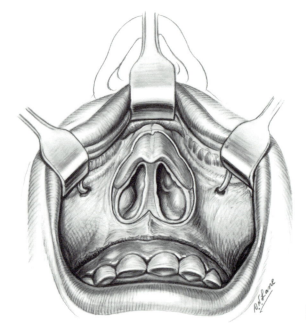

5

Special points of note

1. Nasal deformity may occur if the frontal process of the maxilla is extensively removed.
2. Sachs *et al.*[2] described a modification involving the establishment of a bipedicled flap of lateral nasal wall mucosa fashioned just at the piriform aperture before removal of the remainder of the lateral wall of the nose. Reapproximation of this flap to the vestibular skin at the end of the procedure is said to decrease the occasional complication of vestibular stenosis.
3. Before the resection of any lesion it is important to remove any sharp edges from bony areas that have been resected, particularly if finger dissection of the lesion is contemplated.
4. Considerable retraction is required during this operation and care must be taken to avoid the infraorbital nerve.

After the pathological process has been excised, careful haemostasis is achieved and the resulting cavity packed with ribbon gauze soaked in Whitehead's varnish or other appropriate antibiotic-saturated petroleum gauze. The end is brought out through a nostril. The nasal structures are then carefully repositioned and plain catgut sutures applied accurately around the circumvestibular incision and along the sublabial incision. Care is required with this closure. The midline frenulum of the sublabial incision must be accurately approximated. Routine rhinoplastic taping and splinting helps to reduce facial oedema. A single intraoperative injection of 8–12 mg dexamethasone is given intramuscularly.

Postoperative management

Packing should be removed between 3 and 10 days after the operation depending on the extent of the operative procedure and the type of lesion removed. With the larger resections for lesions such as angiofibroma, the packing may be left up to 10 days and the author's preference for removal of this packing is under a short general anaesthetic; this particularly allows for control of any haemorrhage which may occasionally ensue. The two commonest postoperative complaints are infraorbital numbness and paraesthesia and recurrent crusting of the cavity. The former symptom resolves with time and the latter responds well to the application of saline sniffs up to four times daily. Only occasionally will decrusting be required under a short general anaesthetic during the follow-up period.

Complications

Notable complications are rare with this technique, the commonest being vestibular stenosis which occurs in approximately 5 per cent of patients. Occasional deformity of the nose consequent upon over-resection of the bone has been reported. Disturbance of facial growth in children, atrophic rhinitis, epiphora and oroantral fistulae have not been reported.

References

1. Casson PR, Bonnano PC, Converse JM. The midface degloving procedure. *Plast Reconstr Surg* 1974; 53: 102–3.

2. Sachs ME, Conley J, Rabuzzi D, Blaugrund S, Price J. Degloving approach for total excision of inverted papilloma. *Laryngoscope* 1984; 94: 1595–8.

Prosthetics in head and neck surgery

R. D. Manderson FDS RCS(Ed)
Consultant in Prosthetic Dentistry, Stoke Mandeville Hospital, Aylesbury, Buckinghamshire, UK

Introduction

Maxillofacial prosthetics is the art and science of replacing lost tissue using inert, biocompatible materials to restore the appearance and, where possible, function to the patient.

The prosthetic rehabilitation of a patient following ablative surgery of the jaws or face is an essential part of the management of head and neck malignancy. The objectives, if accomplished, have a dramatic effect on the morale of the patient. Of primary importance in the successful achievement of these objectives is adequate preoperative assessment and planning.

Surgical procedures may be modified to facilitate the design and construction of the most appropriate prosthesis. This may involve removal of more bone at the cut edge, to allow soft tissue to cover these smoothed edges and reduce large unwanted undercut areas which would interfere with the fitting of the prosthesis or require 'blocking out'. The path of insertion of the obturator must be considered as the form of the cavity is assessed towards the end of the operation. This may necessitate the construction of a more complex two-part prosthesis, which can be beneficial for the retention and stability of the definitive prosthesis. Unfavourable undercut areas or conflicting paths of insertion of the denture base and obturator can create problems when attempting to construct a more simple design of prosthesis.

As well as planning the surgery to create a cavity with an appropriate path of insertion with few unwanted undercut areas, horizontal areas which can provide support for the obturator should also be located. In general, respiratory epithelium does not provide suitable supporting tissue. Tissue covered by squamous epithelium from adjacent areas or skin grafts can be used.

Preoperative

When it appears probable that a prosthesis will be required, preoperative planning and discussion between the surgeon, the restorative consultant and the maxillofacial technician should take place as early as possible following diagnosis of the tumour. Dental casts of both jaws (and the face if appropriate), intraoral and full-face photographs and dental radiographs make useful preoperative records, particularly where the facial appearance may be altered postoperatively. Dental caries, periodontal status and the quality of existing fillings, and fixed or removable prostheses are all assessed. Any urgent treatment is initiated and any unsaveable teeth assigned for extraction. Doubtful teeth may be retained and fully investigated later, if radiotherapy is not planned. Fixed bridges which are close to the tumour site may require to be sectioned or removed prior to surgery.

With casts available, the extent of the anticipated surgery is agreed and plans made regarding the design of the prosthesis which will carry the immediate replacement temporary obturator and any reconstructive surgery.

General principles

Anaesthesia

1

A nasal endotracheal tube should be used if possible when maxillary resection is undertaken. This allows access for the immediate replacement obturator without interference from an orally passed endotracheal tube. It also allows the teeth, when present, to be brought together, ensuring satisfactory occlusion, avoiding destabilizing forces on the obturator.

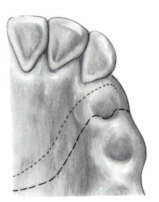

1

Alveolar sectioning

2

In dentate patients, care should be taken to avoid making the bone cut too close to the root of the tooth adjacent to the lesion. The cut should be made at least 3 mm from the abutment tooth through the adjacent socket. The bone should be covered with mucoperiosteal flaps from the buccal and palatal mucosa. This will enhance the healing, preserve bone proximal to the abutment tooth and provide a more appropriate tissue support for the prosthesis.

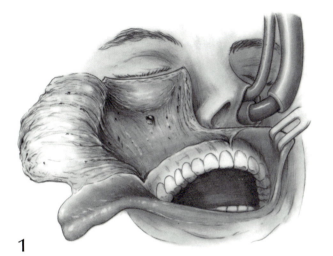
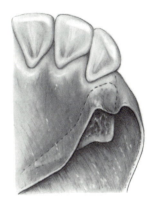

2

Palatal sectioning

3

The sagittal incision of the palate should be designed to allow for the bone edge to be smoothed and covered by mucoperiosteum from the palate, reduced in thickness if necessary and sutured to the nasal mucosa. This provides a more comfortable border to the defect, against which the obturator can form a good border seal.

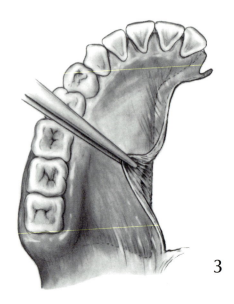

3

Coronoid process

4

Following maxillectomy the coronoid process on the side of the resection may be removed with some advantage to the stability and retention of the obturator. The postero-buccal extension of the obturator can be extended further into the buccal sulcus without the patient experiencing discomfort or displacement during opening or lateral mandibular movements. The more favourable buccal contour of the obturator against the buccinator muscle may provide improved retention.

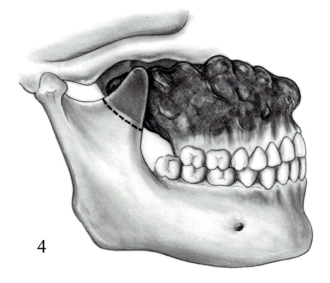

4

Maxillary resection

IMMEDIATE REPLACEMENT OBTURATOR

The ideal objectives of the obturator fitted at the time of surgery should be immediate restoration of speech, deglutition, mastication, appearance and morale. The obturator also serves the function of providing the conditions to hold the skin graft lining the defect in position, and achieve graft take.

Using an existing denture

5

An existing removable prosthesis may be modified to carry the material used to obturate the defect, e.g. black gutta-percha, Stent (De Trey A. G., Zurich, Switzerland) impression compound or silicone putty. The denture base may be modified to increase its support and retention by relining the base by standard clinical and laboratory procedures, or by using a suitable temporary direct relining technique and adding loops of stiff German silver wire to the tissue fitting surface in relation to the defect. This is prepared prior to surgery and fitted in theatre, as described also in the chapter on 'Reconstructive techniques of the oral cavity', pp. 215–240.

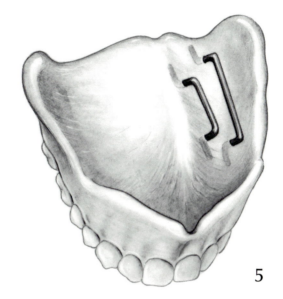

5

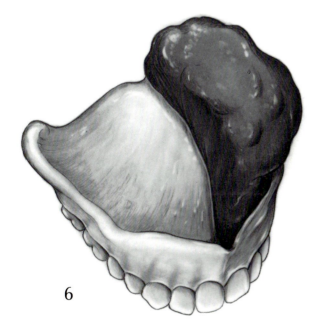

6

6

The tissue surface of the denture is dried and the gutta-percha or other material prepared. Gutta-percha must be heated in near-boiling water for 3–4 minutes to reach its ideal workable state. It is then rolled into a ball and heated with a flame to become tacky in order to adhere to the denture surface and retention loops. The denture with gutta-percha is placed in the mouth and moulded by the tissues to fill the defect. The final shape should be more like an inverted cone than a pyramid.

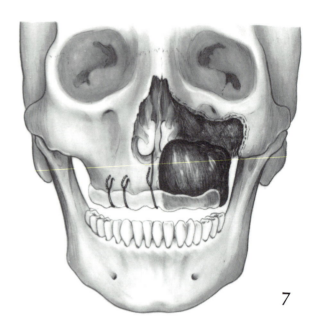

7

Using a simple acrylic dressing plate

7 & 8

A new appliance can be made prior to surgery in the form of a simple acrylic dressing plate without teeth, and with large loops on the upper surface to carry the obturating material and small loops on the buccal surface to attach the ligature wires for peralveolar, circumzygomatic or transnasal wiring. The obturating material is added as before but, as the dressing plate is retained in position by wiring, often less care is taken with the retentive form of the obturator.

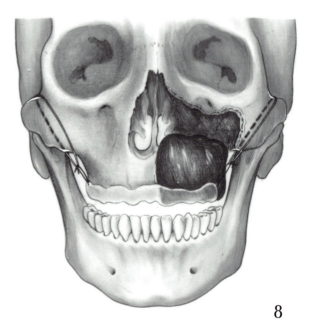

8

Using a new immediate replacement denture obturator

9

As a general rule, if a new appliance is required, it is best to construct an obturator with teeth carried on a correctly extended denture base designed to carry a suitable material, e.g. black gutta-percha, which will completely obturate the defect and provide satisfactory retention and stability without the necessity of surgical wiring. In dentate or partially dentate patients, acrylic bases with stainless steel clasps are used on several remaining teeth.

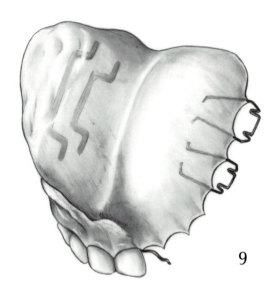

9

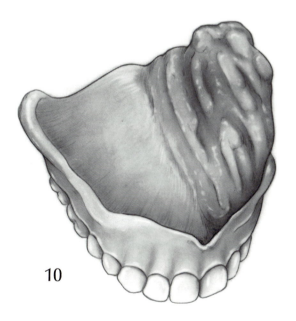

10

10

Care is taken to make an accurate record of the defect in the mouth at the time of surgery. In either event the patient should be restored cosmetically and functionally with regard to speech and deglutition immediately postoperatively, without requiring surgical wiring for retention.

Using a sectional immediate replacement obturator

11–13

A sectional dressing plate can be made which allows the non-obturator section to be left wired in, while the obturator section can be removed separately. The two sections are joined down the centre by a laboratory constructed device which resembles a piano hinge, the central rod of which is removable and may be square or round in section. If a round section rod is used, an antirotation device has to be incorporated on the acrylic base plates. As an additional refinement, small magnets can be incorporated into the base plate and an arch of teeth set up, processed and attached to the sectional base plate by means of these magnets.

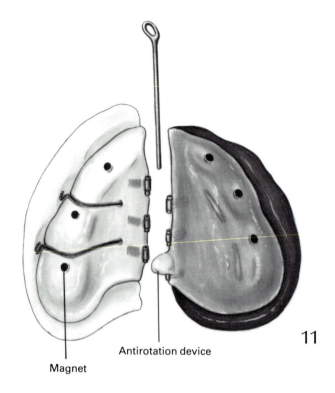

Antirotation device

Magnet

11

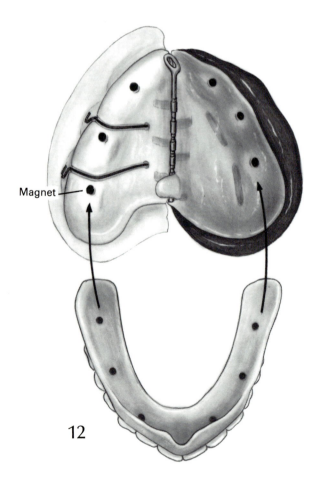

Magnet

12

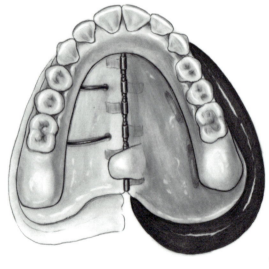

13

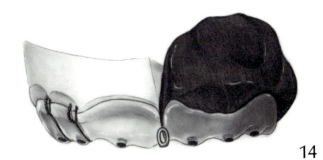

14

14 & 15

The appliance therefore has three main parts, the non-obturator half of the palate retained using peralveolar wiring, the obturator section retained by the hinge-like connection, and the teeth attached to the assembled dressing plate by magnets. To inspect the cavity, the teeth are first removed, exposing access to the central rod of the 'piano hinge' which on withdrawal allows removal of the obturator half of the dressing plate. The other half of the dressing plate remains wired in to provide positive retention for the obturator when replaced. The result is a cosmetic and functional prosthesis with access to the defect, used during the first few weeks postoperatively, prior to the construction of the definitive prosthesis.

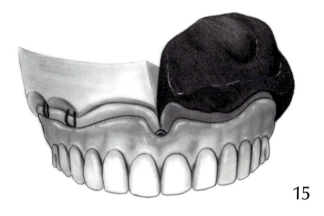

15

Direct obturator technique

16

If no immediate obturator has been constructed, a surgical pack soaked in Whitehead's varnish may be used for a few days and on removal a small elastic obturator can be constructed. Polyurethane foam is cut and shaped to fit the defect approximately following removal of the surgical pack.

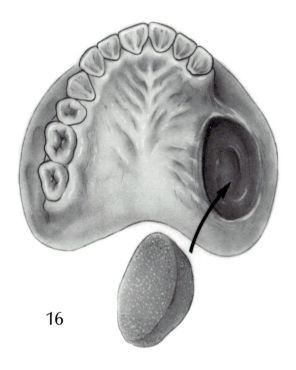

16

17

A sheet of soft metal is cut and contoured to follow the contour of the palate, using the intact palate as a guide.

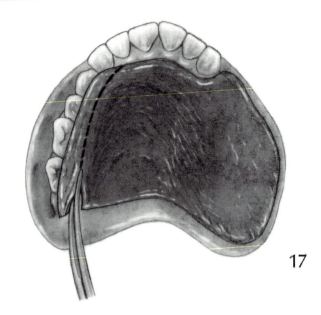

17

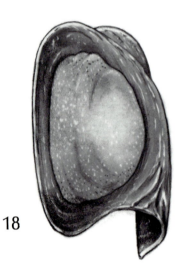

18

18

The foam is then covered with silicone impression material or tissue conditioner, placed onto the soft metal and carried into the defect.

19

When set, the metal is removed leaving a foam elastic obturator covered with an impervious layer of material. This temporary, comfortable obturator fills the defect and restores speech and deglutition.

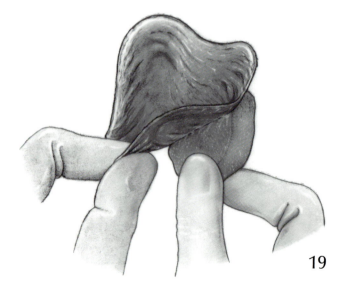

19

DEFINITIVE MAXILLARY OBTURATOR

A number of designs and materials for obturators have been suggested for use following maxillectomy. Materials used are broadly:

1. Hard acrylic: designed as hollow box or open nasally.
2. Soft polymers: latex, plasticized acrylics, silicones, polyurethanes, etc. These are used either in solid or hollow box form, and may be closed or open nasally.

Hollow box acrylic obturator

20

This provides a very satisfactory, lightweight appliance which is easily cleaned. Unwanted undercut areas must be removed surgically or blocked out to allow its insertion. A nasal airway constructed from perspex tubing can be incorporated into the obturator.

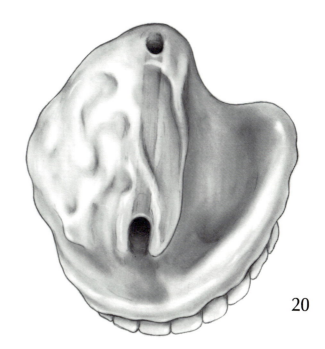

20

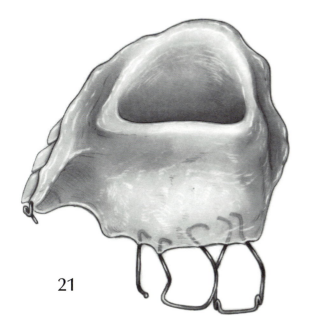

21

Open nasal acrylic obturator

21

These are also hard, light, simple to make and are easily modified, without the risk of perforating sometimes encountered with a hollow box, but they are less easy to clean than the hollow box design.

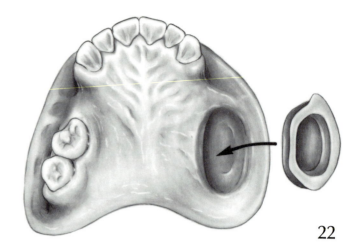

22

Sectional obturators

22 & 23

These are constructed to take advantage of undercuts by using a different path of insertion for the obturator and the denture base. The obturator part may be made of hard or resilient materials and the two parts may be held together using small magnets or precision or semi-precision retainers such as rods and tubes and studs.

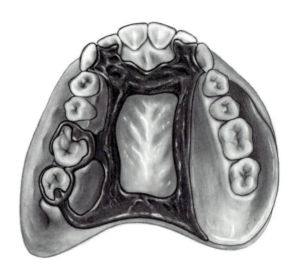

23

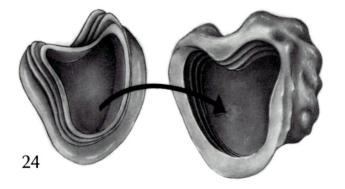

24

24

Another method uses circular grooves around a raised rim of acrylic on the fitting surface of the denture base, onto which a hollow box elastic obturator with ridges fits. The hollow elastic box obturator may be worn at night with a simple removable lid in place of the denture base and teeth.

Springs and swivel-retained obturators

25 & 26

Occasionally it may prove difficult, because of the magnitude of the surgical defect, e.g. total bilateral maxillectomy, or loss of combined palatal and facial tissues, to obtain retention and stability. In these cases, springs may be used. Two coil springs are attached to the upper and lower dentures to keep the maxillary denture up, acting against the mandibular denture. The swivel attachments to which the springs are attached are manufactured or can be made in the laboratory. These are sometimes known as Washington springs after the most famous wearer of dentures retained by these devices, George Washington.

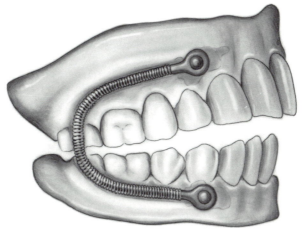

25

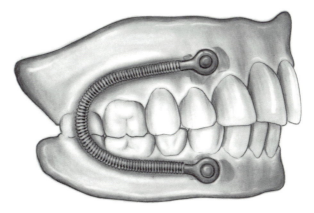

26

Extraorally retained prostheses

27–28

Large combined facial and oral defects may rely to a limited extent on joining the intra- and extraoral parts and using laboratory fabricated attachments, magnets, spectacles or head-straps for retention of the facial prosthesis, which can indirectly stabilize the intraoral element.

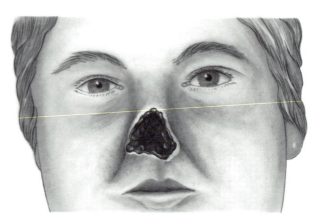

27

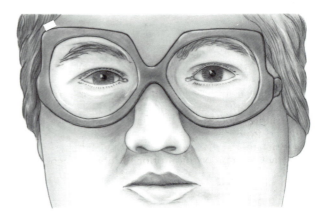

28

Mandibular resection

From the point of view of prosthetics, the major concern following resection of a mandibular tumour is whether the residual defect results in continuity or discontinuity of the mandible.

Edentulous patients

29

When continuity of the mandible has been maintained and the patient has satisfactory dentures, it is often possible simply to modify the mandibular denture by relining the fitting surface to obturate the defect in the mandible with: (a) a periodontal surgical dressing material, e.g. Coe Pack (Coe Laboratories, Illinois, USA); or (b) black gutta-percha, or impression compound, e.g. Stent (De Trey A.G., Zurich, Switzerland); or (c) temporary self-curing acrylic resin designed for direct use in the mouth, e.g. polyethyl methacrylate (Bonar Plastic; WHW Plastics, Hull, UK); or (d) a combination of the above.

The obturator can act as a dressing and support the soft tissues. If used in conjunction with skin grafting or ridge augmentation procedures, it should be retained by circumferential wiring during healing.

Dentate patients

A conventional immediate replacement denture can be constructed with the facility of adding additional material to the fitting surface at the time of surgery. This is fabricated from preoperative dental casts of the mouth, from which teeth are removed and artificial teeth replaced in exactly the same position prior to their extraction and excision of the tumour. If the number of teeth to be extracted is uncertain, it is best to assume the worst and, if surgery proves to be more conservative, teeth and base can then be trimmed from the denture. The conserving of every sound tooth may prove invaluable later in providing support and retention by means of stainless steel clasps.

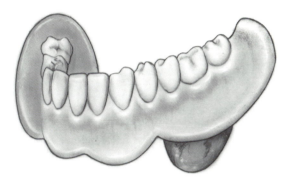

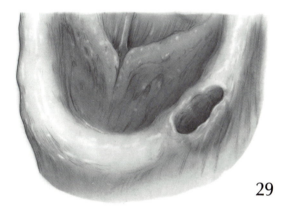

29

Partially dentate patients

Patients with a satisfactory removable partial denture can often have this modified to add teeth and allow for additional material to the fitting surface to obturate the defect. This reduces the laboratory work for the technician and provides the patient with a surgical dressing that feels comfortable and familiar.

SEGMENTAL MANDIBULAR RESECTION

Where continuity cannot be restored following segmental resection, a number of techniques have been used in an attempt to maintain function and reduce mandibular deviation and facial asymmetry. Splinting or interdental wiring initially will maintain the mandibular position in relation to the maxilla. Prosthetic appliances with modified occlusal form or with flange extensions can be used to guide the closing mandible into its centric position. These may include a palatal flange on the maxillary arch, or broad posterior maxillary teeth with long cuspal slopes.

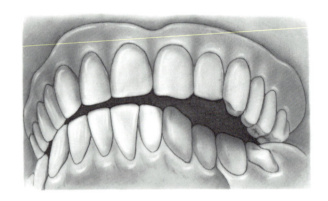

DEFINITIVE INTRAORAL PROSTHESIS

30

This is generally a modification to a conventional removable partial denture, the design of which takes into account the reduced support available from the teeth and the resected mandible. The extension of the base, and the occlusion and the type of clasping, should be designed to provide maximum support and stability without applying damaging forces to the remaining teeth. Similar principles of obturator design apply to partial cases, but the support, retention and stability provided by the remaining teeth are an invaluable asset. Where no bone support exists, it is often best to limit the denture bases to the remaining teeth and saddle areas on the uninvolved side until bone grafting or alloplastic implants have been carried out, if these are technically feasible. Good plaque control and regular dental care are essential for these patients. Carefully designed cobalt chromium denture bases can reduce gingival coverage and plaque formation, but consideration must be given to the flexibility of the clasps, which may often be better constructed from wrought gold or stainless steel and attached to the denture base. The obturator itself can be in a hard or soft material.

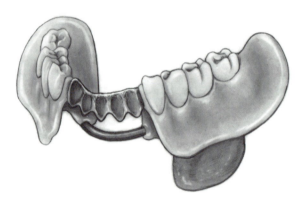

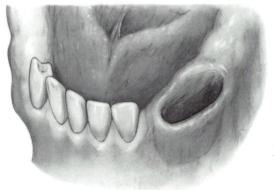

30

Facial prostheses

In general, large defects and those made up of several tissues, or combined intraoral and facial defects are best treated prosthetically. It is now possible to achieve extremely life-like replacements for the nose, ears and eyes with their surrounding tissues.

Conventional facial prostheses

These are made either from (a) hard acrylic resin, coloured to match the skin and held in place by spectacles, straps around the head, or attached to an intraoral prosthesis by means of semi-precision laboratory-fabricated retaining devices, e.g. rods and tubes or magnets, or manufactured precision retainers; or (b) soft resins, usually including addition-cured or condensation-cured silicones, e.g. Silskin (Thackray's Surgical, Leeds, UK), Cosmosil (Cosmed, Cardiff, UK) or Silastic (Dow Corning, Reading, UK). Polyurethane, plasticized acrylics or other polymers may also be used.

These soft materials have much appeal because of their texture, the colour match achievable and the possibility of using medical adhesives to attach them directly to clean, dry skin. Patient acceptance is generally good, but some patients have problems mastering the application and cleaning of the adhesive from the prosthesis. This may result in a build-up of adhesive which collects dirt and spoils the fit and appearance. Over-vigorous attempts at cleaning may cause tearing of the fine edges. As a result,

the life of such prostheses is limited to an average 3–9 months before remaking becomes necessary. For these reasons the longer lasting acrylic prostheses may be preferable in certain sites. The casts of the face used to make the prosthesis should be retained to reduce the clinical work involved when making new ones.

Osseointegrated implant-retained prostheses

The use of Brånemark osseointegrated implants as a means of fixing prostheses has dramatically extended the range of maxillofacial prosthetics. Osseointegrated implants can be used intraorally in oncology patients.

31–32

Their place in extraoral prostheses has proved particularly valuable, providing excellent retention for life-like silicone prostheses without the need for adhesives. Implant retention has extended the life of some prostheses to 4 or more years before remaking is required. Although initial costs are high, maintenance is much less so that, in the long term, implant-retained prostheses are cost effective.

When the prosthesis is being used to reconstruct the eye and eyelids following orbital exenteration, the use of spectacles as shown in the chapter on 'Eyelids', pp. 124–156 is effective in camouflaging the junction line between the prosthesis and its surroundings.

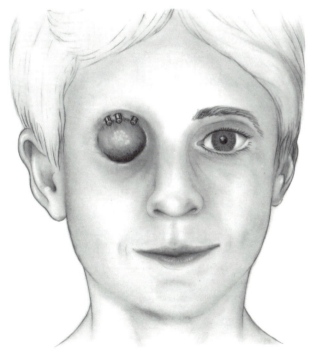

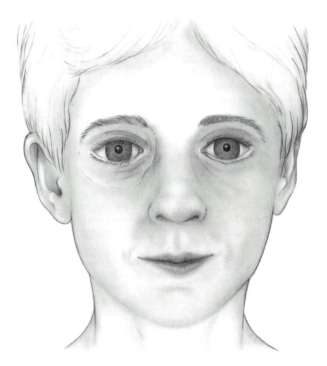

31

32

Surgical technique

33

This is performed in two stages. Following assessment and planning, a temporary wax prosthesis is made to identify the ideal location of the fixtures. A skin flap is raised, the bone drilled and 3 mm or 4 mm flanged fixtures screwed into the prepared sites. They are then covered and left buried to allow osseointegration to take place. The type of bone influences the time interval before the second stage surgical procedure is performed to place the trans-cutaneous abutments to which the prosthesis can be attached. The transcutaneous abutment should pass through thin, hairless skin, which necessitates thinning of the tissues or grafting. The temporal bone, used for auricular prostheses, integrates in about 3–4 months. The bone of the supraorbital ridge, however, seems to require about 6 months to integrate, and it is usually recommended that in irradiated bone, fixtures are placed about 9 months after radiotherapy and are left for an extended period between the two surgical procedures.

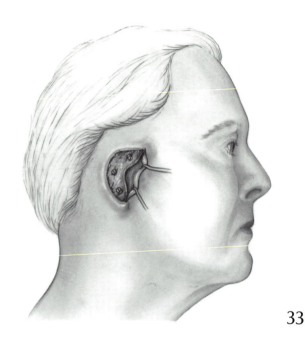

33

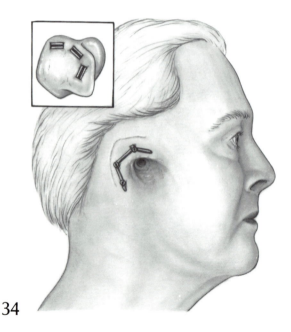

34

34

Following healing after the second stage (about 10 days), the prosthetic procedures may be carried out. Impressions are made of the titanium implant site, using transfer copings, to transfer exact brass replicas of the implants to the cast of the patient's face. On this cast of the patient which contains the brass analogues of the implants, retentive devices for the prosthesis are constructed.

Bars with clips, miniature rare earth magnets or precision attachments are most commonly used for attaching the prosthesis to the implants. The laboratory-fabricated retentive system is screwed directly on to the patient's implants and the prosthesis attached to the bar by clips or magnets.

35

The base colour of the prosthesis will have been matched with the patient's skin at the previous appointment and the final extrinsic colouring added to characterize the surface detail. Because no adhesives are required, the edges of the prosthesis can be made very thin, flexible and almost transparent, to blend and move with the skin.

There is little risk of damage during cleaning, if reasonable care is taken. This ability to clean the prostheses delicately extends its useful life to several years, rather than the few months seen in conventional prostheses, which show rapid deterioration occasioned by the need to clean and reapply adhesive frequently.

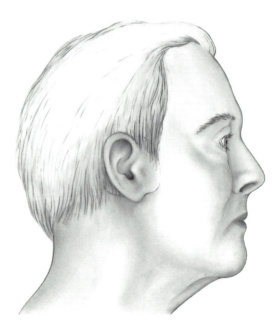

35

Illustrations by Gillian Oliver

Tumours involving the anterior and middle cranial fossae

Ian T. Jackson   MB, ChB, FRCS(G), FRCS(Ed), FACS, FRACS(Hon)
Director, Institute for Craniofacial and Reconstructive Surgery, Providence Hospital, Southfield, Michigan, USA

Introduction

The surgical approach to these areas for the removal of both non-malignant and malignant tumours has changed radically over the past 10–15 years. The advances have come in the areas of exposure, reconstruction, and reduction of complications.

The anterior and middle cranial fossae present their own unique problems. In the anterior fossa, the proximity of the nasopharynx to the extradural space has proved, in the past, to be the 'Waterloo' for patients and surgeons alike. In addition to this, the aesthetics of the face, and their presentation, provide a significant challenge to the surgeon and sometimes the prosthodontist. The middle fossa is an area where exposure is difficult, and the anatomy is complex. Appearance is a less important factor – defects are more easily hidden.

ANTERIOR CRANIAL FOSSA

Frequently, adequate information can be obtained from a standard computed tomography (CT) scan. Occasionally, a three-dimensional CT scan can give additional information as to the position of the tumour and the probable defect after resection.

In the words of A. K. Henry[1], exposure should be 'extensile', in terms of both soft tissue and bone. It was the inability to achieve an extensile approach to exposure which, in the past, led to inadequate resection in this region.

Skin approaches

LIMITED EXPOSURE

1

To approach the ethmoid sinus area when the tumour seems to be confined to the sinus, a limited incision is made in the medial canthal and paranasal areas.

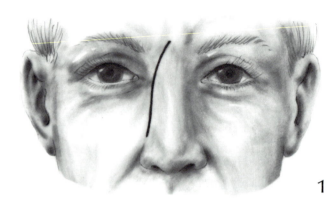

1

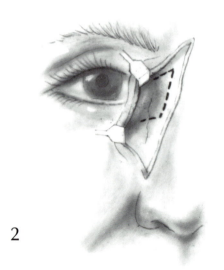

2

2

A subperiosteal dissection exposes the lateral nasal area and the medial orbital wall, and using a side cutting burr, a cut is made in the frontonasal bone over the ethmoid sinuses, outlining a rectangular bone flap based laterally.

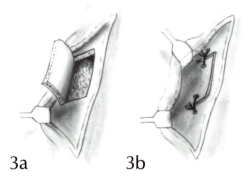

3a   3b

3a & b

The flap of bone is elevated on its laterally based hinge to expose the tumour.

The tumour can then be removed, and the bone flap is replaced and wired in position.

EXTENDED EXPOSURE

4

In tumours of the antrum or orbit extending into the ethmoid sinuses, it may be difficult to be sure of the extent of the superior extension. For this reason an extended Weber–Fergusson skin approach is chosen, the extension being into the glabellar area.

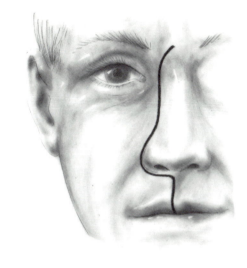

4

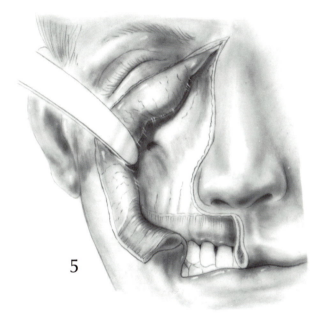

5

5

With the cheek flap elevated and retracted laterally, and the periosteum of the pterygoid fossa raised or incised, good exposure of the medial wall and the floor of the orbit is obtained, together with the nasal cavity and the whole of the maxilla.

6

This exposure allows a total maxillectomy to be carried out.

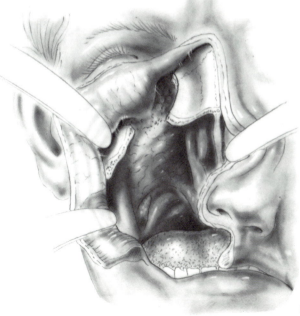

6

7

If there is concern about extension of tumour to the roof of the ethmoid, it is necessary to proceed to anterior cranial fossa resection. The approach to the area is then by extending the skin incision into the frontal region in a W-plasty fashion. The flaps can be of any size according to the surgeon's wishes.

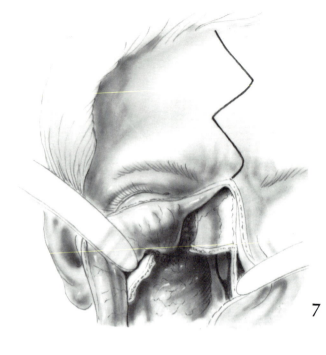

7

8

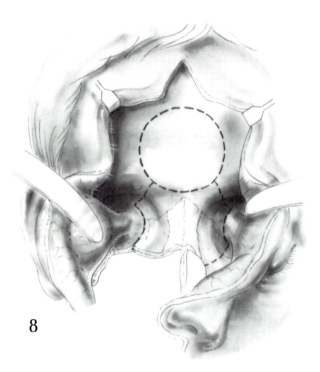

8

With the forehead flaps elevated, it is possible to perform a limited exposure of the anterior cranial fossa, using a midline trephination and a nasoglabellar osteotomy.

9

With this exposure, the frontal lobes can be retracted extradurally and the roof of the sinuses cut around.

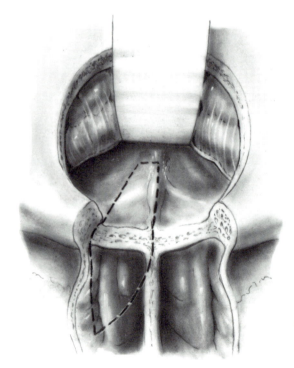

9

10

A total *en bloc* resection of the sinuses can then be carried out.

It is during this manoeuvre, when the dura is being dissected as it plunges down to the crista galli, that a dural tear may occur. Such a tear is sutured directly, or a small graft of temporal fascia is used as a patch. The presence of a dural tear, by providing a connection between the nasopharynx and the subdural space, creates a potentially lethal situation.

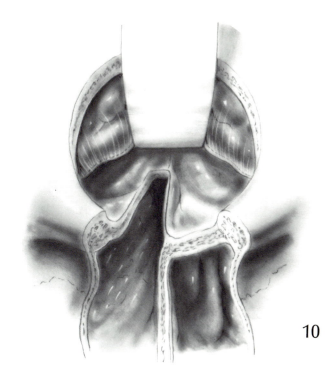

10

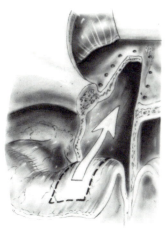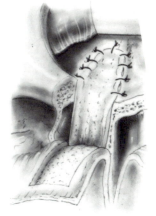

11

11

To deal with this, drill holes are made around the defect of the floor, and a well-vascularized galea–frontalis myofascial flap, described on p. 611, is sutured in such a manner as to totally occlude the connection.

12

The osteotomies are replaced and stabilized with the appropriate number and design of miniplates.

The maxillectomy defect must now be lined or closed. In highly selected cases, a free vascularized tissue transfer may be performed, using one of the flaps described in the chapter on 'Reconstructive techniques of the skin', pp. 45–103. On most occasions, however, the defect is lined with a split-skin graft, using the method described in the chapter on 'Reconstructive techniques of the oral cavity', pp. 215–240.

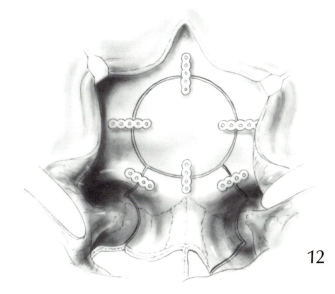

12

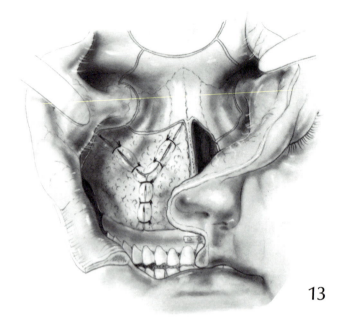

13

13 & 14

A preformed dental plate is wired into position using alveolar wires on the non-resected side. A mould is now made; useful materials for this purpose are gutta-percha and Stent (De Trey A. G., Zurich, Switzerland). Mastisol (Compound Mastic Paint, BPC) is painted on the mould and allowed to dry. A split-skin graft is applied to the mould with its skin surface against the mould, and sutured down as necessary with catgut. The skin graft covered mould is inserted into the maxillary defect and the wound is closed. The area is left intact for 10 days; at this time the dental plate and the mould are removed, and a prosthesis is made and inserted.

In this sequence, the skin approach to the resection site progresses in an extensile manner, while the bony exposure remains limited.

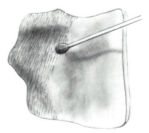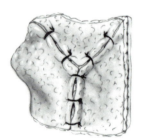

14

BICORONAL FLAP

Using a bicoronal skin flap has virtually become a standard approach to the anterior cranial fossa. In its design and in raising it, certain rules have to be observed to prevent problems from arising and to preserve all the possible reconstructive options.

15

The positioning of the planned incision is most important. It should extend from the superior attachment of the ear across the vertex to the same position on the other side, and continue downward in the preauricular area to a variable extent.

The anterior extension is no longer acceptable. It does not increase exposure, and causes aesthetic problems resulting from the position of the scar, especially if there is poor healing.

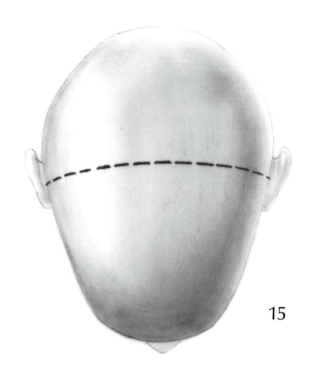

15

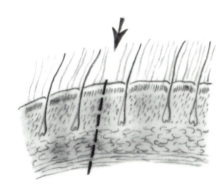

16

16

In making the incision it is important to take note of the direction of hair growth and of the hair follicles, and direct the incision parallel to it. If this is done, the likelihood of significant alopecia is reduced.

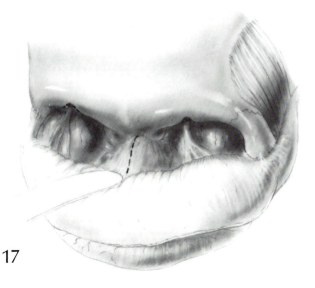

17

17

Unless it is intended to use a temporalis galeal fascial flap (the reconstructive technique described on p. 612, and in the chapter on 'Scalp and forehead', pp. 195–214) in closing the defect, the plane of dissection is between the galea and the pericranium. The plane of dissection proceeds until 1.5–2 cm above the supraorbital rim, continuing in the subperiosteal plane.

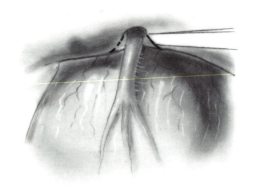

18a

18a & b

The supraorbital vessels are dislodged from their canal and, if the supraorbital notch is a foramen, it is deroofed using a fine osteotome.

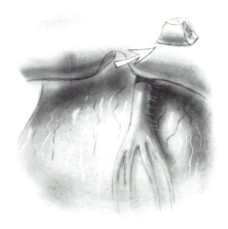

18b

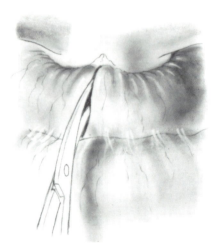

19a

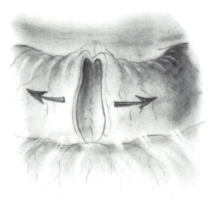

19b

19a & b

In the midline the periosteum is incised vertically and spread with scissors down as far as the distal margin of the nasal bones.

20

Laterally, care must be taken not to become too superficial to avoid injury to the frontal branch of the facial nerve. At the level of the temporal ridge, the lateral extension of the galea is swept off the fascia covering the temporalis muscle, using a Faraboeuf periosteal elevator. Mobilization is continued down to the zygomatic arch, where the periosteum is incised, and the dissection continues in the subperiosteal plane over the arch and the maxilla. Depending on the desired exposure, the medial and lateral canthi may have to be detached from their bony insertions.

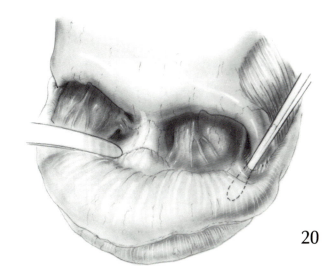

20

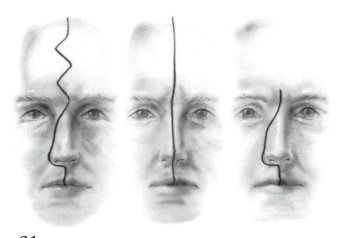

21

21

When further extension of the soft tissue approach is necessary, variations of the facial split procedure are employed. The choice of which incision is used depends on how much exposure is necessary. In this way, virtually the whole anterior skull can be exposed in the sub-periosteal plane.

Bone approaches

As with the skin approaches, the approaches to the bone can be limited or extended.

LIMITED APPROACH

The limited approach, referred to in describing the extended skin approach, is used in resecting midline tumours extending to the posterior wall of the ethmoid sinuses, or into the sphenoid sinus. In these tumours, usually sinus adenocarcinoma or aesthesioneuroblastoma, the posterior extent of the resection is always the posterior wall of the sphenoid sinus. Laterally, the extent of the resection is determined by the position of the tumour, but it frequently involves resection of the medial orbital wall, or walls.

22

Once the bicoronal flap has been elevated as described above, an incision is made through the periosteum, anteriorly in the sagittal plane, stopping short of the glabellar bone, laterally on each side in a coronal direction down to the temporal fossa, and laterally across the supraorbital bone on each side from the anterior extent of the sagittal incision.

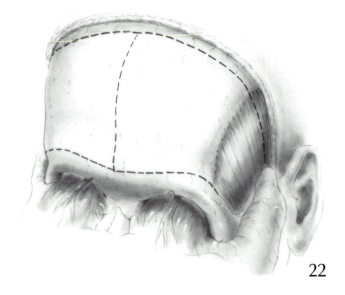

22

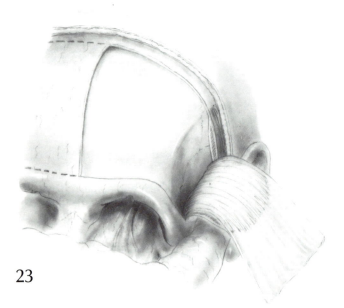

23

23

The periosteum on each side of the midline is now raised as a flap. Constant irrigation applied to the area, and the use of the Faraboeuf periosteal elevator, make the elevation easier. The dissection may end either at the level of the temporal ridge, or continue with elevation of the temporalis muscle from the temporal fossa, the periosteum and the temporalis forming a continuous flap.

24

In the midline, the dissection continues down as far as necessary on the nose and medial orbital walls. The estimated bony exposure is drawn out on the bone with a pencil – the best way of marking the skull.

Using a trephine or a craniotome, a midline disc of the skull is removed. The problem encountered at this point is the frontal sinus, the posterior wall of which has to be cut through. The disc of bone is then gently mobilized and raised with a fine elevator. In carrying out this dissection, the danger areas are the sagittal sinus in the midline and dural adhesions lateral to the sinus. When removal of the disc of bone has provided the cranial window, the frontal lobes can be dissected extradurally from behind the glabellar area and from the floor of the fossa anteriorly. Here the danger area is the crista galli, which can be large and can cause problems during mobilization of the dura.

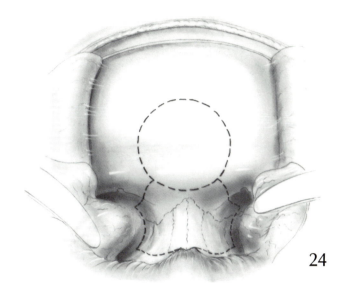

24

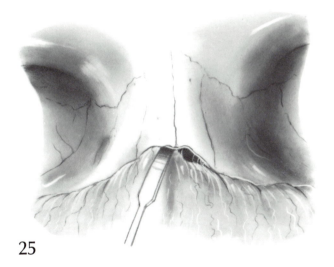

25

25

Attention is now turned to the nose and, with a fine dissector, the domes of the nasal mucosa are swept away from the nasal bones. The nasal mucosa is conserved in this way only where the position of the tumour and its type makes it possible. On most occasions, it is necessary to sacrifice the nasal mucosa.

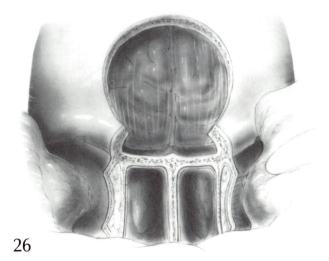

26

26

With the orbital contents protected, an osteotomy of the glabellar segment of bone is carried out, cuts being made through the supraorbital rims, the orbital roof and the medial orbital walls, and across the floor of the anterior cranial fossa. The glabellar bone is then mobilized and removed.

The dura is then dissected from the area of the cribriform plate. If the area is involved with tumour, it is left in position and an incision is made around it, leaving it to be removed as part of the operative specimen. The resulting dural defect is closed with a graft of the fascia covering temporalis or fascia lata. The orbital contents are protected, and the chosen osteotomies are made in the floor of the anterior cranial fossa and the medial orbital walls. The nasal septum is cut with scissors.

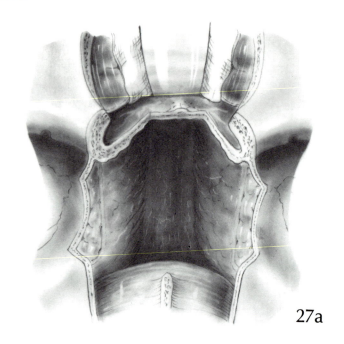

27a

27a & b

The entire block, isolated in this way, can now be mobilized and removed. Any further resection found to be necessary can easily be performed with this good exposure. The sphenoid sinus is usually stripped of its mucosa.

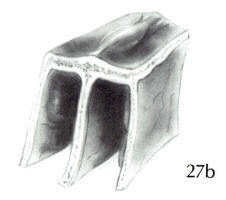

27b

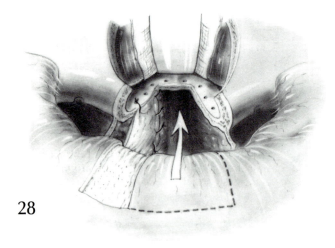

28

28

Vascularized cover is now provided with the galea–frontalis myofascial flap. If there has been damage to the periorbita medially, the orbital wall may be reconstructed with a cranial bone graft, harvested as shown in *Illustrations 62* and *63*, and this is covered with a second galea–frontalis flap. It is not necessary to provide mucosal lining.

The bony segments are now replaced and fixed with mini- or preferably microplates. The periosteum is restored to its original position, and its margins are sutured to one another. The coronal skin flap is closed, usually with staples, and suction drains are placed in both temporal fossae.

EXTENDED APPROACH

29

When the tumour is larger, a frontal bone flap is raised. The flap is marked on the bone with pencil and burr holes are made, one on each side of the sagittal sinus on the vertex and in the frontal area, and two in each temporal fossa.

The cuts between the burr holes may be made with an osteotome; alternatively, the dura may be dissected from the intracranial surface of the skull and the cuts made with a Gigli saw. No matter which method is employed, all cuts are made before the sagittal sinus is crossed, so that exposure and treatment will be immediate if the sinus is damaged.

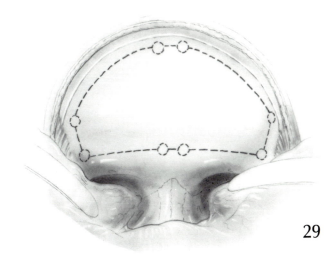

29

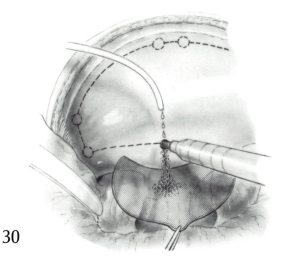

30

30

As the craniotome burr holes are being made, the bone dust is cooled by constant irrigation, and collected on a mesh tray for later use.

When the frontal bone flap has been removed, as much supraorbital rim can be removed as is considered necessary to provide additional exposure, after the frontal lobes have been elevated. This approach provides good exposure when it is considered that it will be necessary to remove the orbital contents in conjunction with an anterior cranial fossa tumour. In such a case, the conjunctiva is located from a posterior approach via the coronal flap, and incised along the fornices. The effect is to free the orbital contents from the face and allow them to fall back posteriorly. A right-angled vascular clamp is placed across the optic nerve and vessels, and they are divided. After the appropriate osteotomies are made, the contents of the orbit and the skull base can be removed *en bloc*.

31

In reconstructing the defect of the orbit, an osteotomy can be made in the lateral orbital wall.

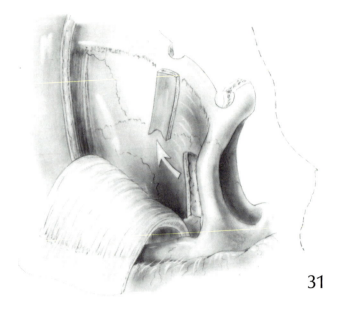

31

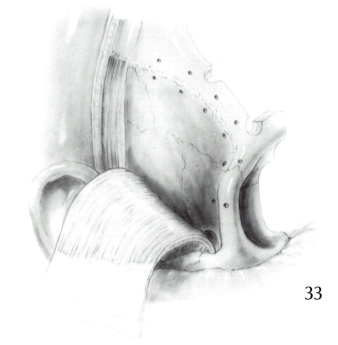

32

32

With the temporalis muscle extensively mobilized, it can be fed into the orbit to provide the bulk which helps with later prosthesis fitting.

The galea–frontalis myofascial flap is used as required medially to seal off any dural defect, and the bone flaps are replaced and fixed in position.

Temporalis muscle reattachment

33

When the temporalis muscle has been raised from the temporal fossa as part of the exposure, it must be carefully replaced to avoid depression of the temporal area. Holes are drilled in the temporal ridge and in the lateral orbital rim, occasionally in the zygomatic arch.

33

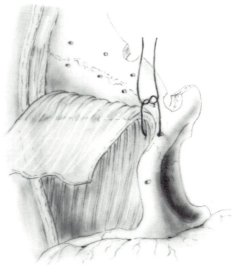

34a

34a & b

Using non-absorbable sutures, the muscle is reattached in its original site. Along the lateral orbital rim the full thickness of the muscle is taken with each suture and it is pulled down to hold it against the lateral orbital wall.

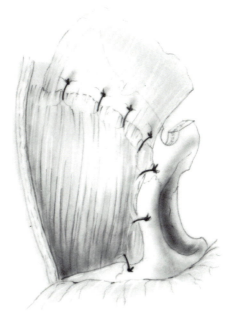

34b

Lateral canthopexy

35a & b

In most cases the lateral canthal ligament will need to be reattached. The ligament is picked up with a haemostat and, by observing on the skin side, it is checked that this is indeed the ligament. Two drill holes are made on the lateral orbital rim, almost at the junction of the supra-orbital rim and the lateral orbital rim. A wire is cut tangentially to give it a sharp point, and it is passed through the ligament. Each end is then passed through one of the two drill holes.

As the wire is twisted and tightened, the ligament comes to lie on the inner aspect of the rim.

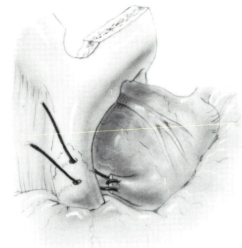

35a

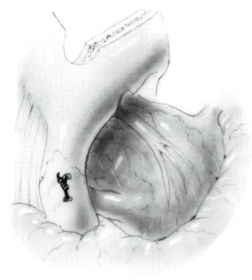

35b

Medial canthopexy

36

In some cases it will be necessary to fix the medial canthus in its correct position. The canthus is identified and its identity is checked as for the lateral canthus. A hole is made in the medial orbital wall in the correct position. Two drill holes are then made through stable bone down to this hole.

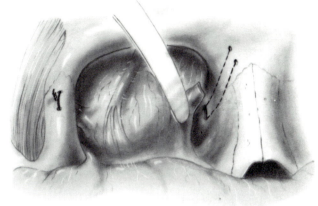

36

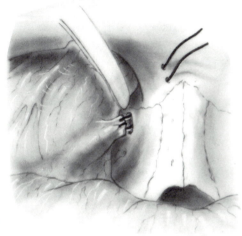

37a

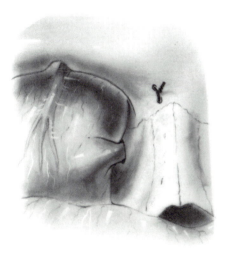

37b

37a & b

The canthal ligament is transfixed with the wire as with the lateral canthus. A Keith needle is passed retrograde through each drill hole in turn, and the wire is put through the eye of the needle. As it is withdrawn, it pulls the wire through the hole.

As the wire is twisted and tightened, the ligament comes to lie in the hole made for it in the medial orbital wall.

FACIAL DISASSEMBLY

38a, b & c

This is the ultimate in extensile exposure. Basically it can be summed up as 'removing whatever bone is necessary to achieve adequate exposure'. The technique is at its most useful in treating tumours far back in the midline or those which lie in both the anterior and middle cranial fossae. Their exposure can necessitate removal of portions of the maxilla, displacement of the maxilla (Le Fort 1), and osteotomies of the orbit or temporal area.

Such an exposure eliminates the need to work at depth in a confined space; instead, the operative field is brought out to the operator. When the resection is completed, and vascularized cover has been provided by the galea–frontalis myofascial flap or the temporal galeal flap, the bony segments are placed back in position and stabilized with micro- or miniplates and screws.

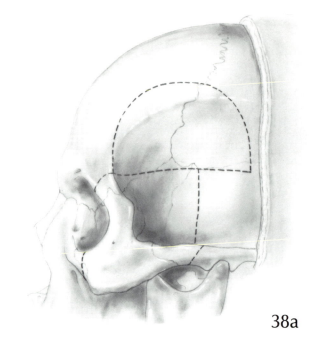

38a

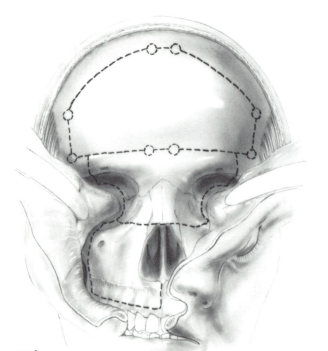

38b

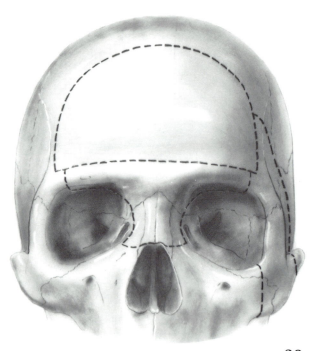

38c

Vascularized tissue reconstruction

LOCAL FLAPS

There are two areas in this region from which tissue having its own axial blood supply can be harvested – the frontal area, making use of a galea–frontalis myofascial flap, and the temporal region using the temporalis muscle.

Galea–frontalis myofascial flap

Prior to the introduction of this technique, surgery in the anterior cranial fossa was hazardous, due mainly to ascending infection from the nasopharyngeal area. As was pointed out on pp. 597 and 604, a connection between the nasopharynx and the extra- and/or subdural spaces is frequently created during the resection. In addition to this, an intracranial, extradural, dead space may be left at the completion of the resection. This predisposes to extradural abscess formation and, in the past, many patients having this surgery did develop lethal infections.

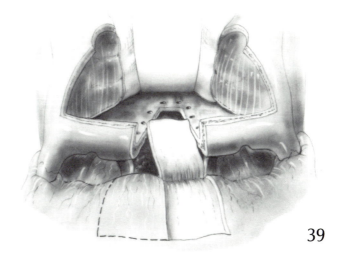

39

39

The best prophylaxis is to fill the area with vascularized tissue, and this can be provided by the galea–frontalis myofascial flap. From the deep surface of the bicoronal skin flap, one or two flaps can be raised, each with its own pedicle, incorporating the frontalis muscle and using as its vascular basis the supraorbital and supratrochlear vessels.

40a & b

The flap is sutured in position using drill holes made around the margins of the defect in the base of the anterior cranial fossa, usually using 4/0 nylon as the suture material. Two separate and identical flaps can be used if two areas have to be covered, e.g. the cranial and medial orbital walls, when a bone graft is being placed in the latter area.

In order to allow the flap to pass to the area requiring cover, a slot is created by trimming the edge of the osteotomy – the 'letter box technique'.

The use of this technique has virtually eliminated intracranial infection associated with anterior cranial fossa tumour resection by eliminating the dead space.

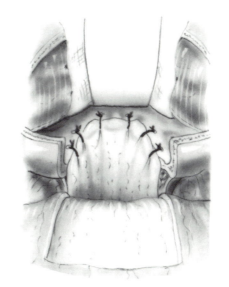

40a

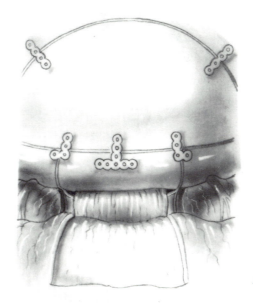

40b

Temporalis muscle flap

The temporalis muscle flap is supplied mainly by the deep temporal vessels, with some additional flow from the superficial temporal vessels. This allows it to be raised on a pedicle just above the coronoid process of the mandible, where the deep temporal vessels enter the muscle. The muscle is raised from the temporal fossa and can be rotated to fill the orbit or cheek area. As with the galea–frontalis flap, it has its 'letter box', provided by an osteotomy in the lateral orbital wall, as shown in *Illustrations 31* and *32*. The flap is capable of filling a good deal of the orbit, and will extend as far as the medial orbital wall.

Temporalis galeal flap

This flap, which has also been referred to as the temporoparietal fascial flap, has been further discussed in the chapter on 'Ear', pp. 178–194. It is based on the superficial temporal vessels, and prior to raising the flap their course should be marked out on the scalp using a Doppler probe. In raising the scalp to expose the site on which the flap will be designed, the plane of dissection is between the hair follicles and the galea. The flap can be raised as far as the midline but not beyond, and its potential width is the entire temporoparietal region. In order to include the origin of the superficial temporal vessels which perfuse it, its base is just above the zygomatic arch. It is capable of resurfacing the orbit and the floor of the anterior cranial fossa.

FREE TISSUE TRANSFER

Where there is an extradural dead space which appears unlikely to fill spontaneously after the procedure, and which cannot be filled by any of the flaps described above, or for which they will provide only a partial solution, a free tissue transfer should be considered. Failure to fill the dead space may lead to an extradural abscess. The galea–frontalis flap will prevent a life-threatening situation, but the lack of contact between the dura and the replaced cranial bone overlying it will lead to eventual loss of the bone with attendant infection. This is seen most frequently in the postirradiation patient. Before this has the opportunity to happen, or as soon as the problem is recognized, a free vascularized tissue transfer should be carried out to fill the dead space, with vascular anastomosis to healthy vessels, e.g. latissimus dorsi muscle or omentum, using anastomosis to the superficial temporal or neck vessels.

With free tissue transfer and local vascularized tissue transfer, most infections in this area can be prevented or combated effectively.

MIDDLE CRANIAL FOSSA

Anterior segment

41

The anterior segment of the middle cranial fossa is most often involved with sphenoid wing meningiomas or fibrous dysplasia. The approach to this site uses a coronal skin incision, displaying the orbit, temporal area, zygomatic arch and lateral maxilla. The temporalis muscle is dissected from the temporal fossa, and the osteotomy lines are drawn out with a pencil on the bone. Part of the temporal bone is frequently involved with tumour and a resection to include this area is planned.

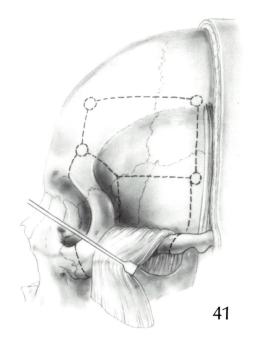

41

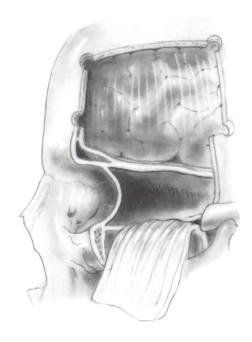

42

42

Using the craniotome, a fronto-orbital craniotomy is performed. This is followed by an orbitozygomatico-maxillary exposure osteotomy, which exposes the anterior cranial fossa, the orbit and the anterior segment of the middle cranial fossa, making it possible to resect the tumour and any involved bone under direct vision, using the operating microscope if necessary.

43

When the resection has been completed, the bone flaps are replaced in position, and the bony defect which has resulted from the resection of the tumour is grafted with a split-skin graft, as shown in *Illustrations 13* and *14*. Solid fixation of the bone flaps and the graft is obtained using a mixture of mini- and microplates.

When the tumour involves the area further posterior in the fossa but anterior to the petrous eminence, especially if it invades or arises from the pterygoid fossa, the approach becomes significantly more complicated because of the presence of important structures which lie in the path of the exposure – the parotid gland, the facial nerve, the ascending ramus of the mandible and the great vessels. There are several possible approaches to this site.

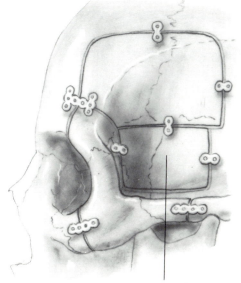

43

Bone graft

LATERAL TEMPORAL APPROACH

This approach is tedious and requires a great deal of dissection. It does, however, provide very good exposure.

44

The skin incision is hemicoronal, curving anteriorly, and continuing down immediately in front of the ear onto the neck as a lazy S.

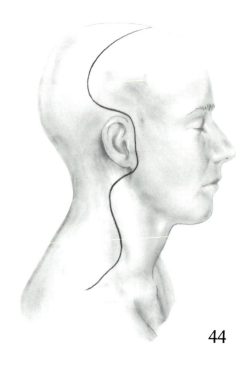

44

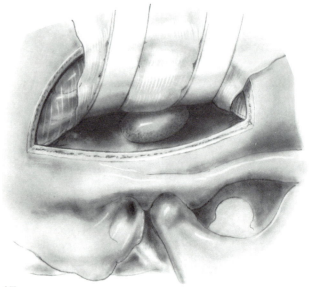

45

45

As an initial step, a temporal craniotomy is carried out, and the temporal lobe is raised, allowing the extent of the intracranial tumour to be assessed. If there is extensive intracranial involvement, resection may not be possible.

46

A dissection of the upper neck is now carried out, primarily to allow an accurate assessment of the position of the great vessels high in the neck. In carrying this out, care is taken to maintain the sternocleidomastoid muscle intact.

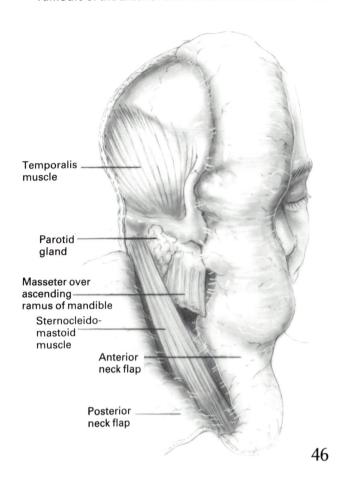

Temporalis muscle

Parotid gland

Masseter over ascending ramus of mandible

Sternocleido-mastoid muscle

Anterior neck flap

Posterior neck flap

46

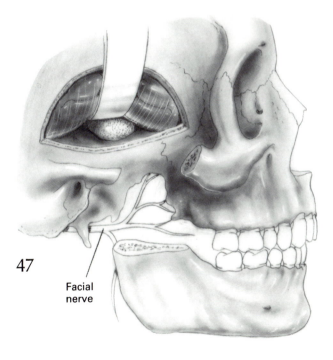

47

Facial nerve

47

Following this, a total parotidectomy is carried out, with preservation of the facial nerve. The ascending ramus of the mandible may be involved by the tumour and, if this is so, it is included in the resected specimen. If it is not involved by tumour, an osteotomy is performed at the angle of the mandible and the ascending ramus is hinged forward on a soft tissue pedicle after freeing of the condyle; alternatively the ramus is removed. The zygomatic arch is osteotomized as a segment, or in continuity with an orbital segment if this is necessary for exposure. The temporalis muscle is now elevated from the temporal fossa. On occasion this may be invaded by tumour, and then resection of an appropriate segment is carried out.

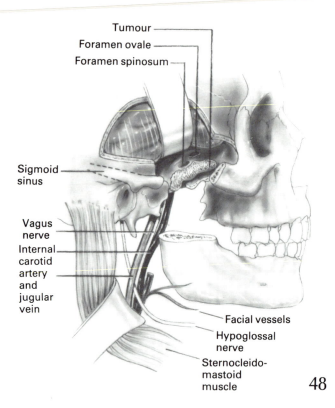

48

48 & 49

It is now possible to proceed with the dissection in a cranial direction, removing the contents of the pterygoid fossa. In the base of the skull an osteotomy is made around the tumour, using a side-cutting drill, and an *en bloc* removal is performed.

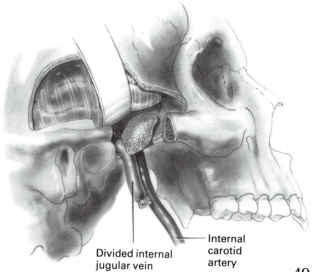

49

50

In order to fill the dead space in the pterygoid fossa region and seal the floor of the middle fossa, sternocleidomastoid is divided inferiorly and elevated, preserving its superior blood supply.

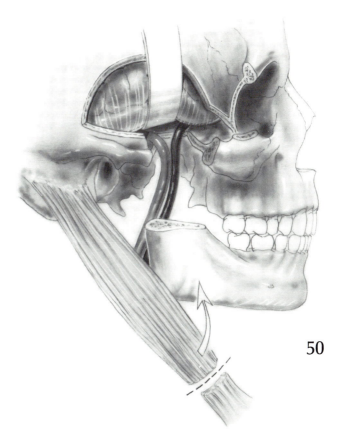

50

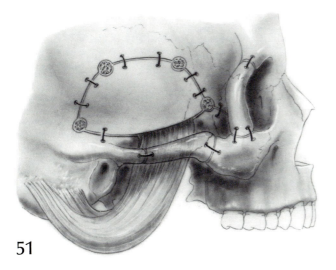

51

51

The muscle is now swung up and sutured, using drill holes, to the margins of the defect in the base of the cranial fossa.

If there is involvement of the internal carotid artery or of the trigeminal ganglion, the tumour may still be 'resectable', but it is unlikely to be curable.

When the posterior aspect of the maxilla is involved by extension from the pterygoid fossa, a maxillectomy in continuity must be performed in the standard fashion, through a Weber–Fergusson incision. It is possible to carry out the necessary maxillectomy leaving the maxilla still attached to the main specimen posteriorly, the entire specimen being removed through the lateral incision.

At the completion of the lateral approach all displaced structures are restored to their anatomical position, the bones being plated securely. If vascularized tissue is required apart from the sternocleidomastoid muscle, as shown in *Illustration 50*, a galeal flap based on the occipital vessels can be used to fill a small volume defect; if a large volume of tissue is required, a free tissue transfer, e.g. scapular flap, can be used.

MANDIBULAR SWING APPROACH

It is also possible to approach the middle cranial fossa using a mandibular swing procedure. This also involves the use of a neck dissection as part of the surgical approach to the site, and is more difficult technically than the lateral approach, the eventual exposure being less extensive.

Petrous temporal bone involvement

Involvement of the petrous temporal bone can occur from skin tumours which extend into the inner ear, from parotid malignancies which spread into the bone, and finally from primary middle ear cancers. These are aggressive lesions, which invade the middle cranial fossa through the tegmen tympani and can rapidly involve the overlying dura.

52

The approach is basically similar to that used for the more anteriorly placed tumours, just described. However, if the pinna is involved, it is included in an island of skin to be excised with the underlying petrous bone. If the pinna is to be preserved, it can be left attached to the anterior or posterior skin flap.

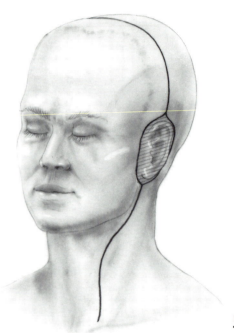

52

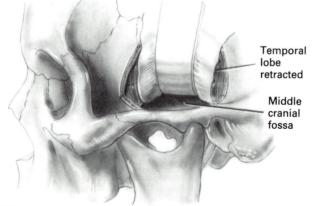

Temporal lobe retracted

Middle cranial fossa

53

53

Before proceeding to make any of the lower portions of the incision, the temporal scalp flaps are elevated and a temporal craniotomy is performed. This allows the middle cranial fossa to be inspected to determine the upward extent of the tumour. If dura has been penetrated, the tumour is probably inoperable.

54

A neck dissection is now carried out, primarily to identify accurately the common carotid artery and the internal jugular vein in their course to the skull base, but also to clear the neck of lymph nodes, possibly sites of metastatic disease. The sternocleidomastoid muscle should be preserved if possible, as a valuable potential source of vascularized tissue for reconstruction.

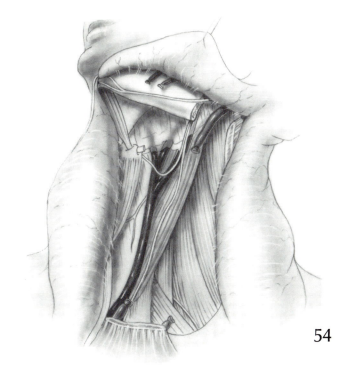

54

PARTIAL PETROSECTOMY

55

If the tumour has extended anteriorly outwith the petrous bone, it may be necessary to resect the ascending ramus of the mandible; when the tumour is purely of the petrous bone, it is sufficient to dislocate it forward. A segment of the zygomatic arch is removed.

When the tumour is of the external ear and the penetration is not too deep, a partial petrosectomy can be performed. In such a resection, the inferior resection line of the bone in the skull base is lateral to the styloid process, and the superior resection line intracranially is through the middle ear. In the temporal fossa the temporalis muscle is displaced anteriorly, and a cut in the temporal bone is made from the anterior portion of the intracranial cut to the anterior portion of the cut in the skull base. Posteriorly a similar joining cut is made, conserving the lateral sinus, but removing the mastoid air cells as part of the operation specimen. The bony block is now freed by placing an osteotome in the intracranial resection line and levering laterally. The block usually comes out cleanly with little bleeding; in the process the labyrinth complex is disrupted.

If a large amount of skin has been resected, it may be possible to fill the gap using a pectoralis major or pedicled latissimus dorsi myocutaneous flap, brought up to the defect deep to the neck dissection flaps. This, however, is only possible if space deep to the flaps is available to accommodate their pedicles when sternocleidomastoid has been resected as part of the dissection. Alternatively, a free tissue transfer, e.g. latissimus dorsi, radial forearm or scapular flap, can be used. Good drainage of the potential cavity is essential to collapse the cavity left by the resection, since the soft tissue may tent over the excisional defect.

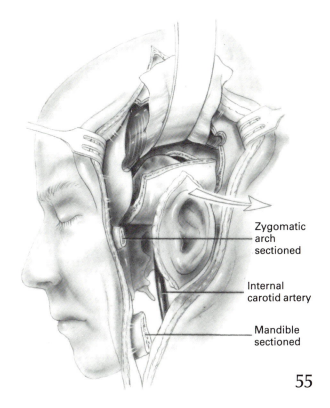

Zygomatic arch sectioned

Internal carotid artery

Mandible sectioned

55

RADICAL PETROSECTOMY

This is a difficult operation, and has potentially lethal complications. The internal carotid artery runs through the petrous temporal bone, and it may be damaged during the resection, with resulting severe bleeding which can be difficult to control. The vessel may go into spasm, with subsequent thrombosis, resulting in hemiplegia and aphasia. The lateral sinus can be traumatized, and this may result in severe venous bleeding which can be difficult to control.

Before starting the procedure, it is wise to have an estimate of the adequacy of cross-flow between the two internal carotid systems. This may be done radiologically with pressure on the vessel or by balloon occlusion; alternatively, radioactive studies can be used. Unless there is extensive skin involvement or in recurrent parotid or external ear tumours, the pinna need not be sacrificed. It is usually kept on the anterior flap.

The first step, as with the partial petrosectomy, is to ascertain whether the tumour is resectable by carrying out a temporal craniotomy and middle fossa exploration. The upper neck is then opened, and the major vessels and associated cranial nerves identified and isolated.

Depending on the extent of tumour beyond the middle ear area, the anterior and posterior subcutaneous resection lines can vary. Anteriorly, resection may include the ascending ramus of the mandible and a portion of the zygomatic arch. The temporomandibular joint may also be involved, and will be included in the resection. Posteriorly, the mastoid and post-mastoid skull is resected. Below, the dissection is carried up to the jugular foramen and to the base of the styloid process. Above, the dissection comes down from the temporal craniotomy into the temporal fossa anteriorly, and posteriorly behind the mastoid, dividing the sternocleidomastoid muscle below it. The lateral sinus is dissected out from its groove in the bone and tied off, a measure which cuts potential blood loss.

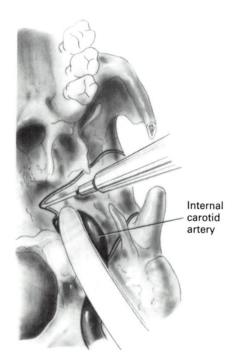

Internal carotid artery

56

56

Anteriorly, a cut is made, continuing the line of the temporal craniotomy, through the temporal bone anterior to the petrous to reach the carotid foramen; posteriorly, the cut is made from the apex of the petrous to the jugular foramen and then up to the temporal bone.

57

Inferiorly, the carotid is dissected from its canal laterally and a cut is made through the skull base. A further cut is made between the carotid and jugular foramen.

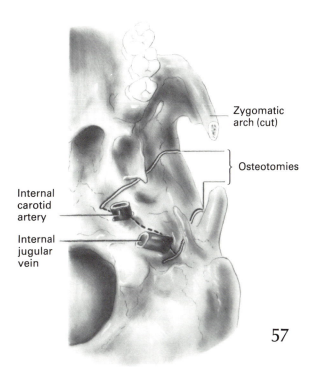

57

58

Intracranially, a cut is made as close to the petrous apex as possible.

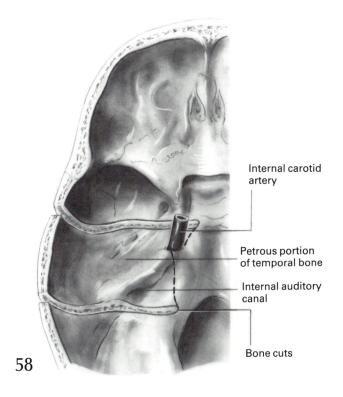

58

59

The petrous bone is now mobile, but needs to be rocked to open the osteotomy medially. As this is done, the carotid is freed from its canal above and below. The fracture of the bone usually takes place through the canal.

It is at this point that severe bleeding has been reported. The separation is likely to be through an area of significant tumour formation, and if this is the case, the remaining medial portion of bone will have to be removed piecemeal. A proportion of cases will be found to be inoperable at this stage. Any dural tears are repaired directly or with a deep temporal fascia or fascia lata graft.

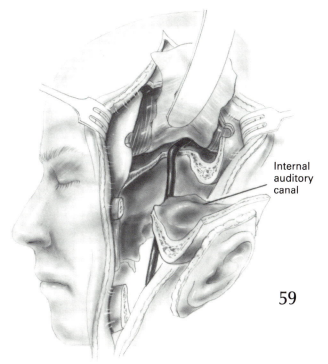

59

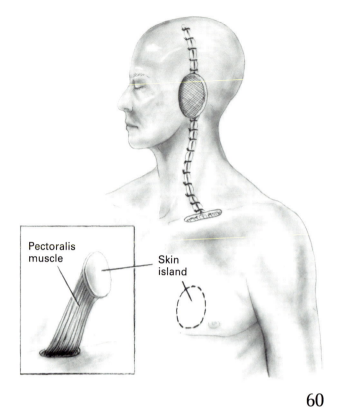

Pectoralis
muscle

Skin
island

60

60 & 61

Large defects are filled with myocutaneous flaps, as
described in *Illustrations 50* and *51*, or alternatively with a
temporalis muscle flap or a sternocleidomastoid transposition if this muscle is still viable. Good drainage of the
site is of paramount importance.

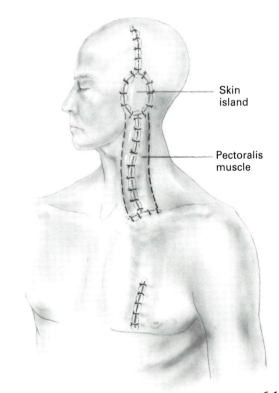

Skin
island

Pectoralis
muscle

61

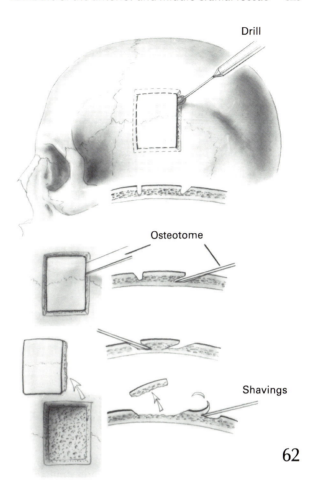

CRANIAL BONE GRAFTS

62

When bony reconstruction is required, cranial bone grafts are used most frequently. The outer table is taken as the graft, using a contouring drill to expose the diploe, and an osteotome to loosen the outer table. Small bone shavings can be used to fill small defects.

63

Alternatively, a bone flap can be removed and then split using a mallet and osteotome. In this way longer plates of bone can be obtained, but this does require a craniotomy.

References

1. Henry AK. *Extensile Exposure*. 2nd ed. Edinburgh: E&S Livingstone, 1966.

Further reading

Jackson IT, Laws ER, Martin RD. A craniofacial approach to advanced recurrent cancer of the central face. *Head Neck Surg* 1983; 5: 474–88.

Jackson IT, Marsh WR. Anterior cranial fossa tumors. *Ann Plast Surg* 1983; 11: 479–89.

Jackson IT. The craniofacial approach to anterior cranial fossa tumors. In: Fish U, Valavanis A, Yasargil MG, eds. *Neurological Surgery of the Ear and Skull Base*. Amsterdam: Kughler & Ghedini Publications, 1989, 285–307.

Jackson IT, Shaw K. Tumors of the craniofacial skeleton, including the jaws. In: McCarthy JG, May JW, Littler JW, eds. *Plastic Surgery*. Philadelphia: WB Saunders, 1990, 3336–411.

Jackson IT. Skull base tumors: methods of approach and techniques to avoid complications. In: Fee WE, Goepfert H, Johns ME, Strong EW, Ward PH, eds. *Head and Neck Cancer, Volume 2*. Toronto: BC Decker, 1990, 365–82.

Jackson IT, Bailey MH, Marsh WR, Juhasz P. Results and prognosis following surgery for malignant tumors of the skull base. *Head Neck Surg* 1991; 13: 89–96.

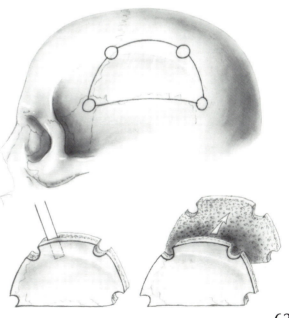

Functional neck dissection

James Yee Suen MD, FACS
Professor and Chairman, Department of Otolaryngology – Head and Neck Surgery,
University of Arkansas for Medical Sciences, Little Rock, Arkansas, USA

Introduction

History

Although neck dissections have been performed for over 100 years, only in the last three decades have modifications begun to surface which attempt to decrease the shoulder dysfunction.

Bocca of Italy was one of the first surgeons to report on functional neck dissections and his technique was first described in 1966[1]. Alando J. Ballantyne of the M. D. Anderson Hospital and Tumor Institute in Houston, Texas has been doing functional neck dissections for over 25 years. His technique is performed completely from an anterior approach, while Bocca's technique uses an approach both anterior and posterior to the sternocleidomastoid (SCM) muscle. Both techniques are useful with each having its advantages and disadvantages. The anterior approach using Ballantyne's technique is not simply an anterior neck dissection as it also dissects out the majority of the posterior cervical triangle.

Principles and justification

The functional neck dissection can remove essentially all of the same lymph nodes in the neck that a radical neck dissection does, but with preservation of the sternomastoid muscle, internal jugular vein, spinal accessory nerve and cervical plexus nerves. Several reports[2–5] in the past 15 years reveal that the control rate for N0–N1 lesions is no different whether treated with a radical neck dissection or a functional neck dissection. This is partly due to the liberal use of irradiation in these advanced cancers where neck dissections are incorporated. Another reason is that lymph node metastasis is predictable. For example, Skolnick et al.[6] have shown that posterior cervical nodes are rarely involved when the nodes in the jugular chain are negative with laryngeal cancers. Therefore, when a lesion is N0 it is not as essential to remove the posterior triangle nodes. Until further studies are completed, it is critical that functional neck dissection follows strict indications and contraindications so that the oncological treatment is not compromised.

The author feels that the present indications and contraindications for a functional neck dissection are as follows.

Indications for anterior approach (Ballantyne technique)

1. Clinically negative neck but significant (greater than 25 per cent) risk of occult nodes; this is considered an 'elective neck dissection'. Included in this category would be involvement on both sides of the neck along with some midline primaries, such as in the base of the tongue and the supraglottic larynx. The modified neck dissection is usually performed in conjunction with resection of the primary.
2. Single node (<3 cm) in patients with thin or medium size necks when surgery is to be followed by irradiation; e.g. T3 or T4, N1M0 of oral cavity, oropharynx or hypopharynx.

Indications for anterior–posterior approach (Bocca technique)

1. N1 neck in patient with short, full neck which is difficult to assess.
2. N2 neck when functional neck dissection is to be attempted.
3. N3b neck where bilateral neck dissections are planned and a functional neck dissection is to be performed on the least involved side. Postoperative irradiation should be given.
4. Papillary carcinoma of the thyroid with neck metastasis.
5. N0 neck in melanomas, level IV or V.

Contraindications

1. Clinically positive nodes when surgery is the only treatment modality to be used.
2. Clinically positive nodes after irradiation of the neck.
3. Clinically positive nodes after previous modified or regional neck dissection.
4. Melanoma with clinically positive nodes.
5. Inexperienced surgeon.

Operations

ANTERIOR APPROACH (BALLANTYNE TECHNIQUE)

Incision

1

The type of incision is not critical as long as it is an acceptable, standard one in which the neck structures are exposed adequately. If the functional neck dissection is performed from an anterior approach only, as described here, then the incision and flaps do not have to be elevated behind the posterior border of the sternomastoid muscle.

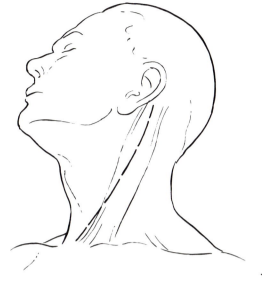

1

Initial dissection

2

A flap of skin and platysma is elevated until adequate exposure is obtained. The mandibular branch of the facial nerve should be identified and preserved as it runs in the submandibular gland fascia. The surgical field exposed should include the ipsilateral strap muscles, submandibular triangle contents, the anterior half of the SCM muscle and the tail of the parotid gland.

Haemostats are used to clamp the thin superficial fascia of the medial half of the SCM muscle and the fascia is retracted medially anteriorly. An incision is made into this superficial fascia along its entire length using a No. 10 scalpel or the Shaw scalpel (hot knife) which works well for this part of the operation. This incision should be anterior and parallel to the superior part of the external jugular vein and then carried inferiorly along the middle of the external surface of the SCM to its lower attachment. The fascia is then dissected off the muscle to its anterior border. Retracting the SCM muscle posteriorly with a gauze pad and hand will facilitate dissection of the fascia.

The dashed line over the fascia of the strap muscles indicates the anterior or medial extent of the neck dissection which is performed toward the end of this operation.

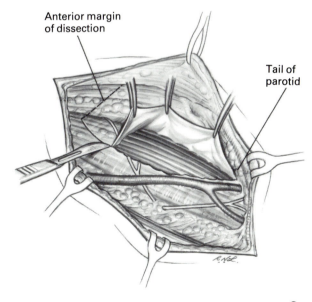

Anterior margin of dissection

Tail of parotid

2

Dissecting underneath the SCM muscle and identification of the spinal accessory nerve

3a & b

The fascia is then dissected from the medial surface of the SCM muscle (an unwrapping manoeuvre). The muscle must be retracted posteriorly, initially using a hand with a gauze pad, then with loop-type retractors. During this dissection small perforating vessels will be seen entering the muscle from the fascia. These can be electrocauterized or ligated as they are encountered. Some of these vessel branches are very close to the internal jugular vein and must be grasped with a clamp or forceps before being cauterized to avoid injury to the jugular vein.

Preservation of the spinal accessory nerve is one of the primary reasons for the functional neck dissection so extreme care must be taken to identify and preserve it. The upper third of the nerve is encountered initially as the fascia is dissected away from the medial side of the SCM at the junction of the upper and middle third of the muscle. The nerve usually divides into the sternomastoid and trapezius branches just before it enters the SCM muscle. Both branches should be preserved.

After identification of the spinal accessory nerve, the fascia dissection should continue inferior to the nerve until the posterior edge of the SCM muscle is noted. The surgeon should palpate the lateral skin of the neck to judge where the posterior edge of the SCM muscle is, so that the dissection will not extend into the posterior triangle skin which is close. The cervical plexus nerves will also be encountered as they wrap around the posterior SCM muscle edge. The upper part of the neck dissection is performed later.

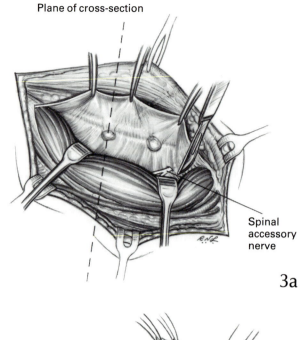

Plane of cross-section

Spinal accessory nerve

3a

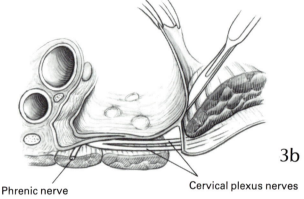

Phrenic nerve

Cervical plexus nerves

3b

Plane of cross-section indicated in Illustration 3a

Posterior cervical triangle

4

This illustration shows the extent of the posterior and supraclavicular dissection with the anterior approach. The inferior limit is at the level of the transverse cervical artery and omohyoid muscle which may be preserved or resected. There is no well-defined stopping point in this area but it is only 2 or 3 cm above the clavicle. The posterior margin is anterior to the trapezius muscle and almost parallel to the lower two-thirds of the spinal accessory nerve.

The author feels that it is unnecessary to dissect to the trapezius and clavicle when the neck is clinically negative. If clinically positive nodes are encountered in the lower jugular or posterior cervical areas the nodes could be checked with frozen sections and if pathologically positive, the dissection should be converted to a radical neck dissection.

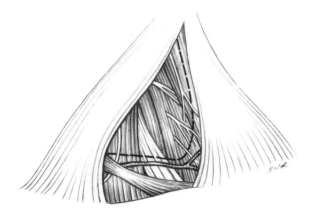

4

Dissecting the posterior cervical triangle

5a & b

At the posterior edge of the sternomastoid muscle, the direction of the dissection is in a 'U' turn and is carried down to the fascia overlying the deep cervical muscles (levator scapulae and scalenes). The cervical plexus nerves should be preserved because the spinal accessory nerve in the posterior triangle usually intertwines with one or two of the cervical plexus nerves and can easily be severed inadvertently. If there is any question as to whether a nerve is the spinal accessory nerve, a nerve stimulator should be used to check it. The second and third branches of the cervical plexus nerves give off branches to the spinal accessory nerve so that stimulation of these nerves will also stimulate the trapezius muscle. Therefore, all of these branches should be preserved.

The fascia, fat and nodes are retracted medially with haemostats and are dissected over the deep neck muscles, care being taken not to injure the spinal accessory, cervical plexus and phrenic nerves. This part of the dissection is performed with a No. 10 scalpel blade. The best way to dissect between the cervical plexus nerves is to dissect out the nerves with a haemostat which will release the fatty tissue between the nerves. The fatty tissue is then grasped with haemostats, placed on traction and dissected off the deep muscles in a medial direction towards the carotid sheath. During sharp dissection it is very helpful for the operator to use his or her opposite hand with a gauze pad to push the tissues medially as the dissection continues.

As this deep layer of fascia is dissected medially, small vessels with accompanying nerves can be noted entering the medial side of the levator scapulae muscle. These neurovascular bundles do not have to be resected and the dissection should be just above these structures.

Dissecting the carotid sheath

6a & b

The phrenic nerve (often two branches) should be identified and preserved as the neck contents are dissected over the trunks of the cervical plexus nerves. The carotid sheath is encountered next. Normally the jugular vein is lateral to the artery but with traction of the fascia and its contents in an upward and medial direction, the jugular vein is almost anterior to the artery. Therefore, the carotid artery is encountered first and the dissection should be directly against this vessel without cutting the artery. Strong traction is important here so that when the knife blade touches the vessels, the fascia and adventitia of the artery and vein are dissected off easily and cleanly. The vagus nerve must be identified between the vessels and preserved. Tributary branches of the internal jugular vein should be divided and ligated next to the vein. This dissection is carried superiorly up to the level of the carotid bifurcation. It is dangerous to use the electrocautery or hot knife around the major vessels.

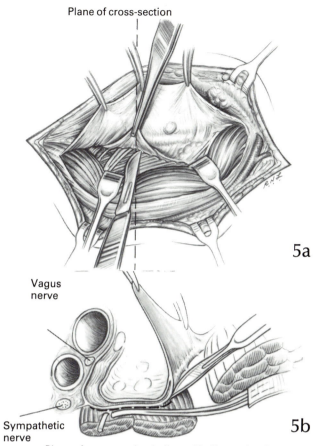

Plane of cross-section

5a

Vagus nerve

Sympathetic nerve

5b

Plane of cross-section indicated in Illustration 5a

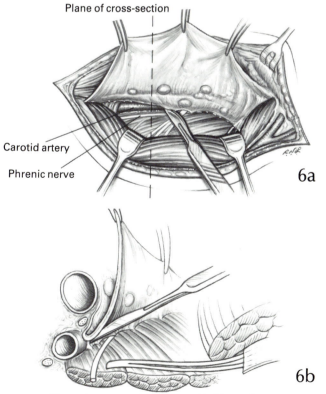

Plane of cross-section

Carotid artery

Phrenic nerve

6a

6b

Plane of cross-section indicated in Illustration 6a

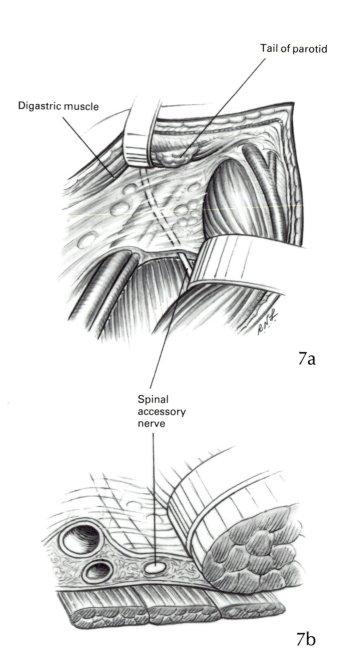

Tail of parotid

Digastric muscle

7a

Spinal accessory nerve

7b

Dissecting the upper neck contents

7a & b

The tissue and nodes remaining in the upper lateral neck are shown in *Illustrations 7a* and *7b*. The superior extent of the dissection is at the level of the digastric muscle. A small amount of the tail of the parotid is included by cutting through it with a hot knife or electrocautery until the underlying digastric muscle is encountered. The posterior facial vein is found in the tail of the parotid and will need to be identified and ligated. The cervical branch of the facial nerve is also located in the tail of the parotid and should be identified. This nerve branch can be divided but the mandibular branch should be preserved with the rest of the facial nerve. The posterior belly of the digastric muscle should be exposed and its fascia dissected off the inferior surface.

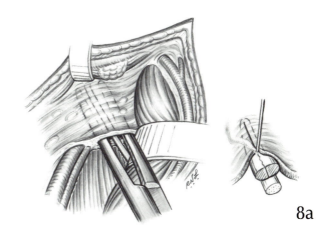

Dissecting the proximal spinal accessory nerve

8a & b

A haemostat is used to follow the spinal accessory nerve superiorly. The tissue overlying the nerve should be divided to expose the nerve, which is protected by the haemostat. The hot knife works well here to avoid troublesome bleeding. At the upper end the nerve goes below the digastric muscle. The jugular vein can be identified immediately beneath the proximal portion of the nerve.

8a

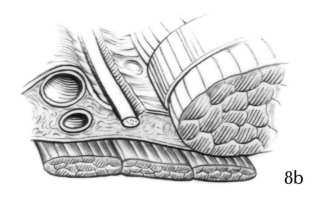

8b

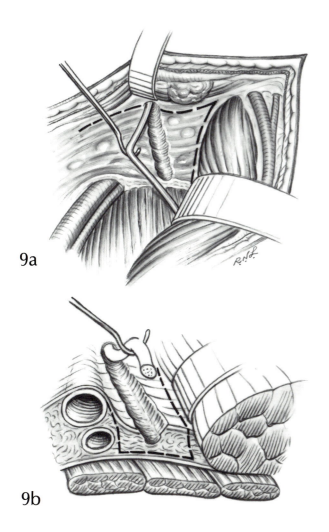

9a

9b

Completing the nerve dissection

9a & b

The nerve is gently freed with sharp dissection. The tissue to be dissected is then identified. The dashed line on the illustrations indicates the tissues to be removed.

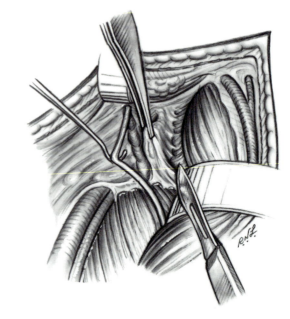

10a

Completing the upper cervical tissue dissection

10a & b

Haemostats are used to grasp this tissue and retract it medially. Retractors are placed on the upper SCM muscle and on the parotid and digastric muscle for exposure. An electrocautery or hot knife can be used to cut through the tissue at the apex until the underlying muscles are seen in the base of the dissection. The spinal accessory nerve should be protected at all times. The tissue is then dissected medially off the splenius capitis and levator scapulae muscles and continued to and underneath the spinal accessory nerve to the jugular vein and internal carotid artery. The posterior occipital artery is in this triangle and this is divided and ligated or cauterized. When near the carotid sheath a No. 15 scalpel blade is used to decrease the chance of injury to the vessels.

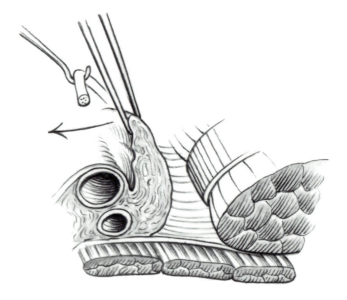

10b

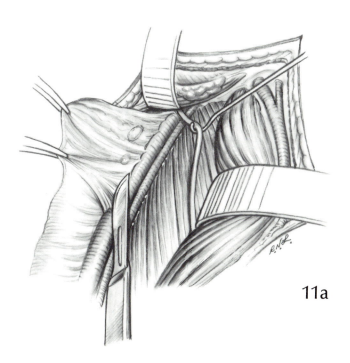

11a

Dissecting over the vessels

11a & b

Using sharp dissection, the nodes and tissues are then dissected over the internal carotid artery and jugular vein towards the submandibular triangle. The posterior belly of the digastric muscle must be retracted superiorly to expose any subdigastric nodes which should be dissected out at this point.

The hypoglossal nerve lies between the artery and vein and crosses the carotid arteries just above the bifurcation. The dissected tissue should be carried over the hypoglossal nerve, preserving it.

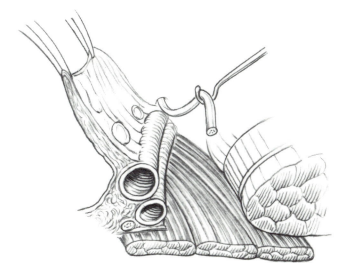

11b

12, 13 & 14

The lateral neck contents are then dissected off the vessels with sharp dissection. The common facial vein and superior thyroid artery can usually be preserved as the dissection is carried to the strap muscles inferiorly and to the hyoid bone and submandibular triangle superiorly. The most medial extent of the dissection is the fascia over the sternohyoid muscle which is cut in a vertical direction and dissected off the muscle up to the hyoid. The anterior jugular vein is usually removed with this part of the dissection. This will complete the neck dissection except for the submandibular triangle.

Submandibular triangle

Dissection of this triangle is described in the chapter on 'Radical neck dissection', p. 636.

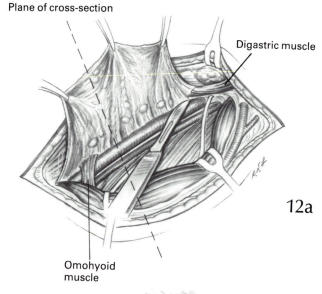

12a

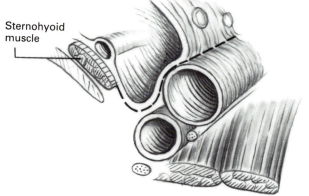

12b

Plane of cross-section indicated in Illustration 12a

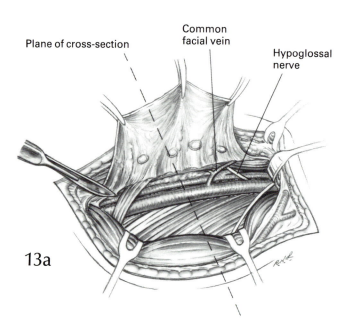

13a

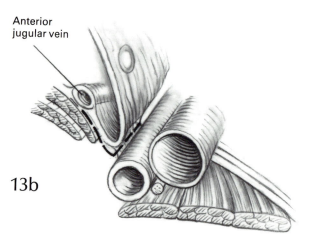

13b

Plane of cross-section indicated in Illustration 13a

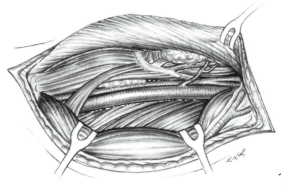

14

ANTERIOR–POSTERIOR APPROACH (BOCCA TECHNIQUE)

Incision

15 & 16

The incision should allow exposure to the same anatomical boundaries as the standard radical neck dissection, i.e. the inferior border of the mandible, trapezius, clavicle and the anterior midline of the neck. This will allow dissection of the posterior cervical triangle separately and carry the dissection under the SCM muscle.

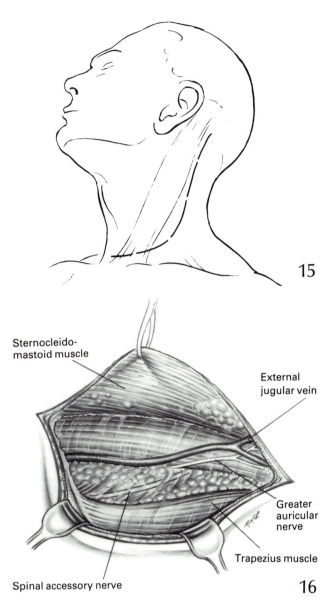

15

Sternocleido-mastoid muscle

External jugular vein

Greater auricular nerve

Trapezius muscle

Spinal accessory nerve

16

Initial dissection

17

An incision is made with a No. 10 knife blade or a hot knife through the lateral superficial fascia of the SCM near the middle of the muscle and carried to its posterior border of the muscle at its inferior and superior attachments. The fascia is grasped with multiple haemostats along its edge and retracted posteriorly while it is dissected off the muscle. The external jugular vein is divided and ligated superiorly but the sensory nerve branches of the cervical plexus nerves are preserved. The fascia is dissected to the posterior border and slightly medially underneath the SCM muscle. The haemostats are then removed.

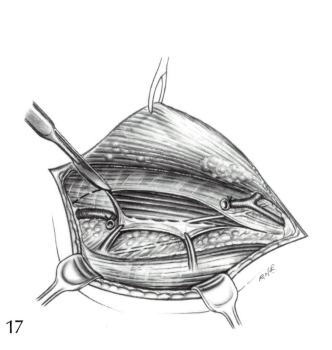

17

Defining the posterior border and identifying the spinal accessory nerve

18

The posterior border of the neck dissection is the edge of the trapezius muscle. This part of the neck dissection is similar to a radical neck dissection except that the spinal accessory nerve must be identified and dissected out carefully. This nerve will run just medial and parallel to the lower third of the trapezius muscle. It can be identified by using a haemostat to dissect in this area until the nerve is found. Once identification of the nerve is confirmed by a nerve stimulator, a haemostat is used to dissect out the nerve superiorly, and the tissue external to the nerve is dissected off with sharp dissection. The hot knife is useful here. The nerve should be dissected free from the lower trapezius area up to where it emerges from the SCM muscle.

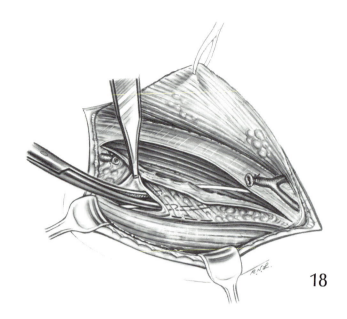

18

Resecting the posterior cervical triangle contents

19

With the spinal accessory nerve protected, the posterior cervical triangle contents can be dissected. Haemostats are placed on the posterior neck contents near the trapezius muscle and are pulled in an anterior and medial direction. The fascia, fat and nodes are dissected down to the levator scapulae and scalene muscles, then the fascia of these muscles is dissected off in a medial direction.

This tissue is carried underneath the spinal accessory nerve and after the nerve is free enough, it is retracted posteriorly so that the dissection can continue medially. In the lower posterior cervical triangle a number of transverse cervical veins will be encountered, and these should be divided and ligated.

The transverse cervical artery should be identified and can be preserved or removed. The supraclavicular branches of the cervical plexus nerves will also be encountered in these areas and can be preserved by using a haemostat to dissect them out. The adjacent tissue is then grasped with haemostats and dissected medially toward the carotid sheath.

The supraclavicular tissue is dissected off the clavicle down to the deep neck muscles (scalenes) and brachial plexus. The lower external jugular vein should be identified, divided and ligated near its entrance to the subclavian vein. The omohyoid muscle can be identified here and divided. A haemostat is placed on the proximal end of the muscle and retracted medially with the rest of the neck contents.

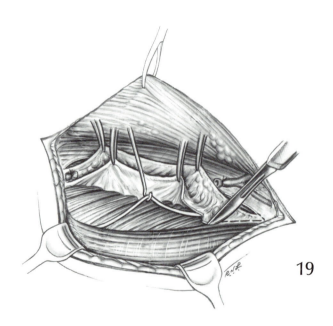

19

Much of the dissection can be made easier during knife dissection if the operator uses a gauze pad in the opposite hand to push the tissue medially. This method makes vessels and nerves much easier to identify and helps to preserve them.

Using the anterior–posterior approach of Bocca, more tissue is resected in the supraclavicular and lower jugular areas than with the anterior approach. The author does not feel this is necessary most of the time. If nodes are suspicious or positive in these areas, he would do a radical neck dissection.

Dissecting medial to the SCM muscle

20

The posterior cervical triangle contents are dissected medially until the dissection reaches the posterior surface or medial border of the SCM muscle. At this stage the posterior dissection can be discontinued. The rest of the neck dissection is done anteriorly as discussed in the anterior approach. When the anterior dissection reaches the posterior part of the SCM muscle, all of the posterior contents can then be delivered underneath the SCM muscle and the dissection completed.

If the transverse cervical artery is divided laterally, it must be divided again just distal to its inferior thyroid artery branch. Large lymphatic ducts at the lower jugular vein area must be recognized and preserved or ligated satisfactorily.

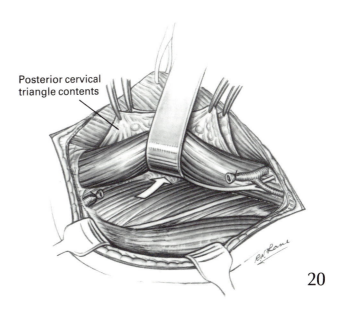

Posterior cervical triangle contents

20

References

1. Bocca E. Supraglottic laryngectomy and functional neck dissection. *J Laryngol Otol* 1966; 80: 831–8.

2. Bocca E. Critical analysis of the techniques and value of neck dissection. *Nuovo Archiv Ital Otol Rinol Laringol* 1976; 4: 151–8.

3. Lingeman RE, Helmus C, Stephens R, Ulm J. Neck dissection radical or conservative. *Ann Otol Rhinol Laryngol* 1977; 86: 737–44.

4. Molinari R, Cantu G, Chiesa F, Grandi C. Retrospective comparison of conservative and radical neck dissection in laryngeal cancer. *Ann Otol Rhinol Laryngol* 1980; 89: 578–81.

5. Jesse RH, Ballantyne AJ, Larson D. Radical or modified neck dissection: a therapeutic dilemma. *Am J Surg* 1978; 136: 516–19.

6. Skolnick EM, Yee KF, Friedman M, Goldon TA. The posterior triangle in radical neck surgery. *Arch Otolaryngol* 1976; 102: 1–4.

Radical neck dissection

Ian A. McGregor ChM, DSc, FRCS
Formerly Director, Plastic and Oral Surgery Unit, Canniesburn Hospital, Glasgow, UK

David J. Howard FRCS, FRCS(Ed)
Institute of Laryngology and Otology, Royal National Throat, Nose and Ear Hospital, London, UK

Introduction

Metastatic spread to regional lymph nodes from tumours of the head and neck is managed surgically by resection of the neck nodes. The detailed pattern of metastatic spread depends on the site of the tumour, and the nodal resections carried out are varied to match the patterns from the individual sites, but they have a 'core' which is common to all. This became stabilized in the classic paper of Hayes Martin in 1951[1], and is referred to as a radical neck dissection.

The dissection area extends from the mylohyoid line on the lingual plate of the mandible to the upper border of the clavicle, and from the midline to the anterior border of the trapezius muscle. Within these boundaries the lymph nodes are resected, together with certain related structures judged to be anatomically dispensable, most markedly the sternocleidomastoid muscle, the internal jugular vein, the submandibular salivary gland and the accessory nerve.

Scope of the dissection

1

The group of nodes into which tumours of these sites finally metastasize is the deep jugular chain, lying alongside the internal jugular vein. From certain of the sites tumours metastasize directly to them but, in the case of the majority, intermediate groups of nodes, lying in a roughly horizontal line, are interposed – the submental in the midline just below the symphysis menti; the submandibular and parotid, each associated with the corresponding salivary gland; and the postauricular and occipital. Of these groups, only the submandibular is resected as part of the standard radical neck dissection.

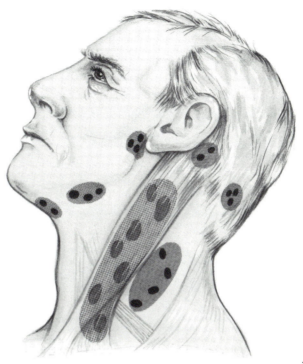

1

2

An additional group of nodes routinely resected as part of a radical neck dissection is in the triangle bounded by the anterior border of trapezius, the posterior border of sternocleidomastoid, and the upper border of the clavicle – the posterior triangle.

It is recognized that, in operable tumours of the oral cavity, larynx and hypopharynx, the group of nodes in the posterior triangle is virtually never involved by metastatic tumour, regardless of whether or not the neck has previously been irradiated. In view of this, the question might reasonably be asked why they are included in the radical neck dissection.

Radical neck dissection, as currently practised, has acquired a status as a result of long usage – in the UK effectively since Butlin's description of the procedure in 1900[2], and in the USA since that of Crile in 1906[3]. Perhaps even more significant is that, in 1951 when Hayes Martin set out the form which a radical neck dissection should take, it was not appreciated that the posterior triangle nodes were not involved when the primary site was operable. This fact has only been recognized relatively recently, and its influence has been more in the direction of providing a basis of surgical respectability for the concept of functional neck dissection, as discussed in the chapter on 'Functional neck dissection' pp. 624–635, than changing the form of radical neck dissection. Certainly, for the vast majority of surgeons it remains the standard procedure for the clinically positive neck.

Radical neck dissection is a well defined procedure and has the virtue of clear-cut margins. Functional neck dissection is less satisfactory in both respects. In particular, the extent to which nodal clearance is extended into the posterior triangle is arbitrarily decided by the surgeon, rather than being dictated by the presence of a recognizable margin such as the anterior border of trapezius.

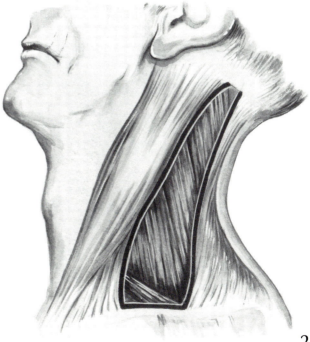

2

Skin incisions

Many skin incisions have been described for use in radical neck dissection, most with eponymous titles, and each representing a particular compromise between good exposure of the neck structures and effective protection of the major vessels by providing adequate skin cover. The skin incisions used prior to 1951 derived from Butlin and Crile but, following the publication of the Hayes Martin paper, the incision which he described became the norm, and it was from it that the more modern incisions were largely developed.

Hayes Martin incision

3

The Hayes Martin incision has a submandibular component which extends from the midline, below the symphysis of the mandible, across the neck onto the mastoid area. The incision consists of two straight lines, the first backwards and downwards to the midline of the neck, the second from there to the mastoid area, enclosing a triangular flap based above on the lower border of the mandible. A comparably designed incision encloses a smaller supraclavicular flap based on the upper border of the clavicle, and a vertical incision joins the apices of the two flaps. The four flaps which the incisions have created are elevated to expose the neck structures.

Of the various incisions which have been described before or since, the Hayes Martin incision provides the best exposure, but its healing properties are unsatisfactory and its capacity to protect the major vessels is inadequate. The site where three points in an incision meet is recognized to be more than usually prone to poor healing and wound breakdown. The Hayes Martin incision has two such points – one supraclavicular and one submandibular – and each, as discussed in the chapter on 'General management and complications', pp. 8–21, is in a site where fluid is prone to collect postoperatively. In the supraclavicular area, breakdown of the wound has the effect of breaking the vacuum seal and suction drainage becomes ineffective. In the submandibular area, the situation has been slightly different because of the practice when the incision was first described of routine hemimandibulectomy. This allowed the submandibular dead space to collapse, and problems of healing arose less often. It has been with the increasing use of conservative mandibular surgery that problems of wound breakdown in the submandibular area have become similar to those of the supraclavicular area. In the 1950s, however, the supraclavicular problems were more troublesome, and it was to avoid these that it was largely replaced by the triradiate incision, either in its simplest form or in one of the modified versions.

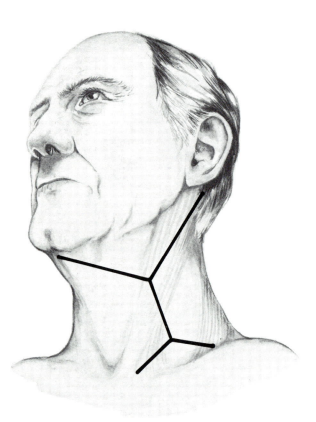

3

Triradiate incision

4

In its simplest form, the triradiate incision has a submandibular construction similar in essence to that of the Hayes Martin incision, but the supraclavicular flap is eliminated by extending the vertical incision down over the clavicle. The submandibular incision can be made with straight lines and an angle at the apex, or as a continuous curve. Neither has any special advantage over the other. The exposure is similar to that provided by the Hayes Martin incision, but the proneness to wound breakdown in the supraclavicular area is largely eliminated.

There are valid reasons for placing the vertical limb of the incision further back in the neck than in the Hayes Martin version. A considerable part of the posterior flap lacks the platysma, and there is no comparably identifiable structure exposed when the flap is being raised. The general laxity of the tissues in the area, even with the head extended and rotated, also prevents the use of traction and counter-traction in dissection, adding to the difficulty of raising the flap with a consistent thickness. It is much the most difficult of the three flaps to raise, and the surgeon will welcome the reduction of the dissection involved by shortening the flap. Positioning the incision further back in the neck also increases the extent of the anterior flap, and this adds to its capacity to cover the major vessels and provide protection for them.

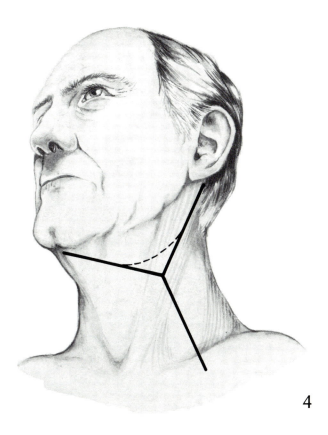

4

5

Variations of the basic triradiate design which have been described include the curving of the vertical incision backwards by Schobinger[4], to add to the protection provided by the anterior skin flap.

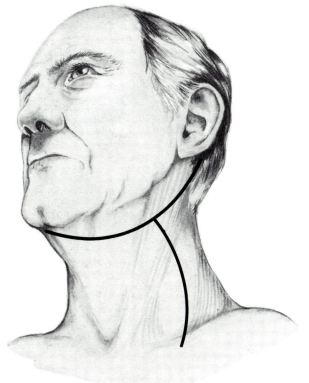

5

6

A further variant, described by Conley[5], converts the anterior part of the submandibular incision and the vertical incision into a single curve which begins at the midline below the symphysis of the mandible and curves over the side of the neck to reach the anterior border of trapezius at its insertion into the clavicle. The posterior element of the submandibular incision meets the curve at a right angle, approximately below the lobule of the ear. The virtues of this modification lie in the considerable reduction of the dissection involved in raising the posterior flap, and the increase in the protection of the major vessels which the extension of the anterior flap provides.

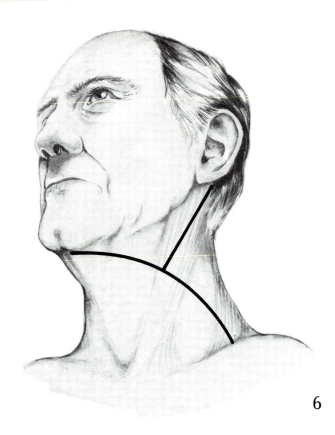

6

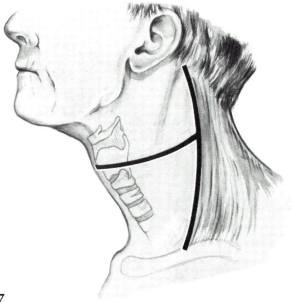

7

7

The vertical limb of a triradiate incision can also be placed along the anterior border of the trapezius muscle, with a horizontal limb joining it at a right angle at its mid-point.

MacFee incision

8

The MacFee incision[6] differs from the others in having no vertical component. Instead it uses two horizontal incisions, one in the submandibular region and one in the supraclavicular region. The bipedicled flap between the two incisions is raised and, retracting the flap upwards to allow access from below, and downwards to allow access from above, the dissection, otherwise standard, is carried out. Although the incisions as illustrated by MacFee are virtually straight, modifications are regularly seen, most often converting the line of the submandibular incision into one which approaches the curving line of the basic triradiate incision and, less frequently, the supraclavicular incision to an upward curve.

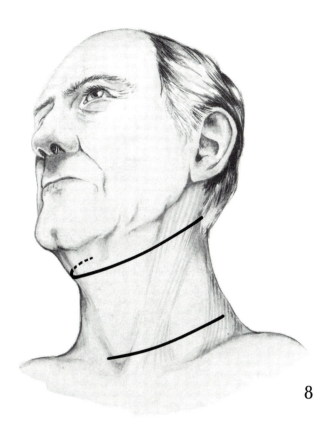

8

9

Incisions for accompanying laryngopharyngeal procedures

Variants of the triradiate incision using a large supero-medial 'apron' flap are used for total laryngectomy combined with neck dissection. They combine excellent access for both laryngeal and pharyngeal mobilization and the incontinuity neck dissection.

9

With supraglottic laryngectomy and neck dissection, the 'apron' is reduced in length to allow the tracheostomy site to be placed through a separate smaller incision in the lower flap.

10

If a previous tracheostomy has been carried out because of extensive laryngeal disease which was compromising the airway, the 'apron' is lengthened, allowing the previous tracheostomy site to be excised as an ellipse, and the subsequent tracheostoma placed directly in the incision.

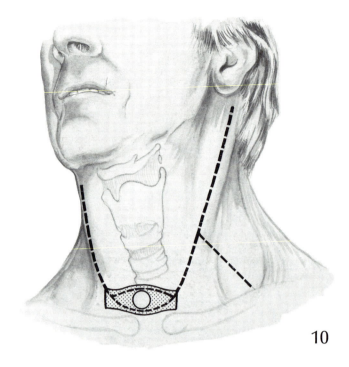

10

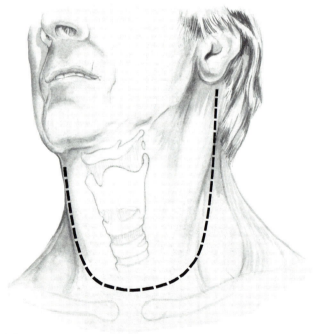

11

11

If the neck has been previously irradiated, the lateral limb of the triradiate incision may be omitted, the entire procedure being then carried out via the apron flap. In this case the length of the 'apron' is increased, bringing its lower transverse limb closer to the clavicle, and the flap is broadened by placing its vertical limb more laterally on the side of the neck dissection.

Comparison of incisions

The Hayes Martin incision has deservedly been abandoned for the reasons already given, and the comparison is really between the triradiate incision in its various forms and the MacFee incision. Their comparative merits are bound up with whether or not the neck has previously been irradiated. As discussed in the chapter on 'General management and complications', pp. 8–21, the probability of wound breakdown is increased if the neck has been previously irradiated. Further, if breakdown does occur, there is a greater probability of the breakdown extending to expose the major vessels, and the likelihood of exposure progressing to 'blow-out' depends virtually entirely on whether or not the neck has been irradiated.

There is no doubt that the MacFee incision provides the greatest overall protection, although even with it breakdown of the upper incision is liable to leave that part of the carotid system exposed. Today, as discussed in the chapter on 'Reconstructive techniques of the oral cavity', pp. 215–240, the pedicled myocutaneous flaps, particularly the pectoralis major flap, used to reconstruct postresection defects of the oral cavity and pharynx incidentally provide a muscle pedicle which protects the major vessels, and this has made the protective element of the argument in favour of the MacFee incision much less valid.

The radical neck dissection carried out using a MacFee incision is technically more difficult than using any of the triradiate variants. The raising of the bipedicled flap at a uniform level is not easy, and the dissection thereafter, with a necessarily limited access, is awkward.

Alleged virtues of the MacFee incision are the better appearance as a result of the absence of a vertical neck scar, and the avoidance of the vertical contracture stated to be liable to develop along such a scar line. Neither of these arguments has any substance. The cosmetic disability which follows a radical neck dissection concerns the contour deformity rather than the neck scars, and the vertical contractural bands which are regularly seen after a radical neck dissection are not related to any vertical scar which may be present in the neck. The bands involve the tissues deep to the platysmal level. If the neck has been previously irradiated, and the reconstruction to be used does not provide the additional protection referred to above, the MacFee incision should be given serious consideration. Otherwise it does not have sufficient virtues to outweigh the technical difficulties which attend its use.

In the absence of the factors discussed above, the triradiate incision in one of its forms is the most generally useful. The placing of the vertical limb further back to reduce the dissection involved in raising the posterior flap is a worthwhile variant, and the still further reduction of the posterior flap which the Conley modification provides, coupled with the protection provided by its extended anterior flap, gives it a real value. It might be felt that the length of the anterior flap would make it difficult to expose the lower part of the neck anteriorly, but this is not found to be so in practice. The triradiate incision in Illustration 7 respects the two main areas of arterial perfusion in the neck, the lower from the subclavian system, the upper from the branches of the external carotid. On these grounds it might be considered to be preferable in the previously irradiated neck.

Modified incisions

It is occasionally necessary to modify further the standard neck dissection incisions when the flap chosen to reconstruct the postresection defect directly adjoins the neck dissection, or when external fungation of a tumour has occurred or appears to be imminent, and the involved skin requires to be resected.

12

The reconstructing flap currently most often involved whose elevation directly adjoins the neck dissection is the pectoralis major myocutaneous flap. The 'defensive' approach to this flap, where a skin incision outlining a standard deltopectoral flap is used (for the reasons discussed in the chapter on 'Reconstructive techniques of the skin', pp. 45–103) precludes any extension of the vertical neck incision over the clavicle on to the chest. The same modification is also necessary when a deltopectoral flap is selected as the reconstructive method. In either event, the vertical neck incision meets the upper border of the deltopectoral flap incision at a right angle.

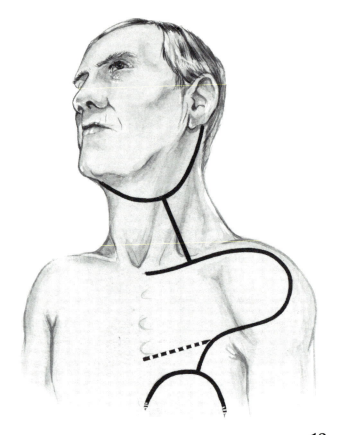

12

13

With a MacFee incision, the upper border of the deltopectoral flap incision serves also as the lower of the MacFee incisions, the effect being to move the line of the lower incision to the level of the clavicle.

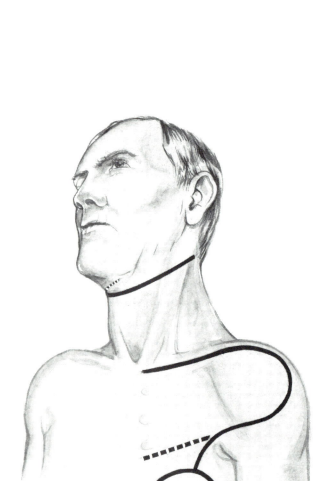

13

14

External fungation of an intraoral tumour most frequently involves the submandibular area, though other sites, particularly in the upper neck, are occasionally involved. Prior to the development of the deltopectoral flap, capable of being raised and transferred without prior preparation, the skin incisions used to expose the neck structures had to be modified to outline a flap which could be transferred to cover the defect after completion of the neck dissection. This was never a satisfactory solution, and with the current availability of both the deltopectoral and pectoralis major flaps it is unlikely to be required. The potential skin sites in the neck are within the range of either of these flaps, and the defects are likely to be of a size with which they can cope.

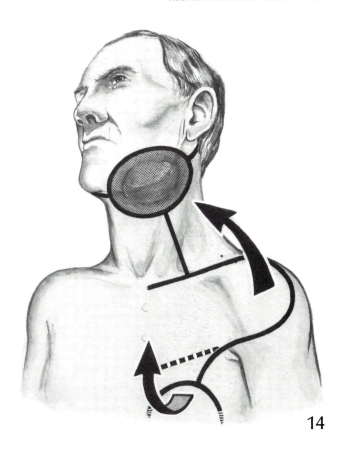

14

Tracheostomy and the dissection

It is good surgical practice to elevate the skin flaps to their full extent, so that the operative field is properly defined before commencing the formal nodal dissection. However, when a tracheostomy is being carried out as a preliminary, the need to make certain that the two operative fields – tracheostomy and neck dissection – remain physically separate from one another is paramount. Failure to maintain separation is likely to result in postoperative contamination of the field of the neck dissection, as the rise of pressure within the trachea with coughing forces tracheobronchial secretions into the supraclavicular area of the neck dissection, making for potential infection of that area, and increasing the likelihood of breakdown of the neck wound.

15

Two steps are available to preserve separation of the two dissections. In the carrying out of the tracheostomy, as described in the chapter on 'Emergency and elective airway procedures: tracheostomy, cricothyroidotomy and their variants', pp. 27–44, dissection laterally should be reduced to an absolute minimum, and in raising the anterior skin flap, elevation should stop short of the tracheostomy dissection.

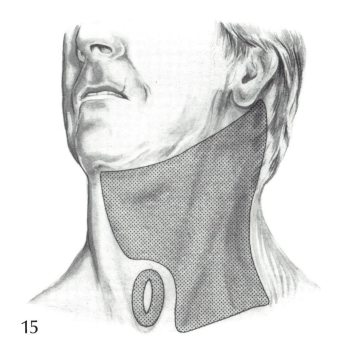

15

Operative technique

In carrying out the neck dissection, two dissection techniques can be used, and each has its protagonists. In one, scissors are used virtually exclusively; in the other, scalpel dissection is the method used. Both techniques make use of the recognized principle of traction and counter traction.

Scissor dissection makes use of blunt tipped scissors, McIndoe's scissors being suitable for the purpose. With traction applied to the tissues in order to define the dissection plane, the scissors are thrust into the tissues in the direction of the dissection plane and the blades are forcibly opened. The plane opened up is then exploited by cutting with the scissors. The rationale of the method is that the resistance provided by fascia against the opening of the scissor blades is less than that of more specialized tissues such as muscle. Probing with the scissor tips is also used to demonstrate vessels and nerves, these structures withstanding the traction exerted by the opening blades better than the areolar tissue surrounding them. The use of scissors in this way confines dissection virtually entirely to fascial planes and, when muscles such as those forming the floor of the posterior triangle are being cleared, the effect is to leave them with a covering of fascia.

Scalpel dissection is completely different, both in the technique used to establish the planes and in the planes themselves. Instead of dissecting in the fascial plane and leaving the muscle covered with a fascial layer, the plane established is between the fascia and the muscle, and leaves the muscle completely bare. With the tissue to be dissected under tension, exerted by tissue forceps when the tissue involved is to be excised, by skin hooks or dissecting forceps when the tissue is being retained, the light stroking of the scalpel blade is sufficient to create the dissection plane. The key to successful scalpel dissection is the use of traction against which the scalpel blade can work. With the blade changed at the least suggestion of bluntness, and allowing it to do the work, stroking the tissues along the plane of dissection, the scalpel becomes highly selective in what it cuts. In this respect it is superior to scissors, which are essentially unselective in what they cut.

Scissor dissection becomes much more difficult when the neck has previously been irradiated, because of the changes radiotherapy produces in the fascia which make it much more resistant both to the insertion of the scissors into it and the opening of the blades to establish the plane of dissection. The virtues of scalpel dissection show particularly clearly in the previously irradiated neck, because it avoids the fascial planes altogether, dissecting instead between the fascia and the muscle.

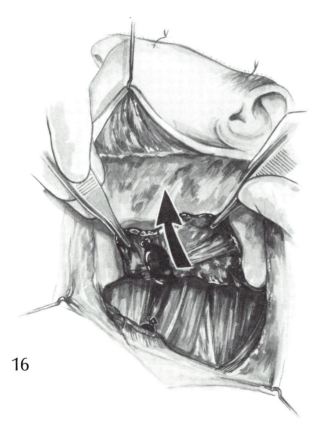

16

Sequence of dissection

16

The dissection, as described by Hayes Martin, was carried out in a general upward direction. Sternocleidomastoid and the internal jugular vein were divided just above the sternoclavicular attachment of the muscle, and dissected upwards together with the contents of the posterior triangle. The submandibular salivary gland with its nodes was incorporated in the resected specimen, and clearance of the vein and its associated nodes was continued upwards as far as the transverse process of the atlas. At that level the internal jugular vein was divided along with the mastoid insertion of sternocleidomastoid, completing the dissection.

This is an adequate way of carrying out the dissection, but it has certain unsatisfactory features. It creates unnecessary difficulty for the surgeon in ligating the upper end of the internal jugular vein, and it does not make the best use of the anatomical features of the major vessels in the neck.

When the Hayes Martin sequence is used, ligation of the upper end of the internal jugular vein is often the most difficult part of the procedure, particularly when the patient has a short, thick neck, and the difficulty is compounded when nodes enlarged with metastatic disease are present in the jugulodigastric area.

17

When the dissection has reached the level of the transverse process of the atlas, the resection specimen, still held attached by sternocleidomastoid and the internal jugular vein, is retracted upwards to expose the vein. From the tissue mass the vein is dissected free using probing scissor dissection. Mosquito forceps are then carefully eased through the path created by the scissors, and the ligating suture is pulled back by the forceps as they are withdrawn. The ligature is then tied and the procedure is repeated until the double ligation with transfixion of the vein wall is completed. The vein is then divided.

In carrying out this manoeuvre, the surgeon has inadequate control of the vessel, and the freeing of the vein over a length sufficient to allow ligation and division is carried out in the least advantageous circumstances possible, with the vein stretched over the convexity of the retracted tissue. In the absence of proper control of the vein, injury to the vessel wall, followed by copious haemorrhage, can be extremely difficult to cope with. In short, ligation of the upper end of the internal jugular vein carried out in this manner is a frequent source of worry to the surgeon.

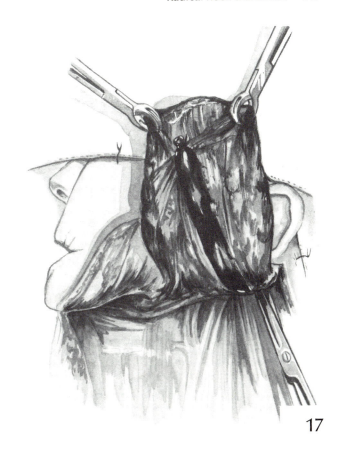

17

18

Altogether more satisfactory is to approach the vein from its superficial surface. This can be done by dividing sternocleidomastoid at its mastoid insertion, elevating its detached upper end and retracting it forward and downward, exposing the posterior belly of digastric which lies immediately under it. The internal jugular vein lies directly under digastric with only the occipital artery between, and retraction of the muscle upwards and downwards as required exposes the vein directly from the surface. Together with the clearance of the vein posteriorly in the standard manner carried up to the transverse process of the atlas, dissection-free ligation and division can be carried out with the vein under direct vision, exposed both superficially and deeply.

The sequence of dissection carried out from below upwards also fails to make use of the anatomical fact that over virtually the entire length of the dissection the major vessels have no posterior branches.

18

19

The occipital and posterior auricular arteries are the posterior branches of the external carotid artery arising under the posterior belly of digastric at the upper extremity of the dissection.

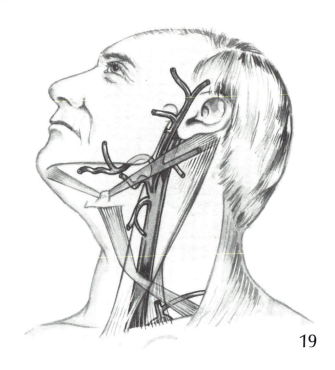

19

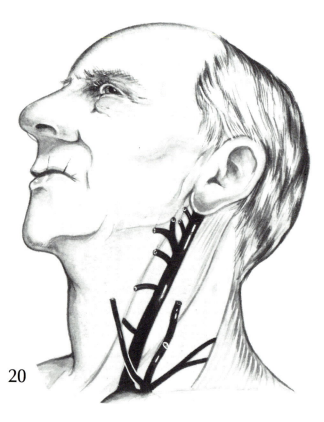

20

20

The internal jugular vein receives a considerable number of tributaries, varying both in number and the size of each, but without exception they join the main trunk from sources anterior to it.

21

These anatomical features can be put to use by carrying out the initial dissection from the posterior triangle, approaching the vessels from behind along much of their length, knowing that no branches – arterial or venous – will be encountered.

The posterior approach has the additional virtue that where there is doubt concerning the operability of the neck because of metastatic involvement of the upper cervical nodes, their state can be assessed early in the procedure. This is preferable to carrying out virtually an entire neck dissection from 'below upwards' only to find tumour involving the internal carotid artery and skull base.

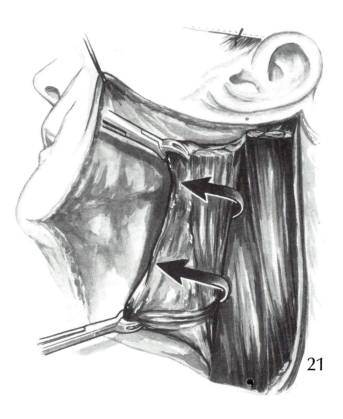

21

Preparation of the patient

22

The standard position of the anaesthetized patient is with neck extended and head rotated to the contralateral side, held in a ring so that the position will be maintained. Extension of the neck can sometimes be increased by placing a pillow under the shoulders, but both extension and rotation are frequently limited in the age group which provides the majority of the patients.

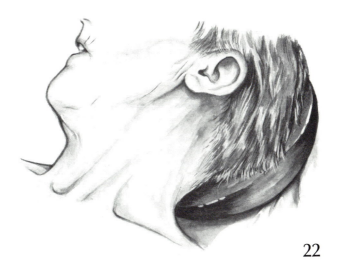

22

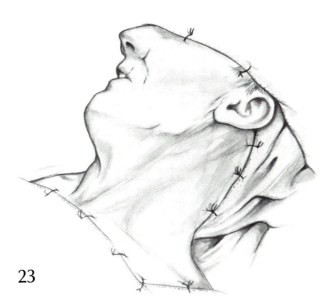

23

23

In towelling the patient, the most effective way of ensuring that the towels stay in position throughout the procedure is to stitch them to the skin.

24

The lines of the skin incisions should be drawn on the skin with Bonney's blue, the line of the submandibular element brought well up onto the mastoid process, and with matching points tattooed on each side of the incision lines. The value of the tattooing of matching points becomes apparent when the wound is being sutured postresection, most strikingly where three points require to be approximated. Failure to prepare the incision in this way makes skin closure unnecessarily difficult.

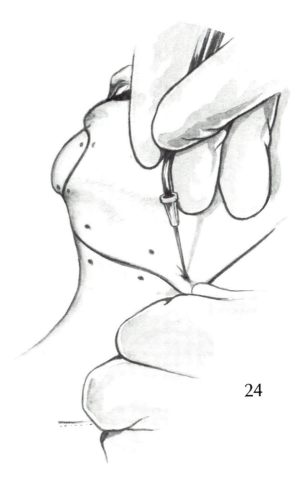

24

25

In making the skin incisions, the assistant and the surgeon together should hold the skin steady and taut on each side of the line of the incision for the stroke of the scalpel, so that the skin will be incised vertically.

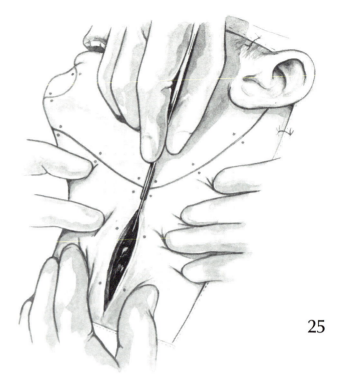

25

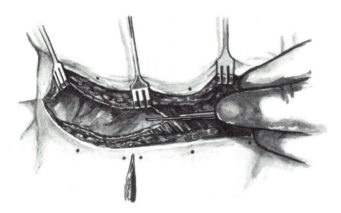

26

26

The surgeon should also ensure that the platysma muscle is cut through completely along the entire length of the incision.

Elevation of skin flaps

The skin flaps are elevated in the plane deep to platysma, making use of its fibres to achieve a uniform level of elevation.

In commencing the elevation, the skin hook or dissecting forceps should grasp the cut margin of the platysma and lift it as the first step in elevating the skin flap. This makes it possible to establish the correct plane of elevation at the outset. In the initial elevation the combined use of the finger and the skin hook to stabilize the flap is an effective way of defining the plane for the scalpel to cut.

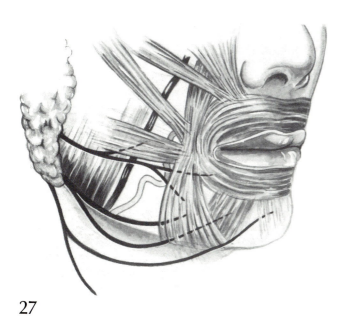

27

27

In raising the submandibular skin flap it is desirable that the mandibular division of the facial nerve should be preserved unless the pathological situation requires its resection. Instructions are regularly given in surgical text books on how to avoid damaging the nerve, but the descriptions of its anatomy which they provide are frequently inadequate. Nelson and Gingrass[7] investigated the course of the nerve during operations in the area, using the nerve stimulator as an aid to identification, and personal experience has been that their account is the most accurate. They found at least three branches of the nerve to be present in every instance. One of the branches was usually larger than the others, and they considered it to be the one most likely to have been identified in other studies as the 'ramus marginalis mandibulae'. It ran slightly above, but sometimes below, the lower border of the mandible, and towards its destination it ascended to run deep to the depressor anguli oris muscle which it supplied. Individual branches supplying the depressor labii inferioris and mentalis muscles were also found below the lower border of the mandible, and further branches were present, one or two in number, above the level of the lower border of the mandible supplying orbicularis oris, depressor anguli oris and risorius.

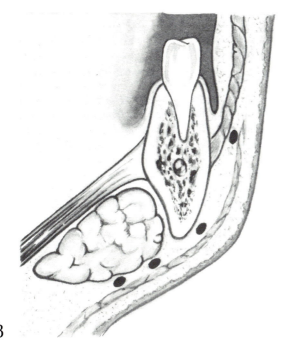

28

28

The branches in the vicinity of the lower border of the mandible run in a thin, rather loose fatty layer of areolar tissue between platysma and the fascia surrounding the submandibular salivary gland.

If these findings are to made use of, the initial skin incision should include and pass beyond platysma to ensure that, when the flap is elevated, the dissection plane is deep to the layer in which the branches lie. The branches themselves are quite easy to identify and preserve, particularly if the surgeon is using loupes.

29

In elevating the posterior flap, the absence of platysma over part of its extent makes it much the most difficult of the flaps to raise, the level of dissection having to be maintained by regularly assessing the thickness of the flap. It is all too easy to make it unduly thick or thin. The laxity of the skin and the tissues filling the triangle, particularly its lower half, adds further to the difficulty of achieving a consistent thickness. A uniform plane is best achieved by holding the flap between the thumb and the fingers. They can be used to exert some traction on the flap against which the scalpel can cut, and also allow its thickness to be continuously assessed.

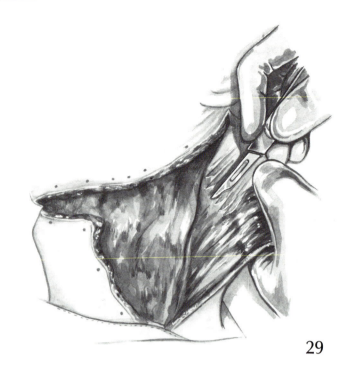

29

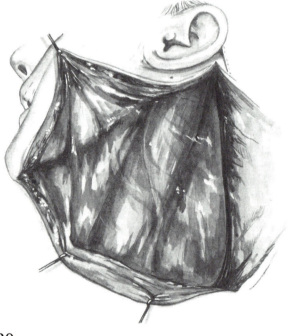

30

The flaps are elevated to the full extent of the dissection and, apart from the anterior border of trapezius, the margins are readily recognized. The extended and rotated position of the head in the anaesthetized patient leaves the trapezius muscle lax, and this adds to the difficulty of finding it. It is all too easy to dissect either superficial or deep to its anterior border. Where the muscle is inserted into the clavicle probably makes the best point at which to make the initial identification, and from there the border can be tracked upwards. Its line should be established over the entire length of the muscle.

30

Clearance of the posterior triangle

The dissection to clear the posterior triangle can commence anywhere along its posterior border, but it is easier, particularly for the surgeon unfamiliar with the operation, to begin at the upper angle where sternocleidomastoid meets trapezius. Here, the distance between the roof and the floor is minimal, and the contents consist of a thin layer of fibrofatty tissue which contains no structures of importance, making it possible to establish the dissection plane without any distractions.

31

At the apex of the triangle an incision is made downwards along the anterior border of trapezius for a short distance, and deepened to expose the floor of the triangle. Forward from the apex also sternocleidomastoid is divided, beginning at its posterior border and through its full thickness.

The line along which the muscle is divided represents the final upper extent of the dissection in this area, and its line should pass across towards the angle of the mandible, even although at this stage dissection does not extend beyond the muscle itself. The muscle belly of sternocleidomastoid varies considerably in thickness depending on the physical type of the patient, thickest in the patient with a short, thick neck. When cutting across the belly with the scalpel and finding it unexpectedly thick, the surgeon who is unfamiliar with neck dissection may have difficulty in believing that there is no structure between the muscle and the posterior belly of digastric, even although it is an anatomical fact. He can avoid much unnecessary worry if he establishes his anatomical bearings clearly before beginning to divide the muscle by making quite certain that he has exposed the anterior border of trapezius up to the apex of the triangle, and by commencing the section of the muscle belly at its posterior border.

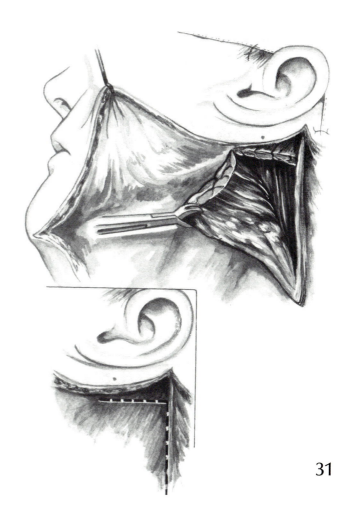

31

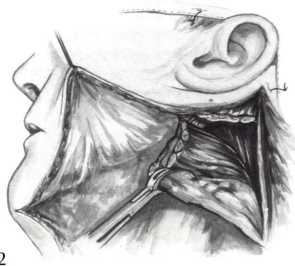

32

32

The triangle of tissue enclosed by the incision along the anterior border of trapezius and the incision dividing sternocleidomastoid is dissected from the floor of the triangle and, firmly grasped with tissue forceps and pulled downward and forward strips bare the underlying splenius capitis muscle, which here is forming the floor. As the division of sternocleidomastoid is extended deeper into the muscle and the tissue dissected free continues to be pulled downward and forward, the exposure extends forward to include the structures deep to sternocleidomastoid, bringing into view the posterior belly of the digastric muscle near its insertion. The muscle is distinguishable from sternocleidomastoid by the different direction of its fibres.

33

With the plane of dissection of the posterior triangle established, the incision along the anterior border of trapezius is extended downwards in stages and the muscles of the floor are serially cleared, first splenius capitis, passing to levator scapulae. As the floor is cleared, further tissue forceps are applied to sternocleidomastoid and the posterior border of the tissue being cleared from the posterior triangle, pulling them forward. Depending on the operative style, as discussed on p. 646, the plane of clearance of the triangle either strips the muscles bare of their fascial covering, or leaves them with a covering of prevertebral fascia. When scalpel dissection is being used, the direction of the scalpel cut is best carried along the line of the muscle fibres, the effect being to leave a cleaner muscle surface.

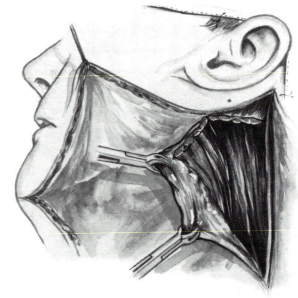

33

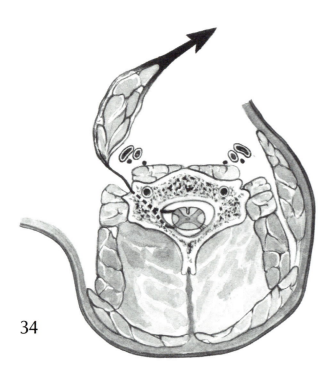

34

34

As clearance of the triangle proceeds downwards, it becomes apparent that the forward retraction of the tissue cleared is being limited by the presence of branches of the cervical plexus as they emerge at segmental levels C2, 3 and 4, just posterolateral to the major vessels. These branches are passing into the layer of tissue being elevated from the triangle, and they form a point of fixation at each exit point of the plexus, preventing further anterior retraction.

35

At this stage further dissection anteriorly can conveniently be stopped, and clearance of the triangle continued in the direction of the supraclavicular area. In this, the lower part of the triangle, its content of anatomically recognized structures is concentrated – the accessory nerve, the inferior belly of omohyoid and the transverse cervical vessels, each traversing the triangle between its anterior and posterior borders. The upper part of the brachial plexus is also just visible.

The accessory nerve emerges from the posterior border of sternocleidomastoid a little above the mid-point of the muscle and passes through the fibrofatty tissue of the triangle, nearer the floor than the roof, to reach the anterior border of trapezius 5 cm from its insertion into the clavicle.

The inferior belly of omohyoid emerges from behind the posterior border of sternocleidomastoid approximately 2 cm above its clavicular attachment, and runs laterally and downwards through the fat in a comparatively superficial plane of its own, disappearing behind the clavicle. Henry[8] described the muscle as having a 'mesenteric' layer of fascia which passes downwards from the muscle and holds it in position. It is a tenuous, barely recognizable structure, seen more as a plane of sorts, noticed in passing as the area is cleared and without significance for the surgeon. The important anatomical fact for the surgeon is that no structure of importance is met superficial to the muscle.

The transverse cervical artery runs in a deeper plane than omohyoid, close to the deep margin of the fat, though still within it. It emerges into the triangle from deep to sternocleidomastoid a little above its clavicular attachment, and passes laterally and slightly upwards deep to omohyoid, towards the anterior border of trapezius, reaching it alongside the accessory nerve 5 cm above the insertion of the muscle into the clavicle.

The transverse cervical vein runs in a more superficial plane than the artery, its course approximately parallel to it, sometimes superficial, sometimes deep to omohyoid, entering the external jugular vein near where it terminates in the subclavian vein.

The brachial plexus, covered with the prevertebral fascia, is just visible between the scalene muscles above the level of the clavicle.

In approaching the clavicle, the roof and floor of the triangle increasingly diverge, the roof passing over the clavicle while the scalene muscles which form the floor at this level pass towards the first rib. The content increases in volume to correspond, becoming less fibrous in the process, softer and more fatty in consistency, so that in the supraclavicular area it consists of soft fat with a tenuous attachment to its surroundings.

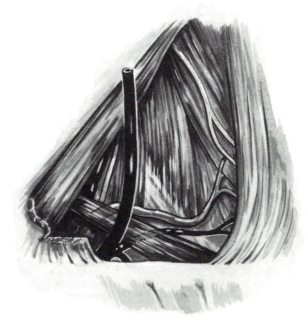

35

When the clearance of the posterior triangle reaches a point approximately 5 cm above the clavicular insertion of trapezius the accessory nerve is divided. The nerve is not consciously sought, its section being recognized by a convulsive contraction of trapezius.

At the same level the transverse cervical artery will be found running laterally across the floor of the triangle. Depending on convenience it can be preserved or divided, as can its associated vein. Both vessels, particularly the vein, have branches which take part in anastomoses along the vicinity of the anterior border of trapezius. These often create a nuisance, particularly in the patient with the short thick neck, with bleeding points which are difficult to catch as they retract into the soft fat deep to trapezius. In the long thin neck they are more easily seen and picked up for formal division and ligation or diathermy.

With the increase in the volume of the fatty tissue, it is liable to become a source of concern to the surgeon unfamiliar with neck dissection. It is difficult to believe that the fat does not contain structures of significance, and awareness that the brachial plexus lies in the depths of the dissection is also liable to add to his concern. By consciously leaving the layer of prevertebral fascia covering the floor intact at this level, he can be certain that the brachial plexus behind the fascia will not be disturbed.

36

Just before the insertion of trapezius into the clavicle is reached, clearance in this area can be stopped and dissection transferred to the supraclavicular area, making an incision along the line of the upper border of the clavicle. In carrying this out, supraclavicular nerves and vessels are divided, the latter often larger than expected.

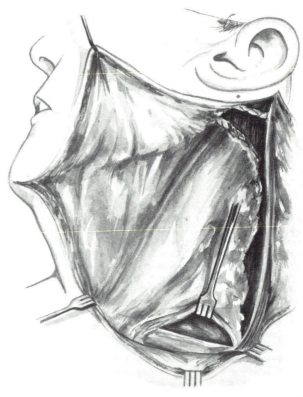

36

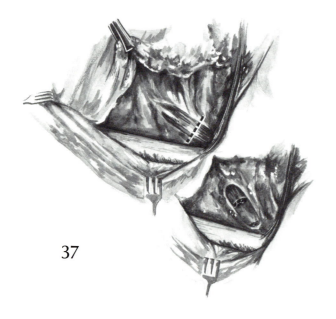

37

37

Taking care that the fatty tissues behind the clavicle are not pulled up into the neck, the soft fat is divided in the same line and retracted upwards until the inferior belly of omohyoid is seen, constant in position but variable in thickness, passing across the field. The muscle is picked up with dissecting forceps and divided, and the dissection is continued deeply to the level of the prevertebral fascia overlying the scalene muscles.

38

The dissection horizontally along the clavicle and the dissection vertically along trapezius can be brought into continuity, and with tissue forceps applied to the fatty content of the triangle, it is cleared forward towards the midline along with omohyoid.

Dissection in the supraclavicular area is easier in the long thin neck, more difficult in the short, thick neck, but with both it tends to be difficult to conduct elegantly. If the surgeon is unhappy dissecting with scissors or scalpel in this area, an alternative is to use dry gauze dissection, and sweep the fat forward and upward. Dissection in this way, however, is liable to tear the transverse cervical vein and its branches, and even the transverse cervical artery.

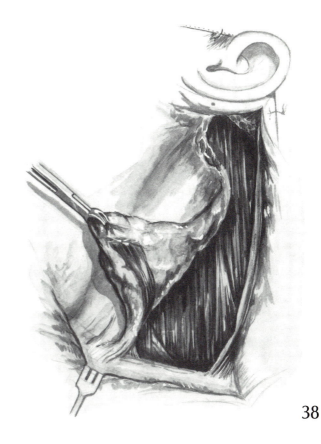

38

39

Continuation of the supraclavicular clearance medially exposes the sternocleidomastoid muscle with the external jugular vein passing round its lateral border. If the vein is required for reconstructive purposes, it is carefully dissected free from its surroundings; otherwise it is ligated and divided.

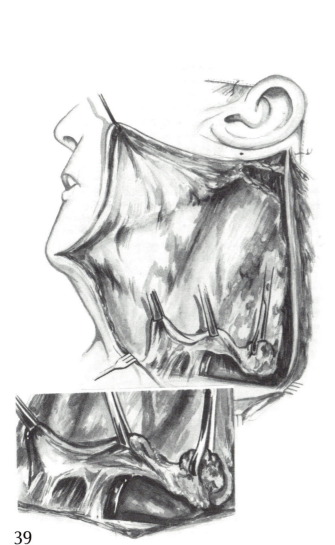

39

Division of sternocleidomastoid

When sternocleidomastoid is reached, it is divided close to its sternal and clavicular origins. The muscle can be sectioned using the probing scissor dissection method, pushing the rounded tip of the scissors under the muscle to isolate it and, with the scissors in place to protect the vein deep to it, cutting the muscle across.

40

An alternative, and in many ways preferable, method is to put the muscle on the stretch with dissecting or tissue forceps, and section it with a scalpel under direct vision, strand by strand. Sectioning the muscle in this way avoids the blind insertion of the scissors into an area close to large blood vessels, at a site low in the neck where control is likely to be difficult if a vessel wall is pierced accidentally. Division with the scalpel might appear to be a more dangerous method, but it is in fact safer. The light stroke of a sharp scalpel blade is sufficient to divide the stretched muscle fibres, a few at a time, and as the fibres are divided the ends retract, exposing fresh fibres ready for the next stroke of the scalpel until it is quite apparent that division is complete. The muscle lies within its own fascial sheath and there is a significant layer of tissue between it and the vein deep to it, though the presence of the vein shows as a bluish line.

While it is usual to divide sternocleidomastoid close to its sternal and clavicular origins, there are occasions when it may be useful to preserve its lower third as a muscle flap, together with levator scapulae as described in the chapter on 'General management and complications', pp. 8–21, to provide protective cover for the common carotid artery and bifurcation when these are considered to be at risk. Use in this way would presume a clinical absence of lower jugular node disease.

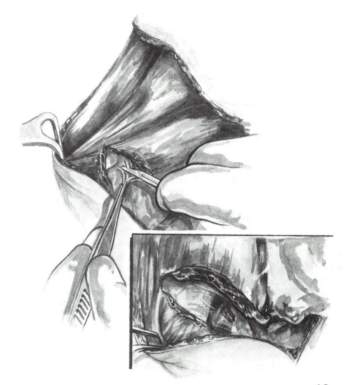

40

Division of internal jugular vein

Reference is made in anatomical texts to a 'carotid sheath' surrounding the common carotid artery, internal jugular vein and vagus nerve, but it is a formalin artefact. The vein, with its associated nodes, dissects readily and cleanly from the artery and the vagus nerve.

41

Using McIndoe scissors and non-toothed rather than toothed dissecting forceps, the vein is carefully dissected free from its surroundings. Even if the surgeon habitually uses scalpel dissection, scissor clearance is preferable in this instance, using a dissection plane close to the adventitia of the vein – a plane which, once reached, is clearly the correct one. The non-toothed forceps are preferred as being less likely to tear the vessel wall. An adequate length of vein should be cleared in this way to allow for easy ligation and division. The upper ligature is tied first, its effect being to cut off flow from above. The vein below the ligature collapses, making the placing and tying of the subsequent ligatures easier. Individual ligation of each end with an additional suture transfixing the wall of the vein, and using a non-absorbable suture material, is appropriate. As a ligature material, 3/0 silk has the desirable quality of good knotting properties, and on this score is to be preferred. It might be felt that the double tie with transfixion is necessary only on the lower cut end of the vein since it will be definitively ligatured at its upper end, but one has only to have the upper ligature slip on one occasion and experience the large and embarrassing haemorrhage to spend the extra moment making certain it does not happen again.

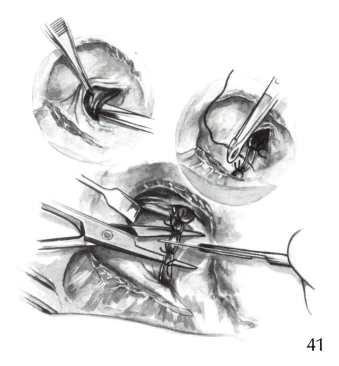

41

In the angle between the internal jugular vein and the subclavian vein, a lookout should be kept on the left side for the thoracic duct. It is rare to see it unless it is being sought specifically but, if clear fluid is seen welling up into the field, the source should be identified and ligated using a non-absorbable suture.

Clearance of common carotid and anterior neck

42

With sternocleidomastoid and the internal jugular vein divided, continuing clearance of the tissue from the posterior triangle with retraction towards the midline exposes the common carotid artery and the vagus nerve and, with dissection of the vein and its surrounding tissue, the upward clearance of the tissue overlying the artery and nerve is begun. The dissection plane is close to the artery and nerve to ensure that the nodes related to the vein are included in their entirety in the resection specimen. Retraction and clearance are continued beyond the carotid onto the infrahyoid layer of muscles, clearing them to the midline and dissecting the omohyoid muscle free as part of the resection specimen up to its insertion into the hyoid bone where it is divided. In clearing the muscles, the anterior jugular vein is met and divided and the ansa cervicalis is destroyed.

While the dissection remains at the level of the brachial plexus there is an absence of branches passing into the resection specimen, in contrast to the region of the cervical plexus from C4 upwards. This allows the dissection to proceed upwards unhindered as the common carotid artery and vagus nerve are cleared. With the resection specimen retracted towards the midline, the middle thyroid vein is seen and divided as it enters the internal jugular vein, and the phrenic nerve is also increasingly exposed up to its origin from the cervical plexus roots, mainly C4.

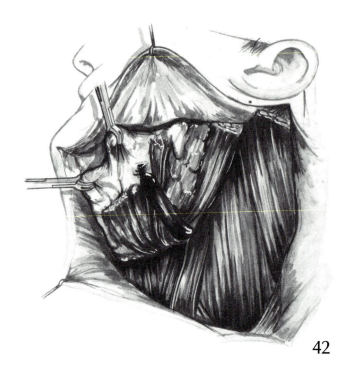

42

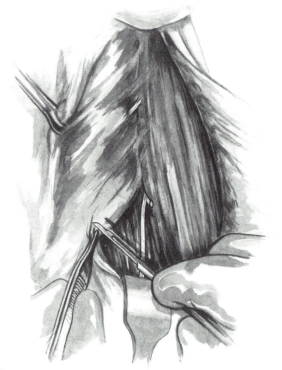

43

43

When upward clearance passes beyond the brachial plexus onto the level of the cervical plexus, forward retraction of the resection specimen puts the lower segmental branches of the cervical plexus, C3 and 4, seen passing into the resection specimen, under tension. Clearly demonstrated in this way, they can be individually divided with the scalpel, at the same time leaving the phrenic nerve intact. Along with each nerve, segmental blood vessels can be seen and these should be picked up for diathermy before the nerves are divided.

44

Division of the nerves allows the specimen to be retracted further towards the midline and brings the internal jugular vein into view from behind. Along with its associated nodes, the process of clearing it from the artery and nerve can be continued upwards without the interference of branches requiring ligation and division. The retraction forward of the vein which is possible decreases towards its upper end, and it is frequently convenient to leave the branch of C2 undivided at this stage.

As the internal jugular vein is cleared it is retracted forward, and tributaries entering its anterior surface from the pharynx are seen and divided, as are the superior thyroid vein and other tributaries reaching it from the hypoglossal plexus. The hypoglossal nerve is also seen as it passes out of this part of the field forward into the submandibular triangle. At this level the concentration of tributaries entering the anterior surface of the internal jugular vein calls for time and care to be taken to ligate and divide each individually. At this level also the common carotid artery is dividing, and the arterial branches of the external carotid artery are beginning to be seen. Unless these branches are involved in the spread of tumour they can be left intact, but there need be no hesitation in dividing them if this is felt to be convenient, even including the external carotid artery itself, making sure of the ligature by an additional transfixing ligature.

Clearance of the internal jugular vein and nodes from the internal carotid artery and vagus nerve, now added to by the presence of the hypoglossal nerve, is continued upwards to just short of the transverse process of the atlas, recognized by the apparent convergence of muscles on its tip as well as by palpation. The final clearance is impeded by the branch of C2, here passing into the resection specimen lateral to the vein. If it is convenient, the nerve can be divided and clearance continued to the level of the atlas. The ease or difficulty of the dissection at this point depends very much on whether the neck is long and thin or short and thick, and also whether or not nodes in the vicinity are enlarged by the presence of metastatic tumour, adding to the problems of retraction and exposure generally. If exposure is cramped, clearance should wait until the vein has been exposed from its superficial aspect and is under more effective control.

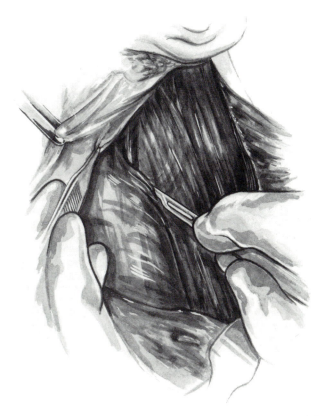

44

Submandibular triangle clearance

45

The clearance of the submandibular triangle concerns the submandibular salivary gland and its associated nodes. Clearance is generally begun at the midline, though if the tumour is in a site where metastasis to the submental nodes is regarded as a possibility, this group is included in the resection specimen, the skin incision being extended beyond the midline and dissection begun at the medial border of the anterior belly of the contralateral digastric muscle. The dissection plane is the superficial surface of the mylohyoid muscle, and as the anterior belly of digastric is met it is also cleared of its coverings.

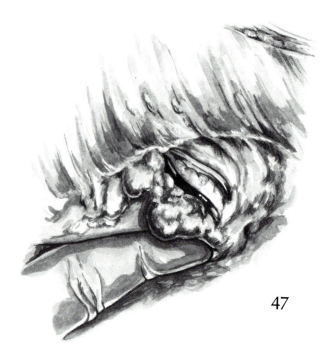

45

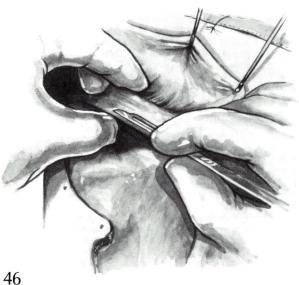

46

46

Behind the mandibular insertion of digastric the fascia enclosing the superficial lobe of the submandibular gland is cleared from its attachment to the lower border of the mandible. This is best achieved by cutting down on the bone along its lower border to the level of its periosteum, and the division can usefully be continued back to the angle. The gland can then be separated from the lingual plate of the mandible using finger dissection.

47

In the process of separating the fascia from the mandible, the facial artery and vein are seen at the anterior border of masseter. Where they are crossing the lower border of the mandible a small node is regularly found. It is felt rather than seen, and can be removed as part of the dissection specimen.

47

48

With the fascial covering of the submandibular gland cleared from the mandible, the gland is dissected backwards off the outer surface of mylohyoid until the posterior free border of the muscle is reached. In the process of this dissection the facial artery and vein are individually met and divided.

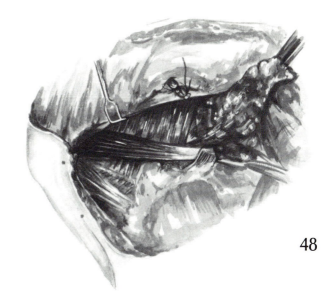

48

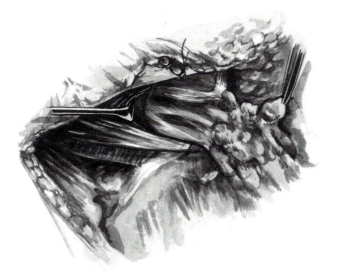

49

49

A retractor is passed round the free border of mylohyoid and the muscle is retracted forward, exposing the deep lobe of the gland with the duct passing forward from it on the surface of the hyoglossus muscle. The lingual nerve above the duct is seen and the hypoglossal nerve below, the former with the submandibular ganglion often visible, suspended from it by two nerve strands. This attachment often results in the nerve being pulled downwards when traction is applied to the gland in the process of dissecting it free. The duct is divided and the entire gland mobilized. In carrying out this part of the dissection the hypoglossal plexus of veins is met, with vessels of a size to be troublesome if they are not formally ligated.

50

With the gland mobilized and retracted, the facial artery is found emerging from the tissue surrounding the external carotid artery and entering the deep aspect of the gland. Traced back to its origin, it is ligated and divided.

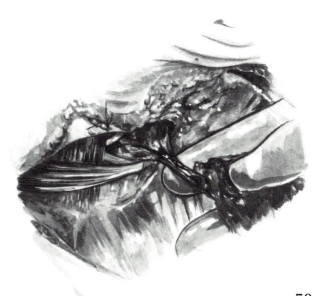

50

51

Separation of the soft tissues attached to the lower border of the mandible is continued back to its angle where it meets the lower pole of the parotid salivary gland. A line drawn from the angle backwards to the divided sterno-cleidomastoid represents the upper limit of the dissection.

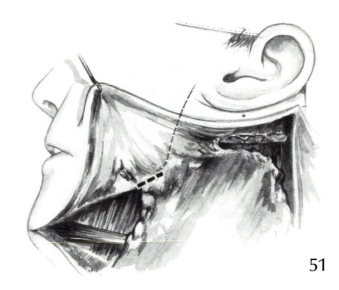

51

52

Upper neck dissection

52

An incision is made along the line of the upper limit of the dissection. Depending on the lower extent of the parotid gland the entire gland may be above this line, but more often it passes through its lower pole. In the latter instance the gland is sectioned along the line and its lower pole is retracted downwards. The gap opened between the two parts of the gland allows the retromandibular vein to be formally ligated before it is divided and separation of the lower pole completed. The level is one which does not endanger the facial nerve and the external carotid artery, entering the deep surface of the gland above this level, is not met.

The next step in the dissection is exposure of the superficial surface of the internal jugular vein at its upper end.

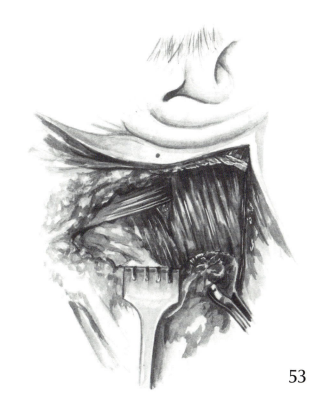

53

53

With the lower pole of the parotid gland and sternocleido-mastoid already divided and retracted downwards, the posterior belly of digastric is seen over virtually its entire length.

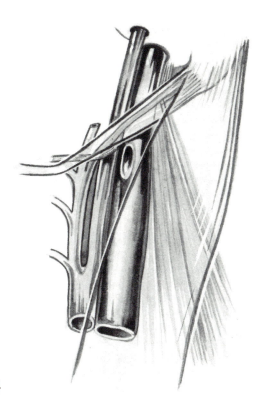

54

The posterior belly of the digastric muscle, normally covered by sternocleidomastoid, with the internal jugular vein and internal carotid artery and their associated nerves immediately deep to it, is the key to dissection in this area.

54

55

The digastric muscle belly is cleared and mobilized from its surroundings. In mobilizing the muscle, a lookout should be kept for the occipital artery which runs parallel to it on its deep surface. It is wise to formally identify it and, if necessary, ligate and divide it since, if it is divided accidentally, the resulting haemorrhage can be considerable. With the muscle retracted upwards and downwards, the internal jugular vein is exposed and its superficial surface cleared.

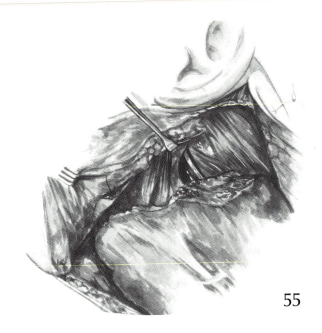

55

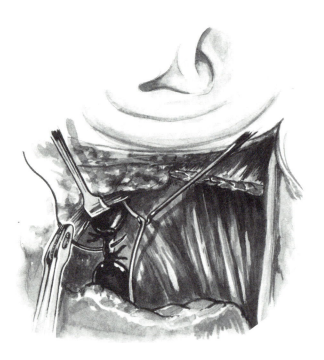

56

56

The vein, cleared on its superficial surface, can be dissected under direct vision using the probing scissor technique. As with the vein at its lower end, the dissection plane is close to the vessel wall. When an adequate length has been mobilized the vein is ligated, with an added ligature transfixing the vessel wall, and divided. Following its division, the accessory nerve is identified and divided. If the vein has already been mobilized posteriorly to the level of the transverse process of the atlas, control is present from both surfaces, superficial and deep, but the excellent control provided by the exposure of its superficial surface makes the need for additional control from the deep surface much less critical.

57

This last step completes the dissection.

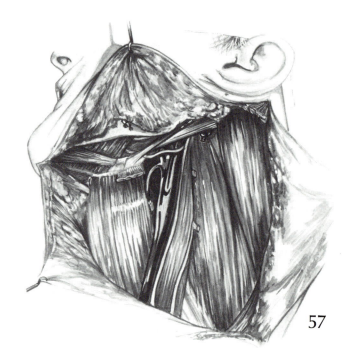

57

Extensions of the standard neck dissection

The standard radical neck dissection is extended on occasion to deal with specific pathological situations. Those which arise most frequently are:

1. When the primary tumour is situated in, or very close to, the skin area of the dissection.
2. When the primary tumour has metastasized to one of the nodal groups which are not part of the standard radical neck dissection – postauricular, occipital, parotid, paratracheal or superior mediastinal.
3. When the primary tumour arises in a site which is in virtual continuity with the dissection site, most frequently the larynx, pharynx, oral cavity or parotid salivary gland.

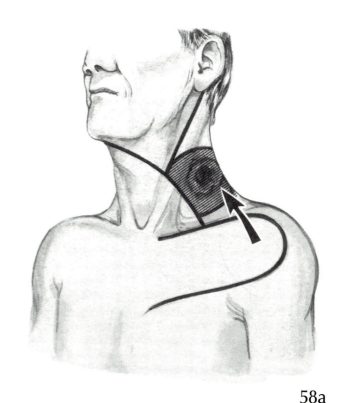

58a

Tumour arising in skin area of dissection

58a & b

When a tumour arising in the neck skin area metastasizes to the nodes underlying it, requiring a radical neck dissection, the skin incisions have to be altered in order to allow the tumour to be resected, but the dissection itself is not significantly changed. Prior to the advent of the deltopectoral flap which could be raised and transferred without prior preparation, the neck skin flaps had to be modified so that one or more could be moved to cover the defect created by the resection of the primary tumour. Today, with both the deltopectoral and the pectoralis major flaps available, the only modification of the skin incisions needed is to make sure that the modified design of the skin flaps leaves them with a blood supply adequate to perfuse them effectively.

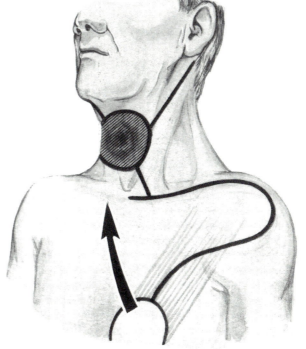

58b

Metastasis to postauricular or occipital nodes

59

When tumour has metastasized to the postauricular or occipital nodes, the dissection has to be extended to include the particular nodal group. The question which then arises on pathological grounds is whether it is safe to clear the nodes without resecting the overlying skin. In the occipital area, the thickness of the skin and its structural similarity to the scalp preclude resection of the nodes except with the overlying skin. In the postauricular site the skin is thinner and more mobile over the underlying bone. It might be felt that there is a marginally greater possibility of resecting the nodes without simultaneously resecting the overlying skin, but even here the risk involved is not acceptable. Clearance of nodes and overlying skin in continuity with a neck dissection is appropriate for both sites. Reconstruction of the resulting defect is most likely to be by a split-skin graft.

Tumour involving parotid gland

Tumour which involves the parotid gland may be primarily salivary, or metastatic from a tumour in the drainage area of the nodal group which is closely related to the gland.

Primary tumour of parotid

When the carcinoma is a salivary one, and a radical neck dissection is required as part of the overall resection of the tumour, the standard preauricular incision used to expose the gland is extended forwards, bringing it into continuity with the submandibular element of the neck dissection incision. The gland is resected as described in the chapter on 'Major salivary glands', pp. 326–348; the extension of the neck dissection concerns the clearance of the upper neck.

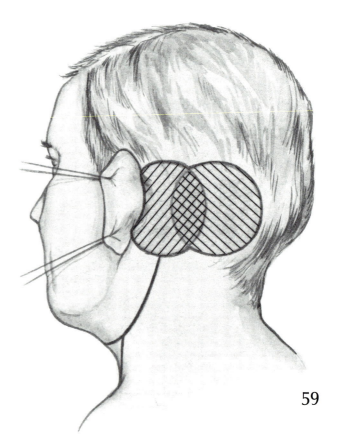

59

60

Above the level of the hyoid bone, the dissection continues initially at the same depth level as below the bone but, beyond the take-off point of the facial artery, the external carotid artery is divided and included thereafter in the resection specimen. The internal carotid artery forms the focal point of the dissection, cleared of the tissues overlying it, though making every effort to preserve the vagus and hypoglossal nerves. This dissection plane passes deep to the posterior belly of digastric and the muscle is resected as part of the specimen, exposing the internal carotid artery and the internal jugular vein. Above this level the clearance carried out is determined by the extent of the local tumour rather than being dictated by potential involvement of lymph nodes, but it is usually carried up close to the skull base before the internal jugular vein is divided.

Depending on the local extent of the tumour, the styloid muscles may require to be resected. If this is considered necessary, there is advantage to dividing the styloid process at its base and removing it along with the muscles attached to it. The effect of its resection is to considerably improve access to the skull base, making clearance of the area technically easier. When the tumour is operable in this area, the looseness of the fascia usually makes clearance easier than elsewhere in the vicinity, although a careful watch has to kept for the glosso-pharyngeal nerve.

Metastasis to parotid nodes

The surgical management of metastasis to the parotid nodes depends on whether the tumour is considered to be confined to the nodes or has spread to the surrounding parenchyma of the gland.

The parotid nodes are described in *Gray's Anatomy* as being 'immediately in front of the tragus, on, or deep to the fascia of the parotid gland', and they have been shown[9] to lie almost invariably superficial to the facial nerve. This is of considerable importance to the surgeon since it indicates that in carrying out a resection for metastatic disease which appears clinically to be confined to those nodes, the possibility exists of saving the nerve.

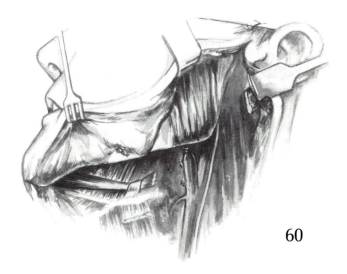

60

When the tumour is confined to the parotid nodes, it presents as circumscribed, mobile nodes. This is the usual situation with non-keratinizing tumours such as malignant melanoma.

When squamous carcinoma involves the nodes, it can present in two distinct ways. In one, presentation is similar to that of malignant melanoma with circumscribed, mobile nodes. In the other, presentation is either as a node with signs of local fixation indicative of involvement by tumour of the adjoining parenchyma of the gland, or as a fluctuant swelling lacking mobility in relation to the gland due to central necrosis of rapidly growing tumour in the node, or liquefaction of keratin in a node filled with well differentiated metastatic tumour.

For the surgeon faced with metastasis to the parotid nodes, the question arises whether to carry out a superficial parotidectomy or a total parotidectomy, and the decision influences the carrying out of the neck dissection.

61

When the nodes are mobile a superficial parotidectomy, clearing the nodes but preserving the facial nerve, in continuity with a radical neck dissection should suffice. In such a dissection the resection plane would be superficial to the external carotid artery and, with the parotidectomy completed to the lower pole of the gland, that part of the resection specimen would become continuous with that of the standard radical neck dissection.

When there is clinical evidence of spread of tumour outwith the nodes into the gland or in the case of the fluctuant swelling a total parotidectomy would be appropriate, in the latter instance almost certainly including the skin overlying the swelling, and in both sacrificing the facial nerve. In addition, a radical neck dissection carried up to the skull base in continuity with the parotid resection in the form described for the primary salivary carcinoma of the gland would be required.

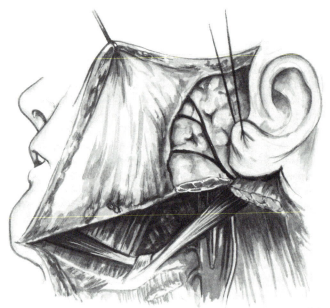

61

Metastases to paratracheal and superior mediastinal nodes

Squamous carcinoma of the larynx and laryngopharynx spreads more commonly to the lower cervical nodes than intraoral sites. It may also spread to the adjacent thyroid gland, prelaryngeal and pretracheal nodes, and all these structures are removed in carrying out a total laryngectomy/pharyngectomy with radical neck dissection. Glottic carcinomas, however, with more than 1 cm of subglottic spread, true subglottic, postcricoid and cervical oesophageal carcinomas commonly involve the lower paratracheal nodes in the upper mediastinum. Inadequate removal of these nodes is a major cause of so-called 'stomal recurrence'. This situation is better prevented than treated, and the manubrial resection and superior mediastinal dissection which is required is described in the chapter on 'Surgery for the prevention and treatment of stomal recurrence', pp. 508–516.

Intraoral tumour site

When the tumour is in a site inside the mouth where its exposure involves dissection in the submandibular nodal area as described in the chapter on 'Access to the mouth', pp. 241–253, bringing the operative field inside the mouth into tissue continuity with the neck dissection, tumour resection and node dissection are carried out as a single procedure in continuity with one another.

In carrying out such a composite resection, the nodal clearance, with the exception of the submandibular triangle, is carried out as for the standard radical neck dissection. Resection of the submandibular gland with its nodal content, and the method by which it is carried out, depends on the site of the tumour in the mouth and the surgical approach used to expose it, and whether it is necessary, because the mandible is extensively involved by tumour, to carry out a segmental resection of the full thickness of the bone.

62

When the tumour is about the level in the mouth of the middle third of the tongue, and a segmental resection of the mandible is carried out, the effect is to leave the submandibular gland between the body of the bone laterally and the resected primary tumour site medially. The three structures are resected as a single mass in continuity with the neck dissection and no attempt is made to dissect the gland as a separate structure.

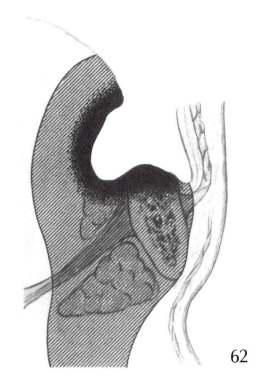

62

63

When mandibular continuity is being maintained and the tumour is exposed using the swing approach, the radical neck dissection is carried out largely as already described, making sure that the submandibular skin flap is elevated only as far as the lower border of the mandible to preserve the blood supply which the bone receives from the soft tissues attached to its buccal surface – the perfusion source on which it will largely have to rely when the resection has been completed. The submandibular gland is mobilized from the lingual plate of the mandible as in the standard dissection, and when the mylohyoid muscle and its overlying mucosa are divided, as described in the chapter on 'Access to the mouth', pp. 241–253, allowing the swing to take place, the effect is to leave the submandibular gland attached to and in continuity with the floor of mouth.

When the tumour is of the lateral floor of the mouth or side of the tongue, the gland is resected as part of the general resection of the primary site in continuity with the neck dissection.

When the tumour is of the retromolar trigone, faucial area or posterior third of the tongue – sites at a distance from the submandibular gland – the gland is dissected free under direct vision when the swing has been completed as it would in the standard radical neck dissection, the continuity between the two parts – primary site and neck dissection specimens – frequently ending up as somewhat tenuous.

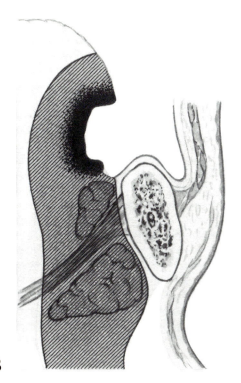

63

Laryngopharyngeal tumour site

64

When either total laryngectomy or laryngopharyngectomy is being carried out in combination with a neck dissection, a base of continuity is maintained medially between the node containing specimen and the laryngopharyngeal complex, extending from the hyoid bone to the inferior lobe of the thyroid gland. The sternohyoid and sternothyroid muscles are divided just above the manubrium of the sternum, their cut distal ends being transfixion ligated, and the ipsilateral thyroid lobe and isthmus are included in the resection. The broad base of continuity is maintained during the submandibular triangle clearance and upper neck dissection which follow.

When a supraglottic laryngectomy is being carried out in combination with a neck dissection, the need to preserve the infrahyoid muscles and the dissection involved in exposing the superior aspect of the thyroid cartilage makes for a narrow pedicle, in continuity only at the level of the hyoid bone. In these circumstances the preservation of continuity confers no benefit, and the nodal specimen is best removed separately for convenience.

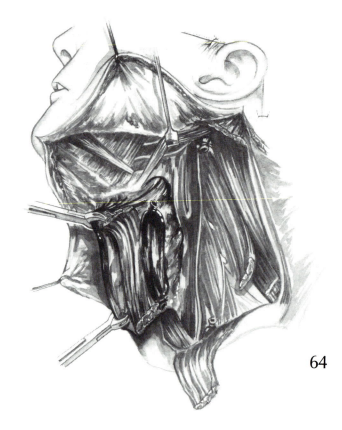

64

Preoperative and postoperative care

Preoperative preparation and postoperative care and complications are discussed in the chapter on 'General management and complications', pp. 8–21.

References

1. Martin H, Del Valle B, Ehrlich H, Cahan WG. Neck dissection. *Cancer* 1951; 4: 441–99.

2. Butlin HT, Spencer WG. *Diseases of the Tongue*. 2nd edn. London: Cassell, 1900.

3. Crile G. Excision of carcinoma of the head and neck. *JAMA* 1906; 47: 1780–5.

4. Schobinger R. The use of a long anterior skin flap in neck resections. *Ann Surg* 1957; 146: 221–3.

5. Conley J. *Concepts in Head and Neck Surgery*. Stuttgart: Thieme Verlag, 1970: 81.

6. MacFee WF. Transverse incisions for neck dissections. *Ann Surg* 1960; 151: 279–84.

7. Nelson DW, Gingrass RP. Anatomy of the mandibular branches of the facial nerve. *Plast Reconstr Surg* 1979; 64: 479–82.

8. Henry AK. *Extensile Exposure*. 2nd edn. Edinburgh: E & S Livingstone, 1957: 48.

9. McKean ME, Lee K, McGregor IA. The distribution of lymph nodes in and around the parotid gland: an anatomical study. *Br J Plast Surg* 1985; 38: 1–5.

Index